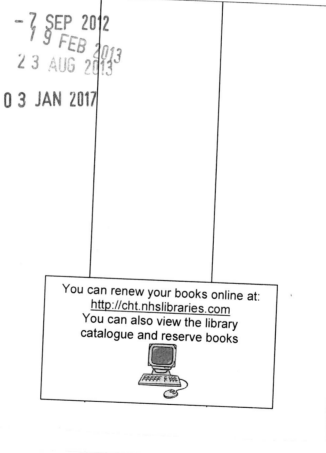

Palgrave Student Companions are a one-stop reference resource that provide essential information for students about the subject – and the course – they've chosen to study.

Friendly and authoritative, **Palgrave Student Companions** support the student throughout their degree. They encourage the reader to think about study skills alongside the subject matter of their course, offer guidance on module and career choices, and act as an invaluable source book and reference that they can return to time and again.

Palgrave Student Companions – your course starts here

Published

The English Language and Linguistics Companion
The English Literature Companion
The MBA Companion
The Nursing Companion
The Politics Companion
The Psychology Companion
The Social Work Companion

Forthcoming

The Anthropology Companion
The Cultural Studies Companion
The Economics Companion
The Health Studies Companion
The Media Studies Companion
The Sociology Companion
The Theatre, Drama and Performance Companion

Further titles are planned

www.palgravestudentcompanions.com

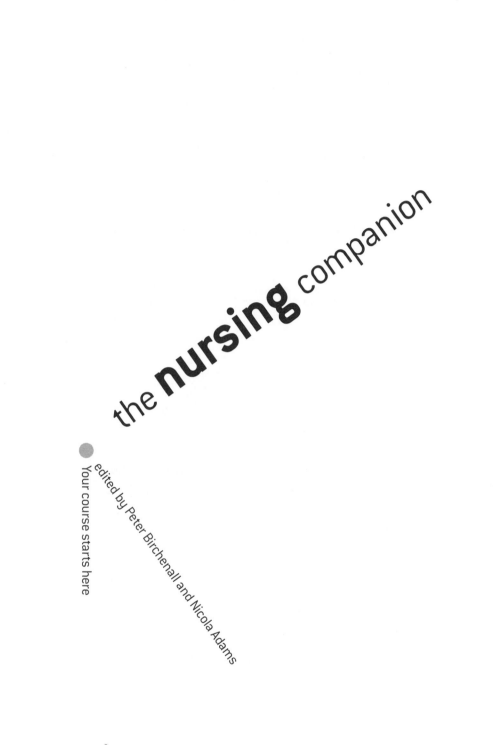

the **nursing** companion

edited by Peter Birchenall and Nicola Adams

Your course starts here

palgrave
macmillan

First published 2011 by
PALGRAVE MACMILLAN

Palgrave Macmillan in the UK is an imprint of Macmillan Publishers Limited,
registered in England, company number 785998, of Houndmills, Basingstoke,
Hampshire RG21 6XS.

Palgrave Macmillan in the US is a division of St Martin's Press LLC,
175 Fifth Avenue, New York, NY 10010.

Palgrave Macmillan is the global academic imprint of the above companies
and has companies and representatives throughout the world.

Palgrave® and Macmillan® are registered trademarks in the United States,
the United Kingdom, Europe and other countries

ISBN 978-1-4039-4188-6

This book is printed on paper suitable for recycling and made from fully
managed and sustained forest sources. Logging, pulping and manufacturing
processes are expected to conform to the environmental regulations of the
country of origin.

A catalogue record for this book is available from the British Library.

10 9 8 7 6 5 4 3 2 1
20 19 18 17 16 15 14 13 12 11

Printed in China

brief contents

contents

acknowledgements

Professor Peter Birchenall wishes to acknowledge the professionalism of Palgrave Macmillan editors Linda Thompson and Kate Llewellyn. Their patience and understanding over the period taken to bring *The Nursing Companion* to fruition is greatly appreciated. He also wishes to acknowledge the unstinting support given to him by his wife Mary Birchenall.

The authors and publishers wish to thank the following for permission to use copyright material: *Nursing Times* for permission to reproduce Figure 5.3, originally from J McLeod Clark (1981) Communication in nursing, *Nursing Times*; Taylor & Francis for Figure 6.1, originally from S Arnstein (1969) A ladder of participation, *Journal of American Institute of Planners*, 35: 216–24; *Ambulatory Surgery* for Figures 10.2–4, originally from MJ Mitchell (2000) Anxiety management: a distinct nursing role in day surgery, *Ambulatory Surgery*, 8(3): 119–28; Quay Books for Table 11.1, originally from B Nyatanga (2008) *Why Is It So Difficult To Die?* (2nd edn), Wiltshire: Quay Books; Catherine Jackson and *Bereavement Care* for Figure 11.3, originally from L Tonkin (1996) Growing around grief: another way of looking at grief and recovery, *Bereavement Care*, 15(1): 10, Cruse: London; Elsevier Limited for Figures 13.1 and 13.2, originally from L Shields and A Tanner (2006) Children and surgery, in *A Textbook of Children's and Young People's Nursing* (eds Glasper and Richardson), Copyright Churchill Livingstone 2006 and also Linda Shields for her personal permission; NHS Employers and the Office of Public Sector Information to reproduce the information in Table 21.2, reproduced under the terms of the Click-Use Licence.

Every effort has been made to trace the copyright-holders, but if any have been inadvertently overlooked the publishers will be pleased to make the necessary arrangements at the first opportunity.

introduction

Introduction

Most of us have experienced the joy of companionship at various times in our lives. Perhaps it has come from human companionship, a pet or even a favourite book. A loyal companion will always be at your side offering support, friendship and advice. This book is intended to be a companion for you on your journey to becoming a modern health professional, offering support and advice whenever you need it. It will be a survival guide and a toolkit, always there to help out with that bit of extra knowledge and understanding when essays are to be written or seminars prepared or just as a source of additional material to supplement a lecture or equip you with transferable and lifelong learning skills.

A guided tour of the book

At this juncture, it should be mentioned that from 2013, the minimum level for pre-registration nursing courses will be raised from diploma to degree standard, so diploma-level courses are being withdrawn. However, the content of this book will remain relevant.

The Nursing Companion is presented in five parts:

> *Part 1 (Chapters 1–3):* The context of nursing is explained before moving on to an in-depth exploration of the pre-registration course.

> *Part 2 (Chapters 4–11):* Core topics that underpin pre-registration nursing education are considered. Here you will find material associated with the social, physical and psychological aspects of caring. The importance of developing interpersonal and professional skills is explored. To be an effective nurse, you must be able to communicate with those you are caring for. It has long been recognised that interpersonal and helping skills form an essential part of the nurse's day-to-day work in caring for sick and vulnerable people. *The Nursing Companion* will give you valuable insight into these skills and in Chapter 10 you will be guided into how to make the best use of 'self' when communicating with patients or clients.

> *Part 3 (Chapters 12–16):* Here you will find chapters on the main branches of nursing:

> ▶ Nursing adults (Chapter 12)

- Nursing children and young people (Chapter 13)
- Nursing people with learning disabilities (Chapter 14)
- Nursing people with mental health problems (Chapter 15).

In addition, it is recognised that the impact of growing old in a modern world is significant for all branches of nursing, therefore a chapter on caring for older people is included (Chapter 16).

> *Part 4 (Chapters 17–20):* Here the focus is on how to appraise evidence to underpin nursing practice and the process of enquiry. You will be taken through the various elements that constitute research and its relevance to the development of safe nursing practice.
> *Part 5 (Chapter 21):* Prominence is given to career development. There is much here to help and guide you into making the right career choices when considering which direction to take and how to prepare for that all important interview.

Lifelong learning

As a nurse, you will experience the reality of lifelong learning and *The Nursing Companion* will assist in forming a sound foundation on which your early professional education and future career can be built. The book is designed and written to light the way towards achieving the knowledge and skills essential to becoming an effective nurse. Should you wish to be more adventurous, the style and layout of each part lets you engage with activities and case studies that reach across the main branches of nursing. The key to success as a student is to develop academic and learning skills such as note taking, essay writing and managing your time. These and other key skills are explored in a straightforward, understandable way in Chapter 3.

Throughout your nursing career, you will need to stay in tune with current developments. There are two areas that cannot be avoided when working in the NHS or the independent sector – politics and research. Chapters 5 and 7 and the research chapters that form Part 4 will encourage you to stay abreast of both of these. As part of lifelong learning, the notion of 'evidence-based practice' is well accepted and *The Nursing Companion* will be on hand to guide you through the processes associated with developing your own practice.

Patients as service users

By reading *The Nursing Companion,* you will discover that, along with changes in the way that healthcare is delivered, there have been changes in terminology when describing people requiring and receiving healthcare. Nowadays patients are sometimes referred to as 'clients' or 'service users'. This moves us away from a passive approach to one that is inclusive and proactive. So, in recent times, health-related information has become more transparent and easier to obtain and has given rise to better informed service users and a greater desire for them to be involved in their treatment and care.

From the outset of your studies, you will be made aware of the part that nursing plays in enabling those you care for to become active participants in their own care. In this context, health promotion becomes important. In Chapter 6 you can explore what is meant by user involvement and why it is important, particularly as day surgery is now a firmly established part of the health services. Chapter 9 describes modern approaches to preoperative and postoperative care and reinforces how user involvement has increased in importance over the past few years. On a daily basis, nurses are called upon to care for or work with people who are in physical or psychological distress and also to bring comfort to those nearing the end of their lives, so Chapters 8 and 11 are part of this companion.

Career development

In Chapter 21, you will discover how pre-registration nursing education is designed to expose you to a wide variety of experiences from which career options will gradually emerge. These options range from clinical, managerial, advanced practice/specialist practice/nurse consultant, pathways to teaching, lecturing and research posts in universities and colleges. Opportunities also exist within the independent sector caring for residents in nursing homes, so it is important for you to be informed on what is available and how to identify what could possibly become a lifelong career pathway. *The Nursing Companion* will advise you on how to move forward and addresses the important process of applying for jobs.

Like all good companions, *The Nursing Companion* is flexible. You can read it from cover to cover or just dip into relevant sections as required. It will be there whenever you need it. We hope you find it useful and enjoyable.

Professor Peter Birchenall and Professor Nicola Adams

1 studying nursing

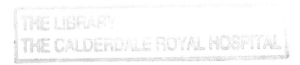

Introduction

This first part of *The Nursing Companion* explores several important factors to be borne in mind when either deciding whether nursing is for you or beginning your career in nursing. It places you at the beginning of what could become an exciting, challenging and fulfilling occupation. Having a caring personality is a good place to begin your professional journey but because nursing is an intensely person-focused profession, you will meet many situations that call for an array of skills and knowledge that take a lifetime to learn. As a student of nursing, you will discover that dedication, motivation and enthusiasm are the building blocks upon which to construct your career.

To be a successful nurse in the modern age, you will have to become adept at applying theory to practice and the structure of your university-based programme will take you systematically through this demanding process. You will be introduced to terms such as evidence-based practice, which invariably means that an inquiring mind becomes an essential part of your skill base. Learning key skills such as how to combine study with a busy work schedule, how to read for understanding and managing time effectively will stand you in good stead as your career progresses. The whole notion of lifelong learning begins right at the beginning, from day one. In this part of the book, you are encouraged to reflect on your strengths and weaknesses, particularly when it comes to balancing study time with recreational time.

University life offers opportunities for meeting new people, making new friends and engaging in sporting and recreational activities. Being at university will develop your outlook and personality in many ways and knowing yourself becomes important. Identifying when you are at your best for study purposes is a key skill. For example, does your brain work best in the morning or later at night? Are you a solitary person or do you work best as part of a group? As well as developing a structured, orderly way of doing things, you will discover the benefits of learning to problem solve, which may from time to time call upon a certain amount of creativity. With this in mind, you are encouraged to think about the activities set out in Chapters 1–3 and then complete them. Review your thoughts during your reading and learning and in this way you start the early aspects of reflection. By doing this you will begin to recognise the value of reflection. You will discover that this advice applies throughout the book and your career.

1 the context of nursing

Nancy-Jane Lee

In this chapter we will explore:

> Becoming a nurse
> Qualities and skills in nursing
> Working in a team
> Learning about nursing
> Key factors influencing the role of the nurse
> Challenges facing nurses

Introduction

Among other things *The Nursing Companion* introduces you to some 'basic' nursing principles. However, the 'basics' are more than the common sense that many people attribute to nursing. They require expertise and experience, knowledge and skill, confidence and compassion, combined with an understanding of the real health influences in people's lives. This chapter introduces some of the basic factors underpinning your role as a nurse, which influence the way you learn about, and practise, nursing.

There are activities and student nurse comments (with full permission) throughout the chapter to help you reflect and begin to develop the understanding you need to be a nurse. So why *do* you want to be a nurse? Hopefully you like learning about people and their lives and want to make a difference for them at profound milestones in their lives. You should love learning, and you need the stamina to combine study with practical **placements**. You should have the enthusiasm to think and read on your own as well as being able to contribute to the work of a group. All these skills are transferable to a multidisciplinary health and social care setting. In choosing nursing as a career, you should be observant and able to identify and respond to people's physical and psychosocial needs. Above all, you should recognise the need for dignity and respect in all nursing care and appreciate the times when healthcare ethics and confidentiality are important.

Activity 1.1

What do you think are the qualities of a good nurse? Compare your thoughts with Sarah and Helen who are third year student nurses:

> A good nurse is compassionate, can do all skills and, unsure about anything, is aware of their limitations, can build therapeutic relationships with anyone from any background; they must possess good communication skills, and have the motivation and enthusiasm to progress.
>
> In my eyes, a good nurse is someone who can listen to a patient, help them as much as they can. A nurse never gives up on anyone or anything. Although caring is important, they must also be independent in their thoughts.

In what situations might nurses apply the skills that Sarah has identified above? While we are more knowledgeable about how social issues such as housing and education, lifestyle issues such as nutrition and mental health, and economic issues such as employment influence health and wellbeing, complex health problems related to lifestyle and societal stressors persist, especially for the vulnerable. How and where you develop and use your skills as a nurse are influenced by these societal factors.

What do nurses do?

Activity 1.2

What do you expect to do as a nurse? List your expectations and when you have done this, watch one of the contemporary nursing and health dramas on television, observing how nursing is presented. Compare your ideas with those in the media and those that emerge from the advert below.

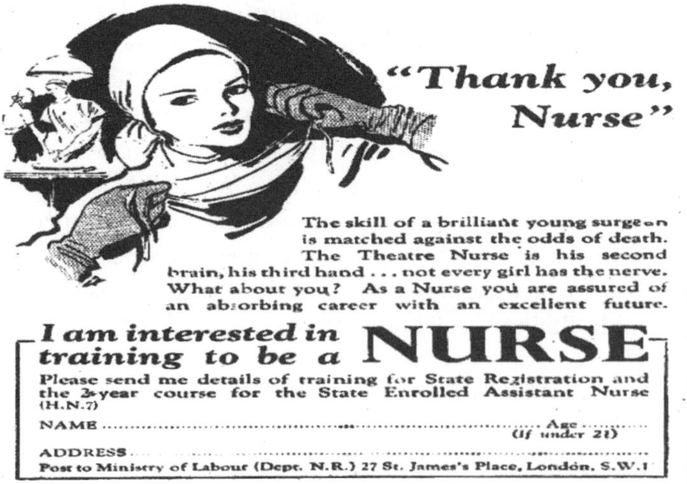

Figure 1.1 *'Thank you, Nurse'*
Source: Ministry of Labour, 1946

To ask what nurses do is to ask the obvious; people expect nurses to care for the sick and help them get better. Historically, nurses have been considered the doctors' handmaiden. This is largely due to gender stereotypes and the status of cure and care; these issues will be explored later in the chapter. The advertisement from 1946 illustrates these perceptions while enhancing the life/death excitement of acute nursing; a favourite feature of nursing on the TV. In contrast, demographic changes, lifestyle and social issues, combined with health economics and policy, mean that your role as a nurse is more likely to focus upon **community care**, health promotion and the management and support for those with long-term conditions. Hospital stays will become shorter, with earlier discharge to care at home, and a focus upon more complex acute and critical care needs within the hospital setting.

Given the shift from hospital-based secondary care to community or primary healthcare, nurses increasingly need the knowledge and skills for community care and understanding of the physical, psychosocial factors influencing health. In addition, earlier discharge from hospital means that community nurses are also dealing with more acute episodes of care in the home. Mental health nursing is also increasingly located in the community, with acute mental health needs being addressed with hospital care. Those patients in hospital are also more acutely ill, requiring increasingly complex knowledge and technical expertise from nursing to manage and deliver care. An increasing feature of nursing work has been that of specialisation. There are, for example, specialist nurses in the areas of palliative care, with Macmillan nurses working in hospitals and the community to provide continuity of care. Other examples of nursing specialisation include those of the breast care nurse, the diabetic nurse and advanced nurse practitioner roles.

Contemporary health policies have meant adaptation to nursing roles in response to changing health needs. For example, the hospital matron was reintroduced to address concerns about hospital hygiene and cleanliness, the increase in methycillin-resistant *Staphylococcus aureus* (MRSA) and infection rates in hospital. The matron's remit also covered standards of hospital nutrition. The role was intended to provide focus and leadership, improve communication and standards and reduce complaints about care.

Consultant nurse roles were introduced (**DH** 1999a) to enhance the career pathway for nurses in clinical practice, as opposed to the pursuit of an education or managerial role for promotion. Consultant roles were also a response to shifting professional boundaries and the extension of nurses' work beyond the original scope of care delivery and management. For example, consultant roles for nurses and other professions such as physiotherapy acted as a focal point for clinical excellence, leadership, education and research to underpin evidence-based practice and quality of care.

As mentioned earlier, the traditional boundaries of health professionals' practice have changed. Roles once associated with medical staff have now transferred to other professions. One example of this is the development of advanced practitioner roles for senior nurses and other health professions following a Masters-level programme of learning. This role incorporates the work of medical staff, junior doctors and registrars in terms of medical history taking, care management pathways, and treatment regimens. Another feature that has changed nursing work is that of non-medical prescribing. This was suggested originally in 1986, and was introduced for community nurses and health visitors. In 2002, it was extended to all clinical areas, with extended and supplementary prescribing following a period of educational preparation.

Activity 1.3

Develop an action plan for your first practice placement to find out about the roles of nurses and health professionals in the multidisciplinary team.

While the nature of nursing is changing, so is the notion of 'who is the nurse?', notably in response to workforce shortages. One solution has been the increased recruitment of overseas nurses and other key health service professionals. This has raised ethical concerns about 'cherry-picking' healthcare staff from developing countries such as India, South Africa and the Philippines. Another solution has been to increase the numbers of student nurses and other health professionals in training. The rise in student nurse numbers has also coincided with government initiatives to widen participation in higher education, beyond the traditional pool of 18-year-olds. This has widened access to nursing in terms of mature students and those from ethnic groups, traditionally underrepresented in nursing.

Technology and nursing

Technology has transformed contemporary nursing, influencing care at the micro- and macro-levels of delivery. For example, syringe drivers, infusion pumps and other equipment have enhanced care delivery, requiring more technical nursing skills and knowledge. Likewise technology has improved diagnostic tests, radiography and keyhole surgery, transforming the nature and location of nursing. Today, surgery that used to require a one-week hospital stay is now carried out as day surgery – transferring nursing care from hospital to community and from nursing team to family and friends, who need nursing support and facilitation.

At the macro-level, technological improvements along with improved pharmacological interventions mean that the patients you nurse in hospital are more acutely ill than ever, with many now surviving where they would have once died. While technology has meant improved interventions in care delivery, it has also had a major impact on care management. Electronic patient records and computerised systems linking hospital departments have enhanced information transfer. Technology has impacted on those receiving care and widened access to health information. Information once in the professional domain is now widely available on the internet. Laypeople can access health information from a wide variety of sources and are likely to want more answers to their questions, and choices about the nature of their care. This proliferation of health information has also led to an increased consciousness of positive health issues such as work–life balance, nutrition and exercise.

Summary of key points

> The nursing profession has historically been subject to stereotypes regarding cure (male oriented) and care (female oriented).
> The nurse's role as a health promoter has become equally important to caring for the sick.
> Nursing has become increasingly specialised; new roles such as consultant nurse have developed as a focal point for clinical excellence.
> Nursing shortages have been partially addressed by increased recruitment from overseas.

Box 1.1 Student nurse likes and dislikes

> I like the caring side and satisfaction when a patient I looked after is happy and received good care.
> I like working with patients and feeling like I have done something to help them, even the really little things; all patients are different and there is always something new to learn or a new problem to solve.
> It makes me happy when I have made a difference during the day, perhaps talked to someone no one else might have.
> I also feel better when I have learned something new, for example a new skill.
> I dislike it when certain members of staff think they are too good to do the dirty jobs.
> As a student nurse, I dislike when the nurses say they have not got time to teach the students. When you're trying to be helpful but you get no feedback from the nurses … it is hard to improve as a student without feedback.
> I dislike the amount of paperwork … as it means less physical patient care.
> I also dislike when relatives are unappreciative of the hard work and knowledge that nurses have to have to care for someone.

How will I learn about nursing?

The history of nurse education: knowing or doing?

Activity 1.4

Talk to friends or relatives who are nurses and ask how they learned to be a nurse. Compare their experiences with your expectations and the information below, looking for similarities and differences.

The kind of education needed for nursing was, and still is, a topic to divide nurses and public alike. There is a perpetual belief that compassion, communication and nursing skill cannot be compatible with an academic education. There are two implicit assumptions in the above. First, that to be a nurse does not require any great intellectual command, and, second, that compassion or any related skill is not commensurate with education. These assumptions are, I believe, wrong on both counts and, if taken to extremes, arguably education for roles such as policing, law, medicine and psychology, for example, would not be needed. These are also people-focused roles requiring the combination of compassion, knowledge and skill/expertise. In relation to gender stereotypes and nursing, the notion that educated nurses are 'too posh to wash' is interesting, as the same anti-education stance is not evident within physiotherapy or occupational therapy, for example. So why is learning to be a nurse different?

There are historical tensions between those who sought to modernise and enhance nursing's professional status, for example Mrs Bedford Fenwick, and those who valued pragmatic, practical nurse training, for example Florence Nightingale (for more insight into the history of nursing, you should read Rafferty 1996). If you were to ask about my nurse education experiences, I started nursing in 1980 and typically of my age cohort, I might discuss 'the training of character and the character of training' (Rafferty 1996, p. 23).

The official way I learned to be a nurse was through direct employment within a hospital setting, developing on-the-job learning and theoretical learning as a student in exchange for contribution to the nursing workforce. In my case, placements of 8–12 weeks were sandwiched between 'modules' of two weeks duration, before and after each placement and interspersed with holidays. A test at the beginning of each new module and placement was used to assess progression towards state registration, and poor performance might result in removal to enrolled nurse training, which was two years as opposed to three years in length, with an emphasis on practical nursing.

The unofficial way of learning to be a nurse was through direct experience of nursing, observation and communication with others and personal thinking and reflection. However, even that was not enough to learn nursing. I truly learned nursing when the experiences I had were combined with wider knowledge of the factors affecting people's lives, experience, personal confidence and, importantly, the curiosity to think about nursing.

It was the advent of *Project 2000* (UKCC 1986) that really accelerated changes in the values and beliefs underpinning nurse education and nursing as a whole, while influencing directly where learning took place and what student nurses did. In summary, there was a shift from nursing as a practical vocation, involving the application of skills and tasks, to a humanistic view of nursing and the development of holistic care based upon education principles. The term 'knowledgeable doer' was used at the time as a shorthand for the educational development required for nurses to be able to question practice and to develop better nursing practice based upon research.

While there was some professional and public disquiet about the separation of university education from the realities of delivering nursing practice, the UKCC (1999) sought to strengthen the links between the two and provide good student support and learning in the practice environment and re-establish the evidence base for nurse education that could develop strong nursing leadership. The Prime Minister's Commission on the Future of Nursing and Midwifery in England was set up in March 2009 to review nurse education and produced a report entitled *Front Line Care* in 2010. Nursing will become an all **graduate** entry profession from 2013, with the phasing out of diploma nurse education programmes (NMC 2008).

Returning to nursing and education stereotypes, Meerabeau (2001) has written about gender and historical issues, and entrenched values and beliefs concerning the nature of nursing as a practical, commonsense skill. For example, it is suggested that media concerns about the quality of nursing and nurses' supposed inability to utilise practical nursing skills as a result of overly academic education strategies are rhetoric and do not take account of the social factors influencing nursing. Notable in Meerabeau's analysis is the arrival of nursing in the higher education sector and the challenges of establishing nursing, traditionally a female role, as an academic discipline in an area traditionally dominated by men.

Training implies the collective learning of procedures and skills that can be learned, refined through experience and followed, and education implies an individualised process, combining knowledge and exploration of values and beliefs with professional practice, and nurse academics, in particular, are sometimes keen to make the distinction. In reality, both have their place in nurse education. There are aspects of nursing practice that require training, for example the acquisition of nursing skills as diverse as hand washing and communicating in sensitive situations. However, both examples need training and education; to develop the skill required, to consider the underpinning knowledge needed and to ask questions and reflect upon what is best practice.

What will my course be like?

Nurse education has traditionally been built upon quite structured teaching enhanced by practical demonstration, observation, practice and subsequent experience. The arrival of problem-based learning (PBL) with *Fitness for*

Practice (UKCC 1999) was designed to bring the best nuggets of learning together. Savin-Baden (2000) has emphasised the central skills of adaptability, problem solving and critique within PBL, which involves learners working in small groups, supported by a facilitator, as opposed to formal teaching or lecturing. Learners work on scenarios drawn from the reality of nursing practice. Contemporary student nurses are likely to study a wide range of topics using PBL, in combination with lectures, personal study, discussion, student-led seminars, practical experience and observation. These reflect the changes in society and the increasing complexity of healthcare. In addition to clinical nursing skills, health promotion issues, public health, healthcare ethics, evidence-based practice and research, along with legal and professional studies are staple components of any nursing programme. Student nurses will be asked to engage in reflective practice – the ability to think over professional experiences and derive learning from them.

As a student nurse, you will be expected to use the internet to study health and nursing issues and you will need good analytical and thinking skills to distinguish the quality of information provided. You will also have access to nursing and health electronic databases and ebooks. Technology has influenced the way that student nurses and other healthcare disciplines learn. Expectations of lectures and seminars are being replaced by the use of virtual learning environments, such as Blackboard. These enable students to have access to course materials, tutorial support and discussion groups anywhere they have internet access.

Box 1.2 Student nurses' good study tips

> I have to be on my own, with no one else around
> I have all my notes in front of me so I know what I have used and what I have not
> Also planning time and organisational skills are very important
> Taking full advantage of the tutors at university and getting feedback on assignments as you go along to keep on the right track
> When writing assignments, always keep a record of references as you go along, as it's much harder to find references again at the end
> Time management is important
> Start early ... plan what you can do within one week, don't stop until you have done it and feel it is your best work. If you finish early that week, have the rest of the week off for enjoyment

Activity 1.5

What kind of learner are you? Make some notes about a time when you enjoyed learning something, and think about where and how you learned, who helped you, and how you could use those principles to learn about nursing.

Student nurses are now more likely than ever to study and deliver nursing and healthcare with other health and social care disciplines. Learning and working with others is important, given successive care breakdowns resulting from professional tribalism and a lack of communication, as evidenced by some high-profile cases.

For example, the problems helping families at risk have been illustrated in the 'Baby P' case. Originally known only as Baby P, this child was subjected to severe neglect and subsequently died as a result of family actions, yet the family was known to the professionals concerned (Fresco 2008). This and other sad situations illustrate the significance of good communication between professionals involved in health and social care, and other agencies, along with the need for excellent assessment strategies to protect the vulnerable within society.

Summary of key points

> Within the history of nursing, gender divisions in labour continue to influence the public's perception of the nursing profession.

> The tension between a professional, university-based education and the traditional skills-based training persists.

> The availability of health information on the internet, along with the use of virtual learning environments, has enabled greater flexibility in the delivery of nurses' education.

> Interprofessional education and practice should be central within nurse education programmes, to promote increased understanding of respective professional roles and enhance professional communication and collaboration.

What factors influence my role as a nurse?

Before reading further, you should tackle the activity below.

Activity 1.6

Factors influencing nursing

Survey as many media sources as you can over a week and list the health and nursing issues you find. You could look at national and local newspapers, TV, radio and the internet.

During your first clinical placement, review your answers, and make a note of the factors you have seen influencing people's lives. You must not include people's names or name any health and social care settings to maintain confidentiality.

Healthcare priorities and nursing

Hand washing, the availability of cancer drugs, obesity, binge drinking, hospital waiting lists, staff shortages, MRSA, influenza and mental health may feature in your media list. All these health challenges, combined with the attitudes of nurses and other healthcare workers, influence our perception not only of health service efficiency but also of healthcare quality.

Health and nursing economics

Today we take the National Health Service (NHS) for granted; there is excellent primary healthcare and freedom to choose where we have hospital treatment. One major challenge for health policy makers and politicians is to manage our demands for healthcare compared to the shrinking resources to deliver; financial, human and other. This situation makes people angry, as they have paid taxes in order to ensure there are essential services such as health for them. The NHS was formed after the Second World War in 1948. Its founding principles were to provide a universal and comprehensive health service, free at the point of use, regardless of users' ability to pay. The NHS was a central feature of the welfare state, developed through the Beveridge Report (1942), as produced by the economist Sir William Beveridge. The welfare state was designed to provide for the population 'from cradle to grave'. Its importance cannot be overstated, as the proposals for welfare were central to postwar reconstruction, and included strategies for education, employment, social services, housing, child and family health. In summary, the welfare state was designed to address the five giant evils – want, disease, ignorance, squalor and idleness.

Before the NHS came into being, people had to pay for healthcare. Those in certain occupations such as coal mining paid a subscription to be a member of a doctor's panel: the doctor was usually employed by the company. Healthcare was usually only available to the breadwinner, at the time this was the man. (For more information, read AJ Cronin's *The Citadel* – a novel that explores the inequalities of healthcare at the beginning of the twentieth century.)

Many people had no access to healthcare at all and were reliant on charity or home remedies. For example, goose grease rubbed on the chest was thought to combat chest infections, while mustard baths were thought to treat colds and chills.

My mother taught me the poem below and it illustrates healthcare before the NHS:

Miss Polly had a dolly who was sick, sick, sick
So she sent for the doctor to be quick, quick, quick
The doctor came with his bag and his hat
And he knocked on the door with a rat a tat tat
He looked at the baby and he shook his head
And said Miss Polly send her straight to bed
He wrote on a paper for a pill, pill, pill
And said 'I'll be back in the morning with my bill, bill bill'.

In the 1980s and 90s, there was better recognition that some client groups had a right to community care and more 'normal' lives as opposed to institutional care which separated them from the community, for example those with learning disabilities and mental health needs. The NHS and Community Care Act 1990 accelerated the development of community services for older people and those with mental health and learning disability needs. There has been an exponential growth in primary healthcare, social care and social enterprises to enable the health and wellbeing of individuals and groups.

The government estimates that health expenditure has increased from £33bn to £67.4bn. The average spending per head is set to increase from £680 to £1,345 per head of population (DH 2004a). The question now being posed is: 'How much health expenditure will be enough'? It would appear that while costs have increased, the benefits are difficult to measure and increasingly slight. For example, pharmaceuticals, surgical interventions and technologies will continue to rise; however, their relative merits may be difficult to determine (Appleby 2006). There is an increasing discussion about the need to evaluate health interventions and determine the effectiveness of treatments and their outcomes. Some of this work is already undertaken by the National Institute for Health and Clinical Excellence (NICE), although there are greater calls for rational decision making in relation to health spending. This issue is highly emotive, as evidenced by media coverage of the cancer drug herceptin and its availability as part of the treatment for breast cancer.

Box 1.3 What are the key challenges according to student nurses?

> Dealing with the death of a patient and the bereavement of family/relatives
> Being there when a patient receives a diagnosis that might not be good news
> Dealing with a medical emergency

> Teamwork
> Health promotion – when patients are admitted to hospital, nurses do very little health promotion. Current health problems like obesity and smoking are not looked at
> I think it is important for nurses to contribute to basic nursing care. You can't fully assess a patient if you only spend a small amount of time with them

NHS scandals

The NHS has been characterised by increasing concerns about quality, public safety and resources, as evidenced by high-profile scandals in the late 1990s. *The NHS Plan* was designed to deal with some of these concerns and reduce growing inequalities in provision and access to services (DH 2000). Public inquiries such as Bristol, Alderhey and Shipman caused scrutiny of healthcare services and the professionals who work in them.

For example, the Bristol inquiry investigated the treatment given to children with heart defects and found high mortality rates for children undergoing surgery (DH 2001a). *The Royal Liverpool Children's Inquiry* was highly critical of senior staff at the hospital who had allowed the collection of children's organs following death without the consent of parents and families, and led to guidelines regarding the way doctors ask relatives for the use of children's organs (DH 2001b). *The Shipman Inquiry* (DH 2005) considered how many patients Shipman had in fact killed, in addition to analysing how the police had conducted investigations concerning Shipman, the management of controlled drugs in the community, practices for the certification of death and the monitoring and evaluation of general practitioners' professional practice.

Public confidence and trust in health services and professionals was so badly eroded by the above that the impact remains in terms of health service scrutiny and critique. While successive governments can develop policies and regulations to try and stop such things happening again, it is up to you, as a nurse professional within the health and social care team, to make a difference and restore the trust and confidence that people want and need. In the final analysis, the majority of complaints are about staff attitude and poor communication. Neither of these requires expensive equipment or financial outlay, they should be within your repertoire as a professional nurse.

Contemporary health policies

To redress imbalances within healthcare delivery, *The NHS Plan* (DH 2000) placed emphasis on reducing health and social inequalities, tackling staff shortages and developing new technologies and media. The development of integrated health and social care services was announced, along with proposals for walk-in primary care centres. A programme of hospital building was announced, along with the provision of more hospital beds.

Organisations within the NHS framework

New statutory organisations were developed as part of *The NHS Plan*. For example, the NHS Modernisation Agency is part of the Department of Health and was created to disseminate good healthcare practice. In order to address health inequalities and the so-called postcode lottery, whereby the nature of care and treatment varied according to geographical region, NICE (www.nice. org.uk/) now focuses on national guidelines for treatment, diagnostic efficacy and pharmacological issues. Public health was incorporated into its function in response to growing concerns about the overall decline in the nation's health.

The Healthcare Commission (www.healthcarecommission.org.uk) is the statutory organisation in England with responsibility for monitoring the overall quality of health services. The resulting information is in the public domain. For some this promotes transparency in terms of quality, while others argue that such league tables do not take account of factors such as social inequalities and other underlying factors that influence health within geographical regions.

Primary care **trusts** are large, community-based organisations that commission health and nursing services from the public and independent health sectors, on behalf of the geographical population they cover. They do this in response to assessment of local health needs, identifying key local health issues and commissioning services accordingly. In addition, they have to take account of stringent government targets and are ultimately accountable to the Department of Health, as well as the population they serve.

Activity 1.9

Google the NHS Modernisation Agency, NICE and the Healthcare Commission and make notes of their key aims and tasks.

Public health and nursing

In addition to care delivery following illness, health promotion and prevention are central to healthcare policies. While health and wellbeing have undoubtedly improved since the Second World War, persistent inequalities remain from childhood to old age. *Tackling Health Inequalities: A Programme for Action* (DH 2003) identified four key areas for action in relation to health:

1 Supporting families, mothers and children
2 Engaging with communities and individuals
3 Preventing illness and providing effective treatment and care
4 Addressing the underlying determinants of health.

Similarly, a report written to coincide with the 60th anniversary of the NHS entitled *High Quality Care for All* (DH 2008a) made recommendations in relation to health promotion and the following areas:

> Tackling obesity
> Reducing alcohol harm
> Treatments for drug addiction
> Reducing smoking
> Improving sexual health.

Given growing concern about the population's health, it is certain that the areas identified above in relation to health promotion will impact upon your role as a nurse influencing nursing care, health education, support and prevention to prevent ill health in the first instance.

Activity 1.10

Do you think the priorities above are the right ones? What are the health issues facing your community and how do you know they are important?

It is important for nurses to understand how social issues impact on the role of the nurse, and National Statistics Online (www.statistics.gov.uk) is a good student resource. Developments in the way we live and work, such as better nutrition, housing, employment and incomes, have improved our health and quality of life. Combined with better health services, these factors have enhanced life expectancy. In 2001, the average life expectancy was 80.4 years for women and 75.7 years for men (National Statistics 2006a). Similarly, childhood mortality from infections untreatable prior to the development of antibiotics, such as diphtheria and scarlet fever, has virtually been eradicated. Diseases such as tuberculosis have declined due to antibiotics.

However, these improvements in society's health have led to several paradoxes. For example, longer life expectancy does not necessarily equate with improved quality of life. It may be associated with more chronic health problems and social deprivation arising from poverty. Antibiotics have done much to improve mortality rates from infectious disease in the postwar era, but they have also led to the proliferation of resistant organisms such as MRSA. While tuberculosis incidence has declined dramatically following the introduction of antibiotic therapy, new and more resistant strains of the infection have evolved. Parental concerns about the safety of childhood immunisation, such as MMR, have led to a decreased uptake, resulting in a reservoir of illness in the population, with the potential for epidemics.

Postwar improvements in lifestyle have been modified by overconsumption of junk food and underconsumption of fruit and vegetables. As a result, obesity in the general population and children in particular is rising. It is estimated that, in 1995, 10% of boys and 12% of girls were obese; in 2002, this had risen to 17% for both boys and girls (National Statistics 2006b). Popular media celebrities have done much to raise awareness of childhood nutrition, while the government advocates changes to food labelling and active health promotion policies (DH 1999b, 2004b). A general decline in childhood exercise, such as walking and cycling to school, has also been considered as a contributory factor in child-hood obesity. It can be seen that while postwar health and social trends have improved, new challenges have arisen as a result. Circulatory diseases are the major cause of death in England, followed by cancers. Diabetes, mental health issues and musculoskeletal disorders are also major concerns.

The sociology of health and nursing

It is also recognised that there is a link between health and social conditions and those experiencing higher levels of social deprivation are more likely to have poor health. This was demonstrated by Townsend et al. (1979) who discussed the health link between social deprivation as indicated by housing, education and employment attainment. This replicated a theme evident since the first social studies conducted by Booth and Rowntree in the nineteenth century. Similar studies by Whitehead (1988) enhanced calls to address health by the reduction of social inequalities, which continue to widen despite health and social policies.

Away from social trends in health and illness, the nature of society is constantly changing. There is now an increased awareness of society's diversity, as illustrated by its multicultural composition. One in twelve people resident in the UK were born overseas. Similarly, migration inwards has increased since changes in the EU composition, with an estimated 223,000 more people migrating to the UK in 2004 for work or study purposes than migrated abroad (National Statistics 2005). Nurses need greater awareness of cultural issues and a greater respect for diversity, individual values and beliefs. Likewise, refugees and asylum seekers have complex health and social needs as they attempt to flee from persecution and integrate into another society.

Another major trend is towards an ageing population, resulting from improved health and living conditions, combined with smaller families and trends for women to have children later in life. Controversially, the ageing population is often portrayed in an ageist manner, with references to the burden of elderly care and the demographic time bomb. Such assertions are damaging, as they miss the richness of wisdom and experience that older people give to society. The implicit stereotypes also suggest that all older people will have health needs. In mid-2004, 16% of the population were over the age of 65 years, and of these, 12% were aged 85 years and over (National Statistics 2006a).

At the same time, opportunities for women in employment have been greatly enhanced by improved education and access to work, resulting from changes in attitude, equal opportunities legislation and the feminist movement. More women are now part of the workforce and are therefore unavailable to assume the caring role traditionally expected of them. Once a family or private responsibility, health and social services now assume an active caring role. However, despite this public sector involvement, it is estimated that 6 million people still provide unpaid care and support to friends and relatives

(National Statistics 2006c). Similarly, complex family networks, including reconstituted families from divorce and remarriage, also have the potential to impact on informal care and nursing practice.

Health in the twenty-first century: the Darzi Review

Professor Sir Ara Darzi, a consultant surgeon, led the Darzi Review (DH 2008b) to consider health service provision and to make recommendations to meet the future needs of the population. Among the many considerations are calls for greater staff empowerment within the NHS and greater choice for patients, especially in relation to GP services. In essence, quality is the key to improved care delivery within the NHS. Darzi recommended that GPs have the ability to commission health services on the basis of the wants and needs of the population they work with. There are calls for more health promotion to address dietary issues and smoking, for example, along with personalised care plans for those people with long-term conditions. There has been discussion of personal healthcare budgets so that those individuals with long-term health conditions can determine themselves how their budget is used to provide healthcare, thus providing more empowerment and choice. (Further discussion on the Darzi Review can be found in Chapter 4.)

While access to such information can be positive, it can also have a negative effect. Expectations of care may be falsely raised. Likewise it is difficult to distinguish between evidence-based practice and dubious information available on the internet and in the media. This is why nurses need good knowledge of research and evidence-based practice, to be able to appraise current knowledge and employ the best skills and techniques, while using health information properly to support patients and their families.

Summary of key points

> The NHS was formed in 1948, to provide a universal and comprehensive service, free at the point of use, regardless of the users' ability to pay.
> Postwar growth in acute services in particular has been influenced by improved diagnostics, surgery and pharmaceutical, sometimes to the detriment of mental health and continuing care services.
> Challenges such as waiting lists, MRSA, staff shortages, along with high-profile inquiries into health delivery, have prompted continuing health reforms.
> Agencies such as NICE, the Healthcare Commission and the Modernisation Agency have been introduced to evaluate the quality of health services.
> Health promotion strategies have been strengthened to address concerns about the overall decline in public health, arising from nutrition and obesity, coronary heart disease and other health problems.

Conclusion

The social influences explored in this chapter shape nurses' own lives and also where and how they work. The makeup of society is an important influencing factor for the location and context of nursing and is closely related to political and economic factors.

Ask yourself again, 'why do you want to be a nurse?' This question started the chapter, and your answers may or may not be the same at the chapter's end. If they are not the same, it is worth reflecting on what has changed and why. If you know you are choosing nursing because it seems to be a stable employment option, or your parents want you to, then you will find it difficult to learn and to be a nurse. Despite the acres of text related to study skills, personal reflection, vocation or whatever, in the final analysis, you will learn to be a nurse because you want to do it – you have a burning curiosity.

Curiosity is the thread running through the education of the nurses and other health professionals I work with; pre-registration to professional doctorate. It is not, as commonly believed, the development of more knowledge and advanced clinical skill relative to professional advancement, seniority or status that helps learning. It is the motivation and desire to learn more about people, from knowledge, from experience, from listening to others, from questioning, from thinking, from reading.

Useful resources

Department of Health www.dh.gov.uk
UK National Statistics www.statistics.gov.uk

References

Appleby, J (2006) *Spending on Healthcare, How Much is Enough?* London: King's Fund
Beveridge, W (1942) *Social Insurance and Allied Services* (Beveridge Report) Cmnd 6404, London: HMSO
DH (Department of Health) (1999a) *Making a Difference: Strengthening the Nursing, Midwifery and Health Visiting Contribution to Health and Healthcare*, London: HMSO
DH (1999b) *Saving Lives: Our Healthier Nation* and *Reducing Health Inequalities: An Action Report* 1999/52, http://www.dh.gov.uk
DH (2000) *The NHS Plan: A Plan for Investment, A Plan for Reform*, Cm 4818-I, http//www.dh.gov.uk
DH (2001a) *The Report of the Public Inquiry into Childrens Heart Surgery at the Bristol Royal Infirmary 1984-1995: Learning from Bristol*, Cm 5207(1), http://www.dh.gov.uk

DH (2001b) *The Royal Liverpool Children's Inquiry: Summary and Recommendations*, HC session 2000-2001012-1, http://www.dh.gov.uk

DH (2003) *Tackling Health Inequalities: A Programme for Action*, http://www.dh.gov.uk

DH (2004a) *NHS Improvement Plan: Putting People at the Heart of Public Services*, Cm 6268, http//www.dh.gov.uk

DH (2004b) *Choosing Health: Making Healthy Choices Easier*, Cm 6374, http://www.dh.gov.uk

DH (2005) *The Shipman Inquiry*: Chair Dame Janet Smith OBE, http://www.the-shipman-inquiry.org.uk/

DH (2008a) *High Quality Care for All: NHS Next Stage Review Final Report* (Darzi Review), http://www.dh.gov.uk/

DH (2008b) *Our NHS, Our Future: Next Stage Review* (Darzi Review), http://www.dh.gov.uk/

DH (2009) *The Prime Minister's Commission on the Future of Nursing and Midwifery*, www.dh.gov.uk

Fresco, A (2008) After 17 months of unimaginable cruelty: Baby P finally succumbed, The Times Online, http://wwwtimeonline.co.uk/tol/news/uk/crime/article5140511.ece, accessed 4/2/2009

Meerabeau, E (2001) Back to the bedpans: the debates over preregistration nursing education in England, *Journal of Advanced Nursing*, **34**(4): 427–35

Ministry of Labour (1946) Thank You Nurse Home Notes, 20 December, p. 46

National Statistics Online (2005) International migration: net inflow rose in 2004, http://www.statistics.gov.uk/cci/nugget.asp?id=1311, accessed 23/7/2010

National Statistics Online (2006a) Trends in life expectancy by social class, 1972–2005, http://www.statistics.gov.uk/downloads/theme_population/Life_Expect_Social_class_1972-05/life_expect_social_class.pdf, accessed 23/7/2010

National Statistics Online (2006b) Eating & exercise:1 in 6 children were obese in 2002, http://www.statistics.gov.uk/cci/nugget.asp?id=1329, accessed 23/7/2010

National Statistics Online (2006c) Caring & carers: 6 million unpaid carers in the UK, http://www.statistics.gov.uk/cci/nugget.asp?id=1336, accessed 23/7/2010

NMC (Nursing and Midwifery Council) (2008) *Confirmed Principles to Support a New Framework for Pre Registration Nurse Education,* available online at http://www.nmc-uk.org/Get-involved/Consultations/Past-consultations/By-year/Pre-registration-nursing-education-Phase-1-/Confirmed-principles-to-support-a-new-framework-for-pre-registration-nursing-education/, accessed 23/7/2010

Prime Minister's Commission on the Future of Nursing and Midwifery in England (2010) *Front Line Care: The Future of Nursing and Midwifery*, London: COI, http://cnm.independent.gov.uk

Rafferty, AM (1996) *The Politics of Nursing Knowledge*, London: Routledge

Savin-Baden, M (2000) *Problem-based Learning in Higher Education: Untold Stories*, Buckingham: Open University Press

Townsend, P, Davidson, N and Whitehead, M (eds) (1979) *Inequalities in Health* (The Black Report), Harmondsworth: Penguin

UKCC (United Kingdom Central Council for Nursing, Midwifery and Health Visiting) (1986) *Project 2000: A New Preparation for Practice*, London: UKCC

UKCC (1999) *Fitness for Practice: The UKCC Commission for Nursing and Midwifery Education,* London: UKCC

Whitehead, M (1987) *The Health Divide*, London: Health Education Council

2 your nursing course

James Richardson and Jackie Davenport

In this chapter we will explore:

> The Nursing and Midwifery Council
> Key access routes into nursing
> Selection of candidates to pre-registration nursing
> Academia
> Practice

Introduction

The Royal College of Nursing (RCN 2003, p. 3) defines nursing as:

> The use of clinical judgement in the provision of care to enable people to improve, maintain, or recover health, to cope with health problems, and to achieve the best possible quality of life, whatever their disease or disability, until death.

Nursing courses are typically split equally into half **theory** and half **practice** and this chapter has been devised to reflect this 50:50 split. You may have already chosen, or are considering, nursing as a career and by choosing to study as a nurse, you are entering a highly skilled profession which is greatly valued by the public and patients and you will be contributing to an excellent health service in the UK. Students of nursing must expect to work extremely hard during their studies because you must study at university while also undertaking a series of different work placements. You might find the course is far more labour intensive than that of other university students who might appear to get long summer breaks and other holidays which you probably don't. On the successful completion of your studies, you will have achieved a formal academic qualification such as a higher education diploma or a degree and become a graduate of your university. You will also have obtained registered nurse status and, in such cases, the university will then notify the **Nursing and Midwifery Council** (NMC, www.nmc-uk.org) that you have met the required standards and that you are eligible for entry onto the nurses register. Your course leader will also complete a declaration of good health and good character on your behalf.

The Nursing and Midwifery Council

Following an NMC consultation and review of pre-registration training in England, from 2013, the minimum level for pre-registration nursing courses will be raised from diploma to degree-level standard, so diploma-level courses are being withdrawn. Wales introduced all graduate training in 2004, Northern Ireland is moving towards degree only from 2011, while Scotland has its own criteria.

Before you can practise as a nurse, you will need to have paid your registration fee before your name is entered onto the NMC register, and only then will you be eligible to practise as a registered practitioner. The NMC's register (NMC 2005) is an instrument of public protection and anyone can check the registered status of a nurse or midwife on their website. A registrant is professionally accountable at all times for their acts and omissions.

The NMC exists to safeguard the health and wellbeing of the public by maintaining a register of all nurses and midwives, ensuring that they are properly qualified and competent to work in the UK. It sets the standards of education, training and conduct that nurses and midwives need to deliver high-quality healthcare consistently throughout their careers. The NMC's (2004) *Standards of Proficiency for Pre-registration Nursing Education* provide the standards of proficiency and education necessary for all pre-registration nursing programmes in the UK and all courses must meet its standards in order to continue delivering pre-registration nursing programmes. There are eight standards in total, which cover the entry to courses, continued participation in courses, and the nature and structure of such courses. Your course must meet these standards and these will determine, more or less, the nature and structure of your course.

Key access routes into nursing

You need to check with individual higher education institutions (HEIs) as to their entry requirements as these can vary. The minimum requirements are normally five GCSEs including Maths and English but if you are applying for a degree course, you will normally need A levels as well. Credit is also given for other qualifications, so you should consult the website of the universities you are interested in applying to or speak to staff in the admissions department who will be able to advise you. Mature students who do not hold traditionally accepted qualifications can also be considered for entry onto the course and should seek advice on an individual basis. Students on nursing courses vary widely in age, come from a variety of backgrounds and have very different qualifications. All have different valuable experiences and skills to offer nursing.

Activity 2.1

Read the following case studies and identify the access point most appropriate for you. ⌐

Case study 1: Jane – foundation degree entry

Jane has just completed a **foundation degree** (FD) in acute care. She had worked for years as a healthcare assistant in various settings and when the opportunity to apply for the course arose, she was encouraged by her manager to apply. She completed the necessary numeracy and literacy assessments and was interviewed by both the **higher education institution** (HEI) and the trust for which she worked. Jane was nervous but excited when she started her course but has found it beneficial to meet others and exchange experiences of working in similar roles with different ways of working.

Her course meant she stayed in her own workplace but with a structured set of outcomes and an identified mentor. Jane says that the FD has changed the way she thinks and she has learned more than she could possibly have anticipated. She now runs her own redressing clinic and is seriously considering doing a degree in nursing, which she could access in the second year because of her FD.

Case study 2: Ann – access course entry

Ann is 47 years old and has just entered the second year of her degree in adult nursing. Ann gave up her job in the tax office when she had her children, and when they left home, she thought she would be too old to pursue a career in nursing, which was what she has always wanted to do. She attended a university open day and was advised that there is no upper age limit. She did not have A levels and spent a year completing an Access Diploma, which meant she was suitably qualified to apply for a nursing degree.

Ann is delighted with her progress on the course. She feels that the skills she gained working in the tax office and also her experience as a mother of three children means she has a lot to offer nursing as well as being able to develop her own knowledge and skills. She has enjoyed the social activities at university, meeting new people and making new friends as much as the learning and is looking forward to the rest of her course and a career in nursing.

Case study 3: Helen – cadet nurse entry

Helen has just qualified as a registered nurse with a Diploma in Nursing. She did not achieve the required GCSEs to allow her access to the diploma but was able to gain access after a two-year course as a cadet nurse (in some areas, this is now an apprenticeship; see www.skillsforhealth.org.uk for further information). This course entailed two days a week in a clinical practice placement where she was supervised by a mentor and the rest of the week studying health-related subjects, numeracy and literacy. Helen then applied for the diploma and went through the interview process successfully.

Helen says her course prepared her for the move into university. She felt that the way the theoretical aspect of her cadet course linked to the things she observed and participated in, in practice, suited her style of learning and gave her confidence to pursue her dream of becoming a nurse.

Case study 4: James – school-leaver

James is in his first year as a student studying for a degree in child nursing. He is 18 years old and gained eight GCSEs including Maths and English. He also got three A levels, which met the 240 **UCAS** points required by the HEI to which he applied. James always wanted to work with children and has found that he has enjoyed all the placements he has had so far. James said he felt apprehensive before his first placement but he has been well supported by his mentor and has grown in confidence. He finds placements easier the more he learns as he says he can really see how the theory helps his practice.

James is living in student accommodation and although it is hard work, he has made lots of new friends, is seeing life in a new city and is thoroughly enjoying the student life.

Work-based distance learning

The Open University offers alternative, part-time, work-based distance learning opportunities for entry into nursing courses, foundation programmes and adult or mental health diplomas, as well as opportunities for registered nurses to top up to degree level.

Selection of candidates to pre-registration nursing

Each university will have its own access-level criteria and requirements, which will be available via their website and all recruitment and selection procedures must comply with relevant legislation including equal opportunities. Best practice would indicate that all candidates will have undertaken face-to-face engagement as part of the selection process; however, not all students need to attend an interview. The selection process should directly or indirectly involve representatives of partner service providers as well as laypeople and nursing or midwifery students, for example giving presentations or meeting with potential candidates. Those involved in the selection process should have received appropriate training, preparation and updating, including training in equality and diversity issues (NMC 2008a).

Good health and good character

Your good health and good character will have been assessed prior to admission to your course via your health declaration and examination, Criminal Records Bureau (CRB) check and your references. Good health can relate to particular health-related problems, which might affect your ability to practise safely and competently, for example epilepsy, drug or alcohol dependency. Good character refers to whether you have been cautioned or convicted by the police, subjected to allegations, investigation or suspension by any regulatory or other body. At defined stages during your course, you will be expected to complete further declarations of good health and good character and again on completion of your course, as you will be responsible and accountable to the NMC for your self-declaration when applying for registration. You must inform your tutors or other designated person immediately of any factors that may affect your good health or good character. If in doubt, talk to them, as it may in reality be nothing to worry about, but by not telling them, you may put your studies in jeopardy. Where it is thought your fitness to practise is impaired, you may be referred to a local fitness to practise panel, which will determine your suitability for practice. The panel outcome will need to be considered by the respective programme leader when deciding whether you can continue on your course or to sign or not sign the student's supporting declaration for admission to the register (NMC 2008b).

Literacy and numeracy

All university applicants must have provided evidence of literacy and numeracy sufficient to undertake nurse education. Evidence of literacy and numeracy is deduced from academic or vocational qualifications, through evidence to meet key skills abilities, or through the university's admissions processes, which may include portfolios or tests for those without formal qualifications. Feedback should be provided to applicants and to those to be admitted to a programme to enable their development needs to be identified and be addressed as part of their programme.

For numeracy, this includes accurately manipulating numbers as applied to volume, weight, and length, including addition, subtraction, division, multiplication, the use of decimals, fractions and percentages and the use of a calculator. For literacy, evidence of the ability to read and comprehend in English (or Welsh for students studying in Wales) and to communicate clearly and effectively in writing including using a word processor is required.

Where the International English Language Testing System (IELTS) is offered as evidence, programme providers should apply the NMC requirements for overseas applicants outside the European Union to the register, although approved educational institutions have the right to set their own standards but they must satisfy the NMC that there is sufficient evidence to meet its requirements. For these applicants, the NMC accepts the IELTS examination (academic or general version) with a score of at least 7.0 in the listening and reading sections, at least 7.0 in the writing and speaking sections and an overall average score of 7.0. The NMC requirements are to ensure, in the interests of public protection, that entrants to pre-registration programmes have a foundation of literacy and numeracy skills from which to develop, for example, proficiency in communication and drug calculation skills relevant to professional requirements (NMC 2008c).

Students with declared disabilities can meet the above through the use of reasonable adjustments, so if you wish to discuss these, the university will be able to help.

Age of entry

There is actually no minimum age entry requirement to pre-registration nursing programmes. The European Council Directive 2000/78/EC established a general framework for equal treatment in employment and occupation, preventing age discrimination in vocational training. The minimum age was removed to meet the requirements of the Directive by way of the Employment Equality (Age) Regulations 2006. Education providers must comply with the Health and Safety at Work Act 2004, which restricts the manner in which young people may be deployed, a young person being defined as 'any person who has not attained the age of 18' (NMC 2007a).

Health or learning needs

The Disability Discrimination Act 2005 does not force you to declare any health or learning needs. Examples of these include dyslexia, dyscalculia, dyspraxia, diabetes and visual or hearing impairment. You are encouraged to share this information with relevant parties such as your lecturers and **mentors** on a need-to-know basis. This information will only be shared with people who need to know in order to help you, and only with your consent; in this way, the staff can make reasonable adjustments to support you. If you don't declare your needs, they cannot be expected to help you. You will often find there are staff members in the trusts and universities who are employed specifically to help people with health or learning needs.

Supernumerary status

While on placement, you will have **supernumerary** status. This means you are not contracted or employed by any organisation to provide nursing care. In effect, you should never be counted in the staffing numbers to make up the full complement of care staff. It does not mean, however, that you are not there to contribute to and get involved in direct care delivery – after all, that is how you learn the skills to become a safe and competent practitioner. Student nurses must never consider themselves 'too posh to wash'. What it does mean is that if learning opportunities arise, you will be free to access them.

Stepping on and off your programme

There may be times during your course where you need to stop your studies for unusual circumstances such as long-term sickness, lack of academic or practice progress, or pregnancy. Your university will have made concessions for this through procedures known as APL (Accreditation of Prior Learning). If you are struggling with your studies for whatever reason, you should consult with a relevant academic member of staff at the earliest opportunity so that supportive action can be taken. You may be able to step back onto the course at a later, convenient date, once the difficulties you experienced leading to the stepping off the course have been remedied.

52 WEEK PROGRAMME FOR THE FIRST YEAR
– STUDENTS WORK A 37.5 HOUR WEEK –

COMMON FOUNDATION PROGRAMME

24 Credit (THEORY/PRACTICE) Introduction to Critical Skills for Nursing Practice

12 Credit (THEORY) Foundations for Professional Practice & Effective Learning

24 Credit (THEORY/PRACTICE) Communications for Well-Being & Health Promotion

24 Credit (THEORY) Human Sciences for Health & Well-Being

12 Credit (THEORY) Introduction to Inter-Professional Learning

24 Credit (THEORY/PRACTICE) Nursing Practice Across Settings 1

– STUDENTS WORK A FULL RANGE OF SHIFTS ON PLACEMENT –

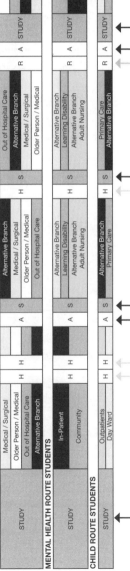

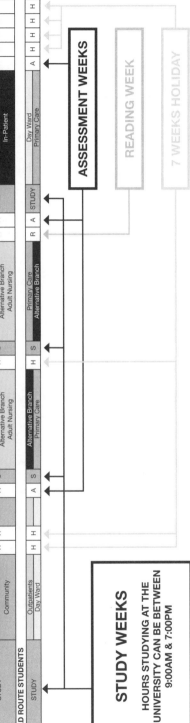

ADULT ROUTE STUDENTS

MENTAL HEALTH ROUTE STUDENTS

CHILD ROUTE STUDENTS

ASSESSMENT WEEKS

READING WEEK

7 WEEKS HOLIDAY

STUDY WEEKS

HOURS STUDYING AT THE UNIVERSITY CAN BE BETWEEN 9:00AM & 7:00PM

Figure 2.1 Example of a nurse training programme

Academia

Typical structure and content of the course

Your nursing programme will be at least three years or 4,600 hours long (50% practice and 50% theory). Full-time students must complete their studies within a five-year time frame (seven years for part-time students) including any interruptions.

The first year of your nursing course is called the **Common Foundation Programme** (CFP) (Figure 2.1). As the name suggests, the CFP is undertaken by all nursing students and provides a base of fundamental nursing skills. Within the CFP, you will gain experience of each of the four nursing branch areas – adult, children's, mental health or learning disability nursing. The end of the first year is a progression point into one of the four branches (Figure 2.2). Usually you will have already decided which branch you wish to progress into when you are accepted onto the course, but there may be an opportunity to change to another branch, another qualification, or even to another university at the end of the CFP. This will depend on many factors and you should not enter a course you do not want to complete in the hope that you will be able to change to another, as this may not be possible.

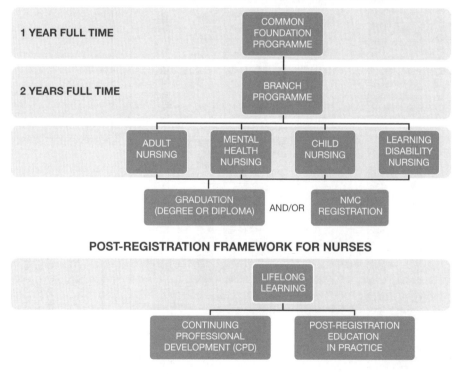

Figure 2.2 Pre- and post-registration frameworks

Your nursing programme will culminate in either a diploma of higher education or a degree along with registered nurse status. The two-year **branch programme** will develop your theory and practice specific to that branch. In order to progress onto the branch, you will have to have met strict progression outcomes as set by the NMC and standards of proficiency during the branch for entry onto the professional register at the completion of your studies.

The different branches of nursing

Adult

Adult nursing involves caring for those from the age of 18 upwards suffering with a variety of medical conditions. Adult nurses constitute the greatest number of NMC registrants and similarly students. The ethos of adult nursing is person-centred care that addresses the different needs, values and beliefs of patients from diverse communities. The qualification obtained is registered nurse (adult), previously known as registered general nurse (RGN) or state registered nurse (SRN).

Mental health

Mental health nurses deal with those experiencing mental distress. They focus on establishing healthy relationships with service users and carers to develop coping strategies to maximise potential for recovery. Previously known as registered mental nurses (RMNs), they are now known as registered nurses for mental health (RNMH). Mental health nurses and their students constitute the next largest number of nurses on the NMC register.

Child

Children's nursing is focused on the principal of family-centred care and that children should be cared for within the home by people they know, as far as is possible. They promote the rights of the child and work within a multiagency team to contribute towards child protection. Previously known as registered sick children's nurses (RSCNs), they are now called a registered nurse for children (RNC).

Learning disability

Learning disabilities nurses work in partnership with people of all ages with a learning disability, their families and carers to help individuals fulfil their maximum health and social potential in all aspects of their lives. They work with vulnerable clients as **advocates** and enable clients to develop their autonomy in exercising their rights and choices and enable clients.

For a complete guide to the content and direction of your programme, you can refer to the following documents: *Requirements for Pre-registration Nursing Programmes* (NMC 2002) and *Standards of Proficiency for Pre-registration Nursing Education* (NMC 2004).

Different approaches to learning

Your course structure will vary depending on which HEI you choose to study in but 50% of your course is theory, so you will spend some time in the university attending various study sessions. Sessions will be delivered in many different ways and these are outlined below.

Lectures

Sessions are delivered to large groups of students in a lecture theatre. You will need to take notes. Most universities run study sessions that you can access for guidance on how to take notes effectively. Lecturers may use PowerPoint presentations to support their sessions and these are often available on the virtual learning environment for you to access in your own time. Lectures usually provide an introduction to, or an overview of, a topic. However, it is up to you to do preparatory reading or expand your learning following the lecture when you have identified areas where your knowledge and understanding need developing.

Seminars

Seminars are small group sessions led or facilitated by one of your lecturers. They are often sessions in which the lecturer or one of the students presents a paper, which then generates discussion and/or further research by the rest of the group (Quinn and Hughes 2007). As a student, you will participate in your own learning, interacting with other students in your seminar group. Your lecturer will guide you in developing the skills necessary to make these sessions effective. For seminars to be successful and beneficial, all group members need to contribute fairly.

Tutorials

Tutorials are sessions given by a lecturer to a very small group or to an individual, and it is usually an intensive session with a particular focus.

Problem-based learning (PBL) or enquiry-based learning

Problem-based learning comprises small group sessions where you will work with other students to address a problem or scenario, which can be presented in varying forms. You will have a facilitator to guide you but the aim is to encourage teamwork in identifying what you need to know and linking the necessary theoretical knowledge to the context of the practice environment. You will then work together with the group to gain the knowledge necessary to address the issues you have identified. PBL is a beneficial way to learn as it is responsive to knowledge developments, promotes teamwork and encourages the use of evidence-based practice (Glen and Wilkie 2000).

Practical sessions

Practical sessions introduce you to, and allow you to develop, clinical skills, such as taking blood pressure, in a safe, supervised environment that poses no risk to patients. At the beginning of your course, these will be simple sessions that allow you to practise basic skills, but by your third year, they may be quite complex scenario-based sessions, which utilise advanced technology that can simulate emergency situations. This allows you to develop appropriate skills and confidence in a supportive and risk-free situation. Before you go onto your first placement, it is essential that you have been prepared in basic nursing skills to ensure you do not put yourself, your colleagues or your patients at risk. These skills may include moving and handling, basic life support and health and safety, including risk assessment, infection control and communication skills.

Directed learning/study

Directed learning/study is study that you will do in allotted study sessions with guidelines from your lecturer about the work you need to do.

Self-directed learning/study

Self-directed learning/study is study that you will do in order to address your own learning needs. The process of reflection will help you to identify gaps in your knowledge and you will then be able to address these accordingly. Self-directed learning may be timetabled or you may need to do this in your own time.

Activity 2.2

List the strategies you need to put in place to be successful in directed and self-directed learning and study.

Core clinical competences: Essential Skills Clusters

Essential Skills Clusters (ESCs) (NMC 2007b) have been incorporated into all nursing programmes since September 2008. They were introduced to clarify the expectations of the public and the profession to address some of the concerns about skills deficits identified in the *Review of Fitness to Practice at the Point of Registration* (NMC 2008d).

The review was undertaken to ensure that newly qualified practitioners were capable of safe and effective practice and reinforced the progression point between the CFP and the branches and addressed potential areas of skills deficit, so the public can be assured that these are assessed in all pre-registration nursing programmes. They have been mapped against Standard 7 of the *Standards of Proficiency for Pre-registration Nursing Education* (NMC 2004). ESCs are a set of UK-wide generic skills statements applicable to all four nursing branches, assessed within the context of the branch field of practice, which identify specific skills to support the achievement of current NMC outcomes for entry to the branch and for the proficiencies for entry to the register.

The ESCs are divided into five themes:

1 care, compassion and communication
2 organisational aspects of care
3 infection prevention and control
4 nutrition and fluid management
5 medicines management.

They identify skills that:
> are under broad headings fundamental to practice
> relate to all nursing fields of practice
> reflect patient expectations of new qualifiers
> complement existing NMC outcomes and proficiencies
> are required to be integrated into all pre-registration nursing programmes
> require specific testing
> require to be demonstrated before entry to the branch and prior to registration
> will be subject to ongoing review and monitoring (NMC 2007b).

For entry to the branch, it has been left to the universities to determine the nature and content of the assessment, so while the ESCs are the same, they may be assessed differently across various HEIs, including assessment via simulation (NMC 2007d). Simulated assessment must include the ability to safely perform basic wound care using clean and aseptic techniques. For entry to the nursing register, all assessment must take place in practice and a 100% pass mark is required for numerical assessment. While the NMC does not stipulate 100% for numerical assessment in the CFP, it would be improper for this not to be the standard that is accepted, as anything less than 100% poses a real risk to the public. Through simulation and coursework, the student is also required to demonstrate knowledge and application of the principles required for the safe and effective supply and administration of medicines via a patient group direction (PGD), including an understanding of role and accountability. Although it is stated that through simulation and coursework, the student demonstrates how to supply and administer medicines via a PGD, a student would never be in a position to partake in dispensing medication via a PGD, as further post-qualification training is necessary.

Practice

Practice experience (placements)

As well as the theoretical component of the course, it will contain a balance of practical instruction to include general and specialist medicine and surgery, childcare and paediatrics, maternity care, mental health and psychiatry (which can include learning disability), care of older persons and home nursing. As a consequence, your placements will include a variety of these specialist areas. There is now a trend to ensure that students experience increasing amounts of placements within the wider community, outside major hospital trusts, and within the private, voluntary and independent sectors. This reflects the changing trends of health service delivery. An example of a database that provides information in advance of practice placements is the Placement Learning Support System (www.plss.org.uk) in Cheshire and Merseyside.

Learning in the practice environment

The NMC's (2005) *Guide for Students of Nursing and Midwifery* gives clear guidance for students while they undertake practice or clinical learning when on placement, which is summarised below. Practice learning accounts for 50% of your student nurse education so must be taken seriously, as during this time you will be working with vulnerable clients with a variety of needs.

Accountability

As a student, you are not yet accountable to the NMC for your actions and omissions. However, the principles underpinning this guidance reflect the standards that will be expected of you when you become a registered practitioner. This does not mean, however, that you can never be called to account by your university or by law for the consequences of your actions or omissions as a pre-registration student.

Identifying yourself

When speaking to patients, relatives or members of the **multidisciplinary team** (MDT), you should always introduce yourself as a student nurse. People can get confused by uniforms and it is a criminal offence for anyone to represent themselves falsely and deliberately as a registered nurse. It is also important to always wear your proper uniform and you should never be on placement without a photographic identity badge (this may be your university card). When answering the telephone, clearly state the name of the placement area, for example 'ward 9 orthopaedics', your name and your status, that is, student nurse. Unless it is a routine phone call, pass the phone over to a qualified member of staff to deal with any enquiries.

The wishes of patients

Patients have the right to refuse to allow you, as a student, to participate in caring for them at all times and you must respect their right to do so. You must ensure that they are aware of your status before giving them any care. You should leave if they ask you to do so. The rights of patients supersede students' rights to knowledge and experience. This includes the manner by which you address patients. Never make assumptions about their personal lives, their lifestyle or how they would like to be treated. For example, check how they would like you to call them, for example 'Miss Jones', 'Mrs Smith', 'Margaret' or 'Peggy'. Don't assume that age differences make someone automatically a son or grandson, and do consider that your patients may be in same-sex relationships. It is all too easy to make a generalised assumption, which may offend them or interfere with the care you are able to give them.

Accepting appropriate levels of responsibility

As a student, you must be aware of working within your limitations, in so much as you should not participate in any procedure for which you have not been fully prepared or where you are not adequately supervised. You must be knowledgeable of local policies and procedures, which will indicate what students are able/unable to do. Some nursing skills require further training and skills development after initial registration and these are known as 'extended roles' and are not applicable to students. If such a situation arises, discuss the matter as quickly as possible with your mentor or personal tutor. Your level of given responsibility will develop as you progress throughout your course, as your skills, experience and confidence develop.

Patient confidentiality

The NMC code (NMC 2008e) provides advice on patient confidentiality, but any information relating to patients must only be used for the purposes for which it was originally provided and it must not be used for any other reason. As a student, you will have access to patient records only when absolutely necessary for the care being provided and you must follow the local policy on the handling and storage of all records. You must never access electronic records using anyone else's password or login as this breaches local data protection policy. If you want to relate an experience of a particular patient for the purposes of a case study, formal reflection or a critical incident report for your studies or portfolio, you must not include any detail that could identify a particular patient and never make a copy of any patient information such as assessment sheets, observation charts and so on.

Handovers

Do not make any written notes that can identify a patient, don't name them or their medical conditions thus breaching confidentiality. It is acceptable to make notes regarding the care or treatment they require and perhaps bed number. If you have any written or printed notes, they must not be removed from the practice area but must be destroyed at the end of each shift.

Handling complaints

If a patient informs you they want to complain about their treatment or care, you should report the matter immediately to your mentor or other appropriate person. Don't ignore the complaint. There will be local procedures for dealing with complaints by patients or their families about the treatment or care they are receiving, and you should become familiar with these. You are in a position to act as a patient's advocate.

If you see another healthcare practitioner doing something you feel is contradictory to the way you have been taught, ask them or someone else about it. Don't ignore it as it may be bad or outdated practice based on previous custom and practice, not in keeping with the evidence-based practice upon which your course is approved. For example, if it was a moving and handling issue, the practitioner could be putting themselves, another practitioner or the patient at risk of harm. In cases where you are not comfortable with what is asked or expected of you, check this out with your mentor or another trained member of staff. Don't put yourself or the patient in danger. Questioning an experienced practitioner's way of doing things can show you are observing and thinking and this may help a practitioner to improve their own practice.

What to expect from practice learning

Your practice area or ward will usually have been notified of your allocation well in advance of you commencing the placement. A named mentor should be allocated prior to you starting the placement. A mentor is defined by the NMC (2008f, p. 19) as 'a registrant who has successfully completed a NMC approved mentor preparation programme, achieving the knowledge, skills and competencies required', and they will have been qualified for at least a year. Your named mentor will not usually be supporting more than three students at a time so they can commit themselves to supporting your learning and assessment. However, note that there may be occasions when they have to prioritise the needs of patients in their care over the needs of the student. The mentor will usually be registered in the same part or sub-part of the NMC register as that part you intend to enter and in the same field of practice, that is, adult, mental health, learning disability or children. Exceptions to this rule are for CFP placements, which are not branch specific, or formative placements where proficiencies/learning outcomes are not being assessed (NMC 2008f, p. 64). Mentors are required by the NMC to maintain and develop their mentor skills, knowledge and competence through regular updating and they must participate in annual updating. You will usually only be allocated to a mentor who has been updated within the previous year and they will coordinate your placement. Students are expected to be proactive in negotiating and planning learning experiences, so in negotiation with your mentor, you will discuss and plan your total learning experience while on placement, and the amount of direct supervision will be determined according to your competence, ability and experience. Most assessment of practice should be done within the practice setting under direct observation. As far as the NMC is concerned, it is the registered practitioners with whom you are working who are professionally responsible for the consequences of your actions and omissions. This is why you must always work under supervision. You must be supervised directly or indirectly at all times, with a minimum of 40% of that time supervised while giving direct patient care. Your 'off duty' should reflect that of your mentor or back-up mentor, so that at least 40% of your time is spent working under their supervision, reflecting their shift patterns as best as possible. It is important therefore that you do not change the planned shift plans without authorisation, as these will have been done to ensure you are working with your mentor. The shifts worked should reflect those of the placement and you are required to demonstrate 24/7 care experience during the course, meaning you are expected to undertake night shifts, weekend shifts, bank holidays and so on. However, if you have specific learning or health needs, this would need to be viewed on an individual basis and a plan of action agreed by all parties. All shifts worked must be recorded on the off duty and in your placement attendance record. In three years, a minimum of 2,300 hours must have been recorded in practice.

Travelling to placements

You will have been informed at your interview or during your course induction that you are expected to travel to and from your placements and make the travel arrangements. In order for students to get a wide range of placement experience and meet the course requirements, is not possible for all students to always be placed near to their homes or within easy travelling distances. You will have to take responsibility for this and may need to be prepared to get up very early for some early morning shifts. Where this is problematic, you can discuss your concerns with the placements department or you mentor/placement manager and some mutual agreement may be possible. Be flexible. Unfortunately, you cannot expect to work 9–4, Monday to Friday for the whole three years of your course, and the NMC does not allow this anyway.

Placement preparation

Be proactive and take control of your learning. Ring up to see if you have had a named mentor allocated and what your off duty will be. You can prepare for each placement by pre-reading information about the practice area beforehand. Learn about some of the common conditions you will encounter, drugs and treatments used and abbreviations for that specialism.

Below is a list of useful hints to make your placement experience enjoyable:

> Ensure you take along relevant documentation on the first day to let the mentor know what your learning outcomes and so on will be. Most areas will provide an induction/welcome pack.
> Use a small notebook to jot down questions you want to ask of your mentor/supervisor. However, you must ensure that patients and their diagnoses are never identifiable as this would breach confidentiality.
> Don't be afraid to ask questions.
> Say no if you don't know how to do a task, or if you are asked to do something that is not correct, or breaches health and safety guidelines, such as lifting a patient without the necessary aids.
> Know your limitations and only work within them.
> Talk to patients – you can learn a lot from them.
> Spend time with the MDT. Interprofessional working is an important part of being a nurse, so take advantage of any available opportunities.

> Ensure that you get regular feedback at regular intervals. This can be formal or informal. Ask for feedback if you do not feel you are getting it.
> Make the most of supervision – be flexible with your working week.
> Ensure that you find out in advance the identities and contact details of the university lecturer and placement link staff.
> Ensure that you accurately record clinical hours and get these signed regularly where appropriate. Don't expect staff to be able to check these for you three months after finishing the placement.
> Attending in-house study days and mandatory training is free so make the most of it where appropriate and with the agreement of your mentor.
> Part-time jobs can cause a conflict of interest – your course must be your priority.
> Reflect on your practice, placement or critical incidents. It is good practice to make reflective writing a regular part of your development. Registered nurses are required to keep a professional portfolio and yours should begin when you start your course. This will continue throughout your career. Your reflections make up an important part of your portfolio and can help to show your progression.
> Know your rights.
> Join a union – they can protect you but also give you access to members services, contacts and support. By joining the **Royal College of Nursing** (RCN), for example, you automatically become a member of the Association for Student Nurses, which lobbies on your behalf. You can also access forums and networks, have free access to online publications and the careers service, which gives guidance on preparation, CVs, interviewing, career planning and so on.
> Make sure you are aware of the sickness and absence policy of the trust and the university. It is important that, if you are unwell and cannot attend either your placement or your university study, you follow policy to ensure that your attendance hours are correctly recorded but also because you should behave in a professional manner.

You will be supported throughout your course by a variety of professionals who are all working towards the same goal, which is to make sure you have a fulfilling education and are a practitioner who is 'fit for purpose, fit for award' by the end of your course. Most of these people will be employed by the university but some may be employed by the trust.

Roles vary between the different HEIs but you will be given information at the start of your course to help you identify where you should seek help with various issues, should they arise. Contact details for the numerous support services available are always readily available via the university website.

Professionalism: how you behave and how you look

You must remember that you are looking after people at the most vulnerable times in their lives and it is important that you present yourself in a way that gives them confidence in your ability. This applies to the way you present yourself in your appearance and your manner. The first impression a patient gets of you may be an important step in helping to build a trusting relationship with them (Arnold and Boggs 2007). The chewing of gum, smelling of tobacco or using a mobile phone while on duty is certainly not acceptable. The NMC (2009) has produced *Guidance on Professional Conduct for Nursing and Midwifery Students* to which you should adhere.

Uniform

There will be a policy that covers the uniform you should wear and how you should present yourself with regards to hair, makeup and so on. You should take pride in your appearance and remember that you are representing a profession. While wearing your uniform, you are an ambassador for your university and the nursing profession, therefore you must always adhere to the uniform policy applicable to any practice area where you are placed. Uniforms are designed to be practical, conform to health and safety matters and as a means of control of infection. Uniforms should not be worn while outside the workplace, and where this is not possible, they should be covered up.

If wearing a uniform outside, the general public might have greater expectations of you in your ability to deal with any emergency situation which might arise, for example if someone collapses or there is a road traffic accident. If this were the case, would you be able to manage within your level of competence? Some general principles apply to uniform policy for health and safety and infection control purposes. Hair should be neat and tied up above and off the collar. Fingernails should be trimmed and not longer than the tips of the fingers, and false nails should never be worn. The only jewellery to be worn is no more than a wedding band and one pair of small stud earrings, and facial or other visible piercings are not allowed.

Most trusts now adopt a 'bare below the elbow' policy, so wristwatches cannot be worn, only fob watches. The excessive use of makeup, fragrances and hair colourings should be avoided. Think about how strong scents could make an unwell patient feel.

Always display photographic identification as part of your uniform as you could be sent home without it. There may be variations to these rules for religious or health reasons.

Where you are allowed to wear your own clothes on placement, for example on some mental health areas or in schools or community homes, smart, sensible dress is expected that is respectful of others.

Footwear

The uniform policy of the organisation in which you work will stipulate the footwear you should wear. Generally, shoes should be flat heeled, closed toe and of a nonporous material (preferably leather). They should be soft soled so that you do not disturb patients.

Ongoing achievement record

For all summatively assessed placements of at least four weeks duration, students are required to provide an ongoing achievement record (OAR). The *Standards to Support Learning and Assessment in Practice* (NMC 2008f, p. 68) require that 'an OAR, including comments from mentors, must be passed from one placement to the next to enable judgments to be made on the student's progress'. The student must therefore consent to the processing of confidential data about them to be shared between successive mentors and with the relevant education providers in the process of assessing fitness for practice. Should the student not consent to the sharing of this data, this would make it incompatible with ensuring fitness for practice and unable to meet the programme requirements (NMC 2007d). The OAR must be given to your mentor at the beginning of any placement to enable discussion of strengths and areas for improvement.

Sign-off mentors

Final placement students will be allocated a **sign-off mentor**. This mentor will be given dedicated time of an extra hour per week to spend with you to ensure that all course outcomes have been met and to help you consolidate your learning. A sign-off mentor is an experienced mentor who is entered on the same part of the nursing register that you are working towards and will be a valuable resource to you as you approach the end of your course.

Conclusion

While nursing is definitely not an easy option when it comes to studies, it will lead to a thoroughly enjoyable and fulfilling career. There is a clear blend of interlinked theory and practice during the course, which is intended to bridge the theory/practice gap. This means that everything you are taught and are expected to practise is based on research and evidence-based practice. Education is a wonderful thing, it helps you to question, appreciate and challenge commonly held beliefs, customs and practices, which are not subject to evidence-based practice.

There will be sadness experienced along the way but also lots of fun and enlightenment. There are many sights that will shock you or smells that dismay you but there will also be experiences that cause joy – patients who recover or are cured, the birth of babies and so on. As a university graduate, you may be the first person from your family to have graduated and you will also have qualified for a profession for life should you choose that path. If not, your academic qualification in itself can be used as a starting point for other studies or professional work. Be proud of your achievements.

References

Arnold, EC and Boggs, KU (2007) *Interpersonal Relationships: Professional Communication Skills for Nurses,* St Louis, MI: Saunders

Glen, S and Wilkie, K (eds) (2000) *Problem-based Learning in Nursing: A New Model for a New Context?* Basingstoke: Macmillan – now Palgrave Macmillan

NMC (Nursing and Midwifery Council) (2002) *Requirements for Pre-registration Nursing Programmes*, London: NMC

NMC (2004) *Standards of Proficiency for Pre-registration Nursing Education,* London: NMC

NMC (2005) *An NMC Guide for Students of Nursing and Midwifery,* London: NMC

NMC (2007a) *Removal of Minimum Age of Entry Requirement for Pre-Registration Nursing and Midwifery Programmes*, NMC Circular 37/2007, London: NMC

NMC (2007b) *Introduction of Essential Skills Clusters for Pre-registration Nursing Programmes*, NMC Circular 07/2007, London: NMC

NMC (2007c) *Ensuring Continuity of Practice Assessment through the Ongoing Achievement Record*, NMC Circular 33/2007, London: NMC

NMC (2008a) *Good Practice Guidance for Selection of Candidates to Pre-registration Nursing and Midwifery Programmes*, NMC circular 13/2008, London: NMC

NMC (2008b) *Good Health and Good Character Guidance*, NMC Circular 08/2008, London: NMC

NMC (2008c) *Evidence of Literacy and Numeracy Required for Entry to Pre-registration Nursing and Midwifery Programmes*, NMC Circular 03/2008, London: NMC

NMC (2008d) *Review of Fitness to Practice at the Point of Registration,* NMC: London

NMC (2008e) *The Code: Standards of Conduct, Performance and Ethics for Nurses and Midwives,* London: NMC

NMC (2008f) *Standards to Support Learning and Assessment in Practice,* London: NMC

NMC (2009) *Guidance on Professional Conduct for Nursing and Midwifery Students,* London: NMC

Quinn, F and Hughes, S (2007) *Principles and Practice of Nurse Education,* Cheltenham: Nelson Thornes

RCN (Royal College of Nursing) (2003) *Defining Nursing,* www.rcn.org.uk

3 key skills for nursing students

Mary Birchenall

In this chapter we will explore:

> Key skills
> Managing time
> Academic skills
> Learning in the practice setting

Key skills

Any student of modern schooling will be well versed in the notion of key skills. Having achieved these skills in core areas of writing, referencing, IT, study and planning and numeracy, perhaps you thought they had been left behind. On the contrary, these key skills form the platform on which the professional skills of nursing can be laid. The foundations for nursing incorporate many elements of the key skills familiar to you and add a few more. As your career progresses, your foundation skills will develop and expand and further core elements will evolve. In this way, the notion of becoming a lifelong learner takes shape and is given some reality. During those early days, it is advisable for the foundations to be laid at the right time, because the old adage 'cart before the horse' is clear in its message that attempting new skills without these foundations is inadvisable.

Early days

For many, the passage into nursing education and university life is paralleled with the newness of living independently for the first time. It is unsurprising then that core skills as a familiar element in education can be put to one side in favour of university life, the more exciting 'new' learning on offer and the anticipation of entering the practice area. However, it is in these early days that most universities offer 'study skills' packages covering introductions to the library, note taking, referencing, the university intranet, literature searching and so on. These are usually core, open to all courses and accessed independently of your course. They are free and very useful, but they are often not found or their significance not realised until it is too late, so do look out for them and try to make use of them. If you have missed them, it is likely that you can access the lecture notes through the university intranet. If you miss these opportunities, consider taking them up in the second year. You could befriend a first year and mentor them through the process of accessing these tutorials so saving face but gaining the learning.

This early warning note about using the resources freely offered provides a reminder of the significance of those core skills and particularly *managing time*. Before engaging with the need to manage time effectively, let us summarise the key skills for nursing students.

The key skills include:

> Managing time
> > Coursework
> > Preparing for assessment
> > 'Knowing yourself'
> > Using the library and internet
> > Practice-related study issues
> > Teamwork
> Academic skills
> > Writing skills
> > Numeracy skills
> Learning in the practice setting
> > Learning by seeing and doing
> > Recording practice
> > Reflective learning

Managing time

Burning the candle at both ends may maximise the use of time but not necessarily manage time. So if you are to enjoy life, study and participate in nursing practice, it is essential to manage time effectively. A core aspect of managing time is to have a clear knowledge of what you have to do and identify a strategy to achieve your goals. The knowing bit should be straightforward as you will have a course handbook that provides you with all the information required to estimate your workload. In relation to the management of time, there is one aspect of academic development that is often overlooked. There is no visible outcome from this activity, in that is often a forerunner to any product. This activity could be labelled 'thinking time'. It is essential, however you work, whether fast or slow, to deadlines or structured diary, that you allow yourself some thinking time. This will include deliberating internally over your reading, examining potential arguments and starting points for your debate or essay. Thinking time can be likened to the proving time in making bread when bread is set aside to raise and become light; in the same way, thinking time allows a maturing process to emerge in the production of a cogent argument. Do not underestimate this activity; the great thing about it is that it can occur anywhere, on public transport, while carrying out mundane household chores or even in the shower. So let us continue now and examine the nature of coursework.

Coursework

It is not unusual to find that course handbooks are filed away and rarely looked at, but this is a serious mistake. Everything you need to know about the nature and demands of your course is in there. There will be hints and tips pertinent to your department and university, contact details for key people who can and will help you, and the rules and regulations for your course. You need to read these and from these regulations identify the must do, the best to do and, if you were perfect, the extra bits. This is an important part of establishing your personal timetable. This latter is separate from the programme timetable and is relevant to you, your lifestyle and preferred approach to study. To take advantage of planning your time, you need some information from the course handbook, in particular the various timetables.

Using the assessment timetable

Alongside the various modules and practice experience timetable, there is an assessment timetable. This timetable forms the structure for managing time throughout any programme you may undertake. It is useful to create a calendar that clearly shows the expected dates for submission of essays and examination dates. Additionally, as you move through your programme, there may be practical assessments and practice-based documentation to complete and submit. A simple table can be helpful at this point. A suggestion is given in Table 3.1; it is not infallible as a structure but the idea is to have something that clearly shows the demands your course makes on you and the clear dates for submission or sitting of an exam. If there are computer-assisted tasks and assessments, there will be specific rules as to when you can access the exam and how long you can work on the task; make sure you clearly understand these rules.

Table 3.1 Planning for first semester assessments

Module	Assessment	Useful activities	Stages of work	Submission date
Intro to nursing practice	1 Reflective diary 2 CAL 1 hour	1 Weekly review 2 IT workshop and student ID		
Intro to biology for healthcare	Unseen exam 1 hour	Review past papers		
Intro to sociology for healthcare	Essay 1,500 words	Check out referencing Clarify titles		
Intro to psychology for healthcare	Essay 1,000 words			

The next stage is to understand how you work, and how best to prepare yourself for achieving the aims of the course.

Knowing yourself

It is likely that during one of your modules, you will cover the topic of learning and leadership types. These can inform you as to the best strategies for you to use to approach work. But this is in the future and you have assessments that require planning and preparation now. Below are some useful questions that, if answered, will help you achieve this important early planning.

Think about how you work. Ask yourself the following questions:

1 Do I work quickly or slowly?
2 Do I need an urgent deadline to stimulate me to work?
3 Can I multitask effectively or do I need to focus on one thing at a time?
4 Am I aware of any shortfalls in my study skills and is there help available?

The answer to these questions will help you plan your assessment strategy. If you are methodical and need to review work continuously, you must start the actual writing and revision processes early. It is fairly common to have assessments clustered around the same week, so planning needs to take this into account. Additionally, if you need to focus on one topic at a time, then you need to create a timetable that gives you the opportunity to get work to the draft stage with sufficient opportunity to review before submission. You may therefore create artificial dates for individual assignments to allow you to stagger your work. You do not need to have completed a module to start the assignment. Usually the assignment requires you to develop knowledge beyond the lecture and show its application to nursing or healthcare.

On the other hand, if the stimulus of an impending deadline is the motivation to work, then you need to recognise this and ensure that during the course of the semester, you maintain your reading and research on the topic and make notes that will be useful at the point of writing or revision. Given that we all require some stimulus to engage in work that may or may not be attractive, consideration must also be given to the speed at which work is achieved. Some people work slowly, others quickly. The slower work is produced, the more time needed to meet deadlines. Hardly rocket science, but not a few students have found themselves in difficulties because they did not marry their speed and approach to work with the timeline developed for that work. Knowing yourself and the way you work can greatly reduce the stress of assessment.

Using the library and internet

Consider the nature of the essential information sites available to you and ask yourself the following questions:

1 How do I navigate through the various information sites and assess their value?

2 How do I tell the difference between researched web-based sites and personal opinion sites?

3 Have I located the IT centre at the university?

4 Have I located the parts of the library that will be most useful to me?

5 Is there more than one library available to me?

The majority of universities are vast and so in those early months finding your way around is no mean task. Locating the library(ies) is important. There is, in this IT-focused era, a temptation to overuse the internet. The problems that will be encountered by an overdependence on the Web are likely to be in accessing seminal work that forms the foundation for the majority of disciplines; the library is an essential tool. Also, current journals are maintained in the library, and it is always useful to know where your discipline keeps its journals and how to use the bound versions of these from past years. Often, having a current reference list is difficult, but efficient use of the journals can bring your references up to date.

Activity 3.1

The table below provides a potential strategy for commenting on the availability of journals and their relevance for your programme over the semester. It is always useful to make notes when visiting a library for the first time, as you may find just what you need but may not find it so easily the next time.

Library	Journal	Location	Key areas of content	Useful for modules

Most universities have several libraries. Visit each one and note the key journals that you may use. It is also useful to visit sections dedicated to subject areas linked to healthcare and explore their journals. You will be pleasantly surprised at what can be used. Do try this out in the early part of your programme as you will get busier as time moves on and assessment deadlines approach. A thoroughly kept **learning journal** will reduce the time spent searching for the right information at your busiest period.

Practice-related study issues

Part of the assessment in a healthcare programme is grounded in practice. This means that at the end of a working day, there is a need to record issues and maintain a **work diary** reflecting on things observed and learned during that day. It is likely that a formal part of assessment will be based on such a

reflective diary/journal. It is easy to put off such recording and feel justified by the hard work of the day in so doing. But this is a dangerous approach. Getting into the habit of making short notes that will remind you of thoughts, feelings and links to theory will not only help your early assessment but will also develop your reflective approach to practice. These short notes can be expanded on a weekly basis and provide the material for a truly reflective journal. Additionally, there are likely to be issues that arise for which you have insufficient knowledge. It is at this point that familiarity with the library and specialist journals will reduce the time taken to source your information. Do take care when note taking from journals, texts or seminal work to highlight for yourself those parts of your notes that are your comments and those that are quotations or close paraphrases from the published authors. Although the old truism suggests that to be copied is to be flattered, in academic terms copying of another's work is labelled **plagiarism**. Plagiarism is an academic 'crime' and, in extreme cases, can be the cause of a student being removed from the course. So take care throughout your student and practitioner life to ensure that you know the difference between your own work and that of others. In this way, you avoid accidental errors.

Teamwork

Few healthcare professionals work in isolation, each discipline works in teams. This is true of studentships also. Some tasks may be given to groups to achieve and working together is required. This is a formal expectation of teamwork. There are key roles in teamwork and knowing your personality type will help you become aware of the role you are likely to take. So if you tend towards the leader role, take care that you do not overload yourself with responsibilities that should be shared. In contrast, if your group is made up of followers who wait to be fed information, again establish clear ground rules for sharing the workload.

Informally, if an area of learning requires extensive literature searching, it is reasonable to share the work between colleagues. If four people each summarise key points from four different articles or chapters in a book, then the key points can be shared. This does not substitute reading the entirety of an article or chapter; it does help get information together for seminars and coursework. The way that each individual uses the material ensures the individuality of the work.

Academic skills

There are specific requirements in every university with regard to the way that assignments are presented and referenced. Also the regulations pertaining to examinations are specific to each university. These regulations and requirements are found in your university handbook and made relevant to your programme in your departmental and programme handbooks. These form your base reference. Within your programme handbook, you should also find the grading criteria used by your assessors to grade your work. These are normally divided into sections showing the criteria used to assess your work. For example, some reference to knowledge and understanding, analytical ability, presentation and style, referencing, and relevance to practice are common in most healthcare programmes. Through reading the grading criteria, you can start to understand the way that marks are achieved and help to improve your grades. At first, it may seem bewildering, but after the first assignments are returned, then do reread the criteria for your grade and this will help you to see where your writing skills and knowledge base are placed. This should help you to improve for the future. The activity below can help you to extend your understanding of the grading criteria and the implementation of this in your written work. Do bear in mind that if you understand properly the relationship between clarity of writing, referral to key sources and discussion of arguments for a seen essay, this will have a complementary impact on writing in unseen assessed work.

Activity 3.2

The table below shows the commonly used criteria for assessment. You may like to change the words for those used in your programme or assessment handbook.

The first column asks you to outline your understanding of these terms. This will help to consolidate your understanding of the criteria and so better enable you to achieve them.

The second column asks you to comment on the way(s) in which you can demonstrate this within your work. This is aimed at helping you to reinforce in a practical way your understanding of these criteria.

Criteria	What I understand this to mean	How I can show this in my essay
Knowledge and understanding		
Analysis		
Presentation and style		
Referencing		
Relevance to practice		

So, having familiarised yourself with the grading criteria, you now need to consider the process of writing an essay. The following section provides some hints and tips on writing an academic essay. The more practised you are at writing, the easier it becomes and you will also be able to apply these principles to unseen examinations. So use your rough notes carefully, practice reviewing articles on a regular basis, and these will be available to you as a ready resource when you write your essay.

Writing skills

This section is most useful in the preparation and review of an essay, but can be applied to unseen examinations also:

> *Structure:* A key issue in writing is structure. This relates to the entire process of writing from the thinking and note-taking stage through to the planning and writing of the essay.
> *Thinking stage:* When you receive your essay title, you need to identify a strategy that will take you to its completion with as little stress as possible. Remember the section above on knowing yourself; you need to put this into play immediately. Here are some pointers you may like to consider:
>   ▶ Do you need the adrenaline surge of the imminent deadline?
>   ▶ Do you like to be organised and methodical in your timetable?
>   ▶ Do you want your supervisor to read a draft section? If so, take this into account when developing your timetable.
> *Reading:*
>   ▶ Organise your library visits
>   ▶ Ensure you make time for computer access
>   ▶ Focus on your topic; avoid digressing because something is interesting. You can always make a note and return when the assignment is finished.

Note taking

Note taking is deliberately presented in note form, using headings, subheadings and bullet points. This helps to simplify reading back and is less time-consuming than having to read whole sentences. It also has the advantage of being quicker than writing mini-essays.

Is your note-taking strategy developed sufficiently so that you will be able to use the material you record from your reading? For example:

1 Each time you start to read a chapter or article, before you start to read, write down the full reference.
2 Create a 'talking to yourself' style of notebook, whether paper or electronic. In this, all references, their value and specific notes can be clearly recorded.
3 Be absolutely clear where your notes end and a direct quotation begins.
4 If you do take quotes, record the page number alongside the full reference.

Ambiguity in note taking in relation to quotations could lead to dire problems. Ensure that you will be able to distinguish between your words and those of the author. The penalties for plagiarism (copying) will be shown in the student handbook issued on registration. It is imperative that you read this, as the penalties can be severe and, at the very least, embarrassing.

Activity 3.3

- Take a new notebook into the library
- Select an article or chapter to read
- Before reading, write the full reference in your notebook
- During reading, note any words you do not understand
- On completion, write a brief comment on the relevance of the article and its relationship to your course or future assessment
- Look up the words in your list and note the meanings
- You have begun to keep a learning journal

Supervision

You will be allocated an **academic supervisor** to support you in your work. It is your prerogative to use this person and it is up to you to organise supervisory meetings. A personal invitation is unlikely to come, so do make appointments and keep them. Avoiding the last-minute approach will help to reduce stress and also ensure that a meeting can be arranged in time to be of benefit to the completion of your assessment.

Planning an essay

Planning will help you to:

> focus on issues that are *relevant*
> keep a *clear* head
> cover all *important* aspects.

These are some general hints:

1 Brainstorm key issues.
2 Organise the ensuing lengthy list into clusters or groups.
3 Check that all the important elements are included.
4 Devise a plan for your essay. There are many ways of doing this. The essential requirement of any plan is that it shows the sequence of points to be covered and clearly identifies the structure. The spider diagram in Figure 3.1 shows some options.

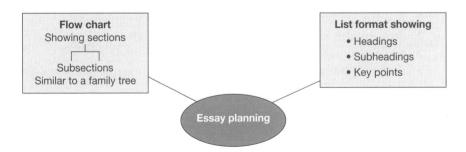

Figure 3.1 Planning an essay with the help of a spider diagram

Read the essay question. What are you being asked to do? You can assess this through the verb that leads the question. For example, the following verbs are often used at some point in an essay question: justify, discuss, critically analyse, and evaluate. A dictionary definition and thesaurus can help you to examine these key verbs and realise the extent to which they influence the accuracy of your approach to answering the question. Your task involves answering the set question, so how you use your hours of reading and thinking is significant. It is unlikely that a question will be set that suggests you should write down everything you know about a subject. Rather, you will be required to present a cogent, balanced academic argument that shows some form of analysis, leading to a conclusion.

Critical thinking

The development of analytical and critical thinking skills is an outcome of undergraduate study, leading to a more open, enquiring and knowledgeable practitioner. Edwards (1998, p. 161) suggests a model for critical thinking that comprises the following components:

> Agreeing
> Presenting a new point of view
> Conceding
> Reformulating
> Dismissing

> Rejecting
> Reconciling
> Retracting or recanting
> Choosing
> Originality.

Edward's (1998) article is particularly useful since each component is defined and illustrated with a model example. If you are uncertain of how to proceed, you can then use such examples as a template to build your confidence and provide time for your own style to emerge.

The essay structure

Paragraphs and stuff

The essay is a total structure, but if that structure is to be coherent to a stranger (your assessor), then each component part of the essay must also have a structure. It goes something like this:

> *Essay:* concerned with the whole issue set out in the question
> *Sections:* each of which deals with a topic that builds towards your essay
> *Paragraphs:* each developing a component of a section topic
> *Sentences:* build up your paragraph and contain a coherent stand-alone statement.

The rules that guide the internal structure of each part of your essay are established within the principles of grammar. Grammatical writing aids clarity in communication. So if you missed out in early education lessons on verbs, nouns, subjects, objects and all the other components of grammar, it would be useful to find an introduction to grammar. Do not be embarrassed to buy something written for schools by publishers such as Usborne, as these are easy to find and relatively inexpensive.

Beginnings and endings

The *introduction* should tell the reader what to expect. The story that goes before the essay starts is a *preamble* and there is rarely space for this in early and relatively short academic essays. It is easy to be trapped into thinking that the process of working your way into a topic is your introduction. This is rarely the case. A sound rule to try out is to omit that early first paragraph and see if anything is lost to your argument. Usually it is best left out. Such a preamble is useful to get you started but not in the presentation of cogent argument.

The *conclusion* should emerge from the arguments that you have put forward in your essay and make some claims as to the significance of your findings. A *summary* is a collation of the key facts that have emerged from your work. Longer essays may have both a summary and a conclusion.

Just to add to the demands of rigorous writing, each section, paragraph and sentence should have a beginning, middle and end. Each section should also have a minor introduction and conclusion, possibly just a sentence in length. It is this strategy that promotes the logic and continuity of an essay. The useful part of this latter strategy is that these mini-introductions and conclusions can retrospectively help you to write a concise and pertinent introduction and conclusion to an essay. Yes, you have surmised correctly, the introduction is best written or rewritten once the essay is finished.

Essay length

The overall length of an essay is prescribed by the assessment criteria. The word extent is given, for example 1,500 words. There is usually an allowance given for exceeding that word limit, often set at 10%, but do check your university's guidelines. Penalties can be imposed if you exceed the word limit. You may think this unjust, but presenting your argument succinctly is part of the challenge set by your examiners, and hence part of the marking criteria used to allocate your grade or mark.

In the case of an unseen examination, the length of time allocated to the question, in conjunction with the weighting for the question, determines how long your essay will be. For example, a question may be in two parts, with a mark of 5 for the first, and 15 for the second. It does not take a genius to realise which part needs the most time spent on it. In turn, if you know a lot about part 1 but not too much about part 2, you may be tempted to reverse the timings. Do avoid this, as the maximum marks that can be gained remain 5 for part 1 and no more, however much you may write. Of course, the speed at which you write in an exam is variable, so the faster you write, the more knowledge you can demonstrate. Set against this, *legibility* is essential, as the examiner needs to be able to read your words in order to allocate the mark.

Additionally, when considering the length of an essay, a hierarchy of importance is needed. Some issues will have greater significance than others and need more space. Using the structure set out above does not require a uniformity of size for each section or paragraph.

Set against this, sentence structure can make or break the *readability* of an essay. Too long and the reader loses the initial point; too short and the feel is abrupt and staccato. A general rule is that each sentence should be complete in itself and provide a building brick in the overall formulation of the paragraph. If your sentence is making more than one point, consider splitting it into two sentences. Alternatively, develop an understanding of the use of semi-colons and colons. If you remain uncertain, try reading a long sentence aloud; if you struggle with breathing, it definitely needs reducing or splitting. Such a strategy will strengthen your arguments.

Evidence

Your assessors are truly interested in what you say, but they also require support for your statements from published literature. Evidence needs to be sound, of significance and relevance to your subject. Additionally, the nature of your supporting material can often determine the depth, accuracy and relevance of your arguments. A strong essay contains information about the nature of the supporting material; for example an indication as to whether the source is a significant research study, an article in an academic journal, or a newspaper report. The more esteemed or valued the source, the higher the significance of the argument. Popular media sources have a purpose if public opinion or trends are an issue of concern, but, generally, source material should have academic rigour guaranteed. After all, it is academic credit that you wish to receive for your work. In relation to the internet, if a source can be added to by the general public, this can lead to confusion as to the accuracy of the content. Therefore, it is sensible to discriminate and use websites that are dedicated to the subject and maintained by authorised individuals rather than general subscribers.

Presentation

The presentation of your essay is more than cosmetic. Accurate spelling, clear type face or handwriting, complete sentences, page numbering and clear instructions to the reader are essential components of your final work. The grammar and spellchecker are useful but not in isolation from your own careful review. How many times has the spellchecker *mist* a correctly spelled word despite its inappropriate placement? Editing your own writing is a useful means through which to develop your writing skills. Always leave time between completion and the final read through, as this will help you to take the editing process seriously, and result in feeling less pain. You may find that if you can let some time pass between completion and review, you will find positives that you did know were there and can confront and rectify the negatives. The key is to read your work as though you were the stranger; such a strategy ensures that you read what is on the page, not what is in your head. It is not unusual to find that the point you intended to make is not entirely made clear in the actual words written on the page; if part of your evidence remains in your thinking rather than your writing, then it cannot contribute to your argument.

Levels and marking

The grading criterion used to assess work, normally found in the student hand-book, was mentioned earlier. This criterion provides helpful indications as to the standards necessary to achieve particular grades. If you combine a thought-ful approach to your planning, reading and writing, in conjunction with insights gained from the marking criteria, then you can strengthen your posi-tion in relation to successful academic achievement. Frequently, students say, 'I'll be happy just to pass!' but is this a true sentiment? When hard work and time has been put into something, a good mark is felt to be the only just reward. So thoughtful application of the principles outlined here will help. Safety first suggests that rather than aiming for a pass, it is best to aim for the highest mark, ensuring that failure will not be possible.

Numeracy skills

We have travelled a lengthy journey considering writing skills. Next, in order to ensure safety in the practice area, we will consider numeracy skills. For some, this is basic knowledge comfortably held through schooling. For others, it is embarrassing to admit that it is an alien field. Again, there are likely to be opportunities in the early days at university to consolidate maths learning and these should be noted.

Numeracy in nursing is an essential key skill. The administration of medi-cine, reading of tests, recording routine observations, such as temperature, pulse, respiration and blood pressure, all require mathematical awareness. These skills will emerge in the early days and develop further with the use of more sophisticated tests in later years. A quarter of legal claims are due to mistakes made in prescribing and administering drugs (DH, 2004). Since 2008, the NMC requires that all students have their numerical skills assessed. This must happen during the first year of the Common Foundation Programme (CFP) to enable progression to your chosen branch of nursing. Practice place-ment in the branch programme must include achievement of an assessment of numerical skills to enable registration with the NMC. So it is essential that numbers can be recognised.

Activity 3.4

Some important facts are given in the table below. You are asked to reflect on the implications of these. As you progress through your first year, for each placement area, consider:

- The impact of numeracy in all aspects of your work
- Personal learning needs
- The significance of numeracy for your future.

Key issues	Examples	Reflections
Use of calculator	The NMC (2007, p. 24) makes this clear statement about using calculators when making drug and other calculations: 'The use of calculators to determine the volume or quantity of medication should not act as a substitute for arithmetical knowledge and skill'	
Estimation	For example: If a calculation asks you to multiply 4 by 2.5; an estimate will tell you the answer must lie between 8 (4 x 2) and 12 (4 x 3). Estimation has an important place when doing a calculation as this can prevent *large mistakes due to decimal point errors*	
Due process	Identify any processes that nurses are required to follow in each practice area	
The future	You could be expected to complete a numeracy test when applying for posts at the end of your training and for senior positions. Also, nurses in senior roles use numbers to calculate staffing ratios	

As a student, you are free to ask for advice and help. An in-depth review of numeracy in nursing is provided in a number of texts (for suggestions see the recommended texts at the end of this chapter). You will find such a book extremely useful, especially if numeracy is an area that you consider with apprehension. To assist you to identify numeracy needs or reassure yourself that you can transfer school-learned mathematics to nursing practice, complete the following activity.

Activity 3.5

Carry out the tasks in the table below: record your experiences in your learning journal and, significantly, identify any learning needs now.

Numeracy in practice	Calculations	Reflections
Drug doses	Select a frequently used medication in your practice area: • Identify the daily dosage • Calculate the quantity required at each point of the medication regime • How will this vary if taken twice as opposed to three or four times daily? • Seek out the dosage in both solid and liquid forms if possible • Have your calculations checked by your mentor	

Fluid intake and output	Over a period of three education-based days:
	• Complete a fluid balance chart for yourself
	• Consider problems you experience:
	  • ensuring accuracy
	  • measuring from non-standard containers
	  • remembering and recording elimination
	Over a period of three practice days:
	• Complete a fluid balance chart for one or more patients/clients
	• How will you ensure accuracy for self-recorded measurements?	

Future placements may require you to record measurements that are more complex than the examples given. It is essential therefore that basic calculations are mastered at the beginning of your learning	Find out about: • Body mass index • Risk scores for malnutrition • Degrees of burns	

Developing IT skills

A linked area to numeracy is that of IT. Modern approaches to communication mean that familiarity with the internet is a given. There are specific requirements for nursing students.

Visit www.palgrave.com/glasper to read the online IT skills chapter from Glasper et al. (2009) *Foundation Skills for Caring*: 'It offers top tips and advice on information management and Web technologies and will help prepare you for study in the digital age.'

Learning in the practice setting

Student nurses are required to demonstrate at least 50% of their course time in practice or practice-specific activities. This means that there is a complex demand made on novices from the onset of the programme. Before you feel too hard done by, you are not alone. Many programmes have practice-specific components. You will meet many other learners in healthcare and if you are university based, you may also meet student teachers, speech therapists, social workers and engineers to name but a few. All these students will struggle to balance academic theory with knowledge-based practice. So you have scope to share some dilemmas with others and learn from them too. Many universities now share work-based learning modules that each programme tailors to suit the needs of that particular area of practice. Through such modules, common aspects of learning in the practice setting can be shared and problem solving becomes energised, as each discipline shares their perspective on managing learning through reflecting on practice. Of course, this does not make your learning task simpler. The following section offers a potential map through the sometimes rocky terrain of work-based learning.

Learning by seeing and doing

Practical learning has many variations. Initially, there will be mock-up situations in the teaching environment; these may take place in a clinical laboratory or a classroom. This is an early opportunity to carry out everyday activities of living and nursing in a safe and non-threatening environment. Ultimately, and usually not soon enough for most students, you will move into a practice-based experience. Here it is unlikely that the focus of the nursing staff is teaching students, rather it is patient care.

So it becomes essential that you start to use your eyes and listen attentively to interactions to create learning opportunities for yourself. No one is being lazy or neglecting their responsibilities here. Active learning is a core feature of nurse education. This means that you are the active partner rather than a passive observer. Even when your role is that of observer, you need to be an active learner. This sounds a bit confusing, but observing is an action on your part. Making use of those observations determines the depth of your learning and your preparation for future nursing practice.

Mentors

In each practice area, there will be a number of identified mentors or clinical supervisors. Whatever term is used, you will be supported in your clinical learning from two dimensions. First, and most significantly, within the practice area, you will be allocated a mentor who will be responsible for determining the extent and success of your clinical placement. This qualified practitioner will have a dual role. They are first and foremost a practitioner and have responsibilities to patient and client care. Their educational role is secondary. You should not feel displaced here, rather take from that division of labour the notion that the patient or client is at the centre of care and this becomes your role model. In turn, you are entitled to expect some set aside time for discussion of clinical problems, skill development and commentary on progress. Set against this, there is your responsibility as an active learner to make use of your observational, library and university taught times to create links between theory and practice. The mentor is there to help rather than replace personal learning. A good mentor–student relationship enhances learning and promotes a positive experience of care for you and for the patient or client.

The second dimension in your support as a learner is based within the university itself. Here there are several key people who will provide support: the programme leader, the module leader and your personal tutor. The macro-area of the programme is the responsibility of the programme leader. Module-focused issues belong to the module leader, although if you are part of a large programme, you may have a specific academic supervisor identified by the module leader to assist you with the assessment process. Personal tutors provide a more generic support role and should be approached with any personal difficulties, particularly those that could impinge on your learning.

Recording practice

The essential link between the observation of practice and reading the literature is your personal record keeping. There are many ways of referring to this document, for example reflective journal, daily diary or learning log to mention but a few. The universal purpose is to act as a record of observations in practice that enables you make links to the taught theory.

Once you begin to carry out nursing procedures, whether basic daily care or more technical clinical procedures, your thoughts and feelings can be recorded. If kept properly, the reflective journal can show your development in practice, remind you of dilemmas faced and help you to problem solve future nursing work. With the reflective journal, you can make notes to yourself to check particular theories you have read about and now need to reread with these new insights from practice. It is likely that some form of reflective documentation will be part of the assessment process. Early notes can be beneficial here in helping you develop strategies for the recording of practice.

If, in the early stages of learning, you establish a routine that fits your lifestyle, this will be advantageous in the future. A learning pattern of practice, recording and review within a set weekly or daily timetable is a good habit to develop. Leaving practice records until some future date is problematic, not just because of the resulting volume required but because of the possibility of flawed and false memories of events.

In relation to making these practice records, think back to the note-taking tips given above. Take the same disciplined approach and ensure that your records are accurate. Ensure that the date and time is the first thing you write down. The time, in particular, may be significant in that support is easier to find at certain times within a 24-hour day. You will think of other areas that time of day is significant.

Reflective learning

The challenge for nursing students is to undertake new theoretical learning and apply this to the clinical setting. Nursing theorists are often practitioners and seek to move forward the knowledge base of nursing through research and literature review. The student nurse is required to learn new subjects, sometimes of a perplexing nature, and then take this learning and see how it fits into the 'real' world: a tall challenge for even the most adept of learners and practitioners.

Naturally a direct and neat fit between theory and practice is rarely found, creating what has been termed the 'theory–practice divide'. The reality is that practice without theory can be dangerous and theory that lacks grounding in real-life situations is less than helpful to practitioners. The novice learner needs to combat this tension and bring the two centres of learning, theoretical and practical, into some alignment.

The answer to this is reflective learning. My task here is not to create a chapter on reflective learning but rather to take the study skills outlined above and apply them to practice and so provide you, the student, with the tools to commence the task of reflective learning. This latter phrase is somewhat overwhelming, so let us examine it.

A practical example of reflection is the bouncing back of an image, for example in a mirror. It is not a wholly exact image, in that it is reversed and is dependent on the quality of the mirror. So here we have two things interacting (more if you bring in light and refraction, but let's keep it simple for now), each dependent on the other in terms of quality. But the image itself provides a useful guide when checking individual appearance. In the same way, observations, whether of actions or interactions, can be regarded again through notes, thoughts and discussion.

In nursing practice, there is another dimension that we know as 'self-reflection'. Through consideration of your feelings and emotions, you can perceive your personal impact on the patient's experience of care. Rote learning, ritual and tradition have their place, but not in isolation from review both personal and also through the literature. Questions raised and answers sought through a cognitive exploration of recent experiences will form the basis of your reflection. When you engage in any form of practice, there are social, physical, psychological, spiritual and intellectual consequences. These may not always be obvious and do not have equal value or impact at all times. But they are key aspects of being human and need to be taken into consideration when practising as a nurse. The activity below offers a process through which you may start to analyse a practice event. Through asking yourself these four questions, you engage in an early form of reflection. It is particularly important to carry out this simple process in the early stages of practice and retain your observations so that you can measure your growth as a practitioner and learner. Of course, the first time you carry out any procedure is difficult to replicate, so do complete some form of reflective account during those exciting early days.

Activity 3.6

The outline below is an early guide to help with the process of reflection.

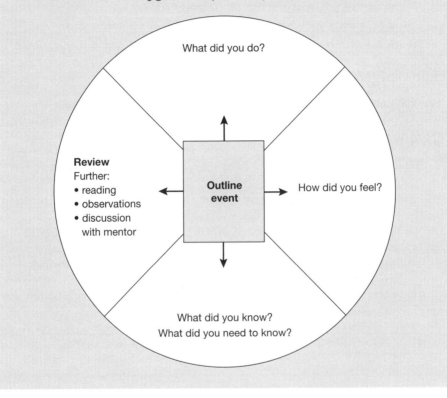

Conclusion

The process of learning is dependent on the individual. This chapter has outlined some strategies to help you find your way through the academic maze, in particular the process of studying, using the libraries and preparing for assessment. The culmination of a good approach to study skills is the completion of a learning journal. Such a journal will form a resource throughout your programme and indeed into further education. Clarity of thought is encouraged by a planned approach to study and assessment, so do take up the advice in this chapter to know yourself and your study style, be aware of the assessment timetable, become familiar with the library and, perhaps most of all, enjoy your studies.

Further reading

To continue your learning, there are a number of books published on study skills, reflective practice and grammatical presentation. The following are recommended.

Bulman, C and Schutz, S (eds) (2008) *Reflective Practice in Nursing*, London: Blackwell

Chapelhow, C and Crouch, S (2007) *Nursing Numeracy: A New Approach*, Cheltenham: Nelson Thornes

Gimenez, J (2007) *Writing for Nursing and Midwifery Students*, Basingstoke: Palgrave Macmillan

Glasper, A, McEwing, G and Richardson, J (eds) (2009) *Foundation Skills for Caring: Using Student-centred Learning*, Basingstoke: Palgrave Macmillan

Mason-Whitehead, E and Mason, T (2008) *Study Skills for Nurses*, London: Sage

Strunk, W Jr and White, EB (2000) *The Elements of Style* (4th edn), London: Allyn & Bacon

Acknowledgement

The input by Sheila Dunbar to the numeracy section of this chapter is recognised.

References

DH (Department of Health) (2004) *Building a Safer NHS for Patients: Improving Medication Safety*, London: TSO

Edwards, S (1998) Critical thinking and analysis: a model for written assignments. *British Journal of Nursing*, **7**(3): 159–65

Glasper, A, McEwing, G and Richardson J (eds) (2009) *Foundation Skills for Caring Using Student-centred Learning*, Basingstoke: Palgrave Macmillan

NMC (Nursing and Midwifery Council) (2007) *Essential Skills Clusters for Pre-registration Midwifery Education,* circular 07/2007, annexes 1, 2 and 3, London: NMC, available online at http://www.qub.ac.uk/schools/SchoolofNursingandMidwifery/Mentorship/filestore/Filetoupload,136972,en.pdf, accessed 18/6/2010

part 1 glossary

Academic supervisor The educator appointed as your guide for a particular assignment. Often this person will also mark your work. This is an important relationship and you should always attend these sessions having completed some advance preparation, so maximising the potential help you could receive.

Advocate As a nurse, you will be an advocate for the patient and this means that you will always represent their best interests.

Branch programme Having met all the criteria necessary to progress from the CFP, you will begin the first of two years of your branch programme where learning will be directed towards the specific area of nursing you have chosen, that is, adults, people with mental health problems, people with learning disabilities, and children.

Common Foundation Programme (CFP) This is the foundation year of your course, which is common to all nursing students regardless of which branch of nursing you have chosen. All nursing students share learning in the first year and gain experience and insight into other branches of nursing before progressing into their chosen speciality.

Community care This loosely defined concept encompasses the care and support offered to a person within the community. It can involve caring within a person's own home, within a care home, hostel, nursing home or a family placement. It can also include respite and daycare within a community-based facility.

DH The Department of Health

Foundation degree (FD) A degree-level qualification designed in conjunction with employers and combines academic study with workplace learning to equip people with the relevant knowledge, skills and understanding to access higher level qualifications.

Graduate Someone who has been granted an academic degree or diploma.

Higher education institution (HEI) This is usually a university.

Learning journal A structured set of notes that records learning, both formal and informal. The significant use of this journal builds a record of reading and learning that can be of use throughout a programme and into further education.

Mentor A registered nurse who will supervise and assess you in clinical practice and who meets the NMC requirements for a mentor. This role is a significant link between education and practice. In some academic and practice settings, practice-based assessment may have a tripartite role involving clinical mentor, academic assessor and yourself.

Multidisciplinary team (MDT) As a nurse you will work as a member of a team of professionals with different knowledge and skills in order to attain the best possible care for patients. Examples of MDT members may be nurses, doctors, physiotherapists, social workers, dieticians, occupational therapists, community nurses and many others.

Nursing and Midwifery Council (NMC) The organisation set up by Parliament to protect the public by ensuring that nurses and midwives provide high standards of care to their patients and clients. They do this by:

> Registering all nurses and midwives and ensuring they are properly qualified and competent to work in the UK.
> Setting standards of education, training and conduct for all nurses and midwives.
> Ensuring that nurses and midwives keep their knowledge and skills up to date and uphold the standards of their professional code.
> Using fair processes to investigate allegations made against nurses and midwives who may not have followed the code.

Placements An area of practice to which you are allocated to gain work experience.

Plagiarism The unattributed use of another's work, whether this is published, web based or another student's. Penalties for plagiarism are outlined in university regulations and can range from significant reduction in marks to removal from the programme.

Practice The part of your course where learning takes place in the clinical area and you develop your knowledge, skills and attitudes in contact with patients and practitioners. The definitions from the *Oxford English Dictionary* (2008) that apply to nursing are:

> The actual application of a plan or method, as opposed to the theories relating to it
> The practising of a profession
> The action or process of practising something so as to become proficient in it.

Reflective diary/journal A record of practice, showing elements of problem solving, personal reflection and links to theory, which is an essential aspect of practice-based learning. A journal such as this is encouraged throughout your professional life, and in some areas is a required aspect of continuing practice.

Royal College of Nursing (RCN) The only nursing-specific union in the UK.

Seminars Interactive sessions of learning, facilitated by an educator but usually led by a student. These sessions require all members of the group to undertake a minimum amount of reading and participate in discussion based on the leader's presentation.

Sign-off mentor A mentor who has met additional criteria and, in nursing, spends extra time with you as a student in your final placement and is able to 'make judgements about whether a student has achieved the required standards of proficiency for safe and effective entry to the NMC register' (NMC 2008).

Supernumerary This means that you are not counted in ward staff numbers but are in addition to the staff complement. You should therefore be able to pursue your learning needs without it being at the expense of ward work. It does not mean you do not participate in patient care or work as part of the team. Supernumerary status was introduced to facilitate students to 'become increasingly self-directed as the educational programme progresses and ... explore areas of skill and knowledge on an individual basis' (UKCC 1986, p. 55).

Theory The *Oxford English Dictionary* (2008) defines theory as:

> A supposition or a system of ideas intended to explain something, especially one based on general principles independent of the thing to be explained.
> An idea accounting for or justifying something.
> A set of principles on which an activity is based.

In nursing, these definitions all apply, and theory is that which is applied to underpin all you do in practice.

Trusts The organisations that manage either the hospitals you will work in (acute trusts), the services in the community such as doctors, dentists, pharmacists, walk-in centres and many more (primary care trusts), or health and social care for people with mental health problems (mental health trusts).

UCAS Universities and Colleges Admissions Service.

Work diary A useful strategy to employ as a planner for reflective learning. This diary or log records actual events as soon as possible after they happen to ensure accuracy when engaging in a reflective learning cycle.

1

References

NMC (2008) *Standards to Support Learning and Assessment in Practice,* London: NMC

UKCC (1986) *Project 2000: A New Preparation for Practice*, London: UKCC

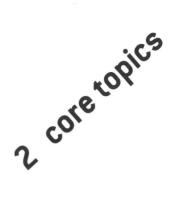

2 core topics

Introduction

The second part of *The Nursing Companion* introduces you to core topics associated with contemporary nursing practice. Chapters 4–11 cover key areas of skill, knowledge and understanding that relate to many different elements of the nursing course. For example, the professional skills and methods introduced include health promotion, communication, interpersonal skills and the involvement of people who use the NHS.

Modern nursing courses make strong connections with the social sciences, so this part will help your understanding of the role of psychology and sociology in nursing practice and how these areas of study underpin practice.

Finally, this part will introduce core areas of knowledge for nursing practice, including the management of pain, caring for people before and after surgery and the care of those near the end of life.

By working through the chapters and completing the activities, you will develop an understanding of the relevance and relationships implicit within the psychological, social and physical aspects of healthcare.

4 health promotion and public health

John Clayton and Peter Birchenall

In this chapter we will explore:

> Health promotion and health education
> Strategies for health promotion
> Individual versus societal approaches
> The nurse's role in promoting positive public health

Introduction

The promotion of good health and positive physical and mental wellbeing are important agenda items in the modern delivery of healthcare. That this statement is true can be evidenced when one considers the willingness of recent British governments to shift healthcare provision from a largely **curative** approach to one that incorporates an increasingly preventive agenda. The Labour government, for example, continually set out its focus on health promotion in such important documents as the White Papers *Saving Lives: Our Healthier Nation* (DH 1999) and *Choosing Health: Making Healthy Choices Easier* (DH 2004). This chapter will discuss the modern developments that are pertinent to this changing shift in healthcare provision and discuss the nursing contribution.

Health education versus health promotion

The two concepts of **health education** and **health promotion** are interrelated and not necessarily in competition as the title of this section implies. However, in the wider agenda of public health, there has been some debate about the **efficacy** of health promotion in general and health education specifically.

A reasonable place to start this debate is to define what is meant by the terms 'health education' and 'health promotion'. Health education involves those activities in which information is given to individuals to empower them to make positive choices about their own health. It demands that professionals with greater knowledge on health issues transmit the information to a member of the public. The nurse working in antenatal care who advises pregnant women of the dangers of cigarette smoking to her unborn baby is an example of how clinical knowledge can inform health education. Other examples are when community nurses advise elderly clients about diet or how to avoid falls or when they give young adults and teenagers information regarding safe sexual practice to reduce the incidence of teenage pregnancy and chlamydia infections. Still further examples are when nurses, working with clients who have mental health problems or are learning disabled, make use of their specialist knowledge to advise on important aspects such as medication, social activities or sexual health.

Activity 4.1

Research the bacterial infection chlamydia. You will find that it is one of the most common sexually transmitted diseases to affect adolescents and young people.

Produce a short leaflet that can be given to university and college students informing them of the risk posed by this infection and giving them the information they will need to avoid becoming infected.

Make your advisory leaflet clear, precise and professional but make it eye-catching and appropriate for your target audience.

Box 4.1 Chlamydia

Chlamydia is a sexually transmitted disease caused by the atypical bacterium *Chlamydia trachomatis*. The symptoms vary from asymptomatic carriers to severe infections and genital sores. *Chlamydia trachomatis* is incriminated in neonatal eye infections, which can cause blindness if cases are untreated.

The incidence of sexually transmitted chlamydia, especially in adolescents and young adults (under the age of 25), has so concerned the Labour government that it responded by introducing *The National Chlamydia Screening Programme* in 2002, and has continued to target chlamydia in subsequent legislation.

In 2002, the Department of Health discovered that 10.1% of women and 13.3% of men, under the age of 25, who were screened for chlamydia were found to be positive for the infection (DH 2002).

Health promotion is a broad, multifaceted concept. To use the World Health Organization's (WHO 1986) definition, it is a process that enables people to increase control over and improve their health. It suggests that people should reach a state of complete physical, mental and social wellbeing. Health promotion encompasses health education but additionally accepts that improvement in a person's health must consider the social and cultural contexts in which people live. For this reason, it requires an interrelated approach to health improvement demanding that, within society, genuine health promotion requires the involvement of government, the local community and the individual. This interrelated approach is the one put forward by the Labour government in *Saving Lives: Our Healthier Nation* (DH 1999): '[Promoting healthy living] will require action by Government, by local organisations and by individuals.'

Although there is a growing international consensus that modern health-care needs to focus on health promotion and education, it is noticeable that both have received criticism. Health education, with its focus on 'informed decision making' is criticised for relying on a deficiency model (Naidoo and Wills 2001, p. 282). In other words, a deficiency of knowledge or skills is identified in the 'patient'. A professional with greater knowledge who informs the patient rectifies this. The patient is a passive recipient of the information, who subsequently changes their lifestyle accordingly. For the patient not to change is inappropriate. This tends to undermine the essence of health education, which is to inform people to make a choice about their lifestyle, and can lead to the patient being blamed or labelled for not agreeing to follow the professional's advice. In her seminal study *The Unpopular Patient*, Felicity Stockwell (1972) sought to demonstrate traits displayed by patients that resulted in them being labelled as either 'popular' or 'unpopular'. For example, being of foreign nationality, having been in hospital for more than three months, and having a psychiatric diagnosis are three of a number of traits originally described by Stockwell (Porter 1998). Johnson and Webb revisited this work in 1995 and found that the notion of popular or unpopular was more fluid than previously demonstrated by Stockwell. They say:

> Labels are pluralistic. By this we mean that patients were incapable of being evaluated on more than one level by the same individual. Physically they could be unpopular because of the difficulties involved in performing their care, but interpersonally they were liked, perhaps because they were stoical or humorous. Labels were uncertain in another sense, that there was no true consensus over the evaluations. Frequently nurses would suggest privately they really liked someone who had been defined elsewhere as 'unpopular'. (Johnson and Webb 1995, p. 472)

Another criticism of health education is that it does not take into consideration social and cultural contexts. For example, it may be sensible to recommend that the general public as a whole take more exercise and eat a healthy diet in an attempt to reduce the incidence of coronary heart disease (CHD). However, it may be more difficult for people living in socially deprived areas with low incomes to make these changes even if they accept the advice given, particularly now that a minimum of five portions of fruit and/or vegetables a day is considered to be an essential part of a healthy diet.

Despite these criticisms, the Labour government showed a willingness to accept that health inequalities exist in the UK. It supported the *Independent Inquiry into Inequalities in Health* (Acheson 1998) and accepted its findings. In *Saving Lives: Our Healthier Nation* (1999), the government displayed an awareness that 'the better off were more likely to act on health information'. In addition, it indicated that a partnership approach was required to support disadvantaged citizens, stating:

> The Government recognises the importance of individuals making their own decisions about their own health but equally recognises the steps the Government can take to help support these decisions. (DH 1999)

The following section will consider strategies for health promotion.

Strategies for health promotion

The realisation that increased expenditure on curative healthcare did not lead to improvements in health persuaded modern governments, including the British government, to change healthcare provision from a curative approach to a preventive one. Fuelled by an economic recession in the 1980s, together with the demographic demands of an increasing older population, governments began to search for strategies that could prevent people from becoming ill rather than develop expensive ways to treat sick individuals.

The health promotion strategies that began to be formulated broadly fitted into one of three categories:

1 Strategies that prevented people from becoming ill in the first instance, for example the introduction of the 'flu jab' to older and at-risk citizens.
2 Strategies with the ability to identify disease at an early stage. These have the potential to increase the chances of survival through early intervention, for example the cervical screening programme.
3 Strategies that aimed to assist the morbidity/disability of citizens who were already suffering from an incurable disease, for example palliative care for citizens with terminal cancer (Caplan 1969).

Currently, the development of the preventive approach to healthcare has led to a diverse range of health promotion strategies. These are intended to meet the government's targets on health improvement, as specified in *Saving Lives: Our Healthier Nation* (1999), in the areas of CHD, cancer, mental illness and accidents, and also in the range of National Service Frameworks (NSFs) introduced since 2000, which offered 'long term strategies for improving specific areas of healthcare' (DH 2000).

Health promotion includes local initiatives as well as government policies; it encompasses specific conditions such as screening for sickle cell disease and large-scale areas of health improvement such as the immunisation programme of the UK, and targets individual groups or whole populations. Despite this great diversity, the range of strategies can be classified using theoretical models such as the ones set out by Tannahill (1985) and Ewles and Simnett (1999).

Tannahill's (1985) model sees the strategies as lying within three overlapping circles of health prevention, health promotion and health education. Within these overlapping circles, there are seven possible areas of health promotion (Naidoo and Wills 2001, p. 293; Davies and Macdowall 2006, p. 17):

1 *Preventive services,* such as immunisation
2 *Preventive health education,* such as information given to empower smokers to stop smoking
3 *Preventive health protection,* such as the banning of British beef in the 1990s because of the BSE scare
4 *Health education for preventive health protection,* such as drink-driving campaigns or campaigns aimed at a specific target groups (for example adolescents) to include a range of relevant health concerns such as alcohol abuse, smoking, healthy diet and teenage pregnancy
5 *Positive health education,* such as education to encourage citizens to exercise regularly
6 *Positive health protection,* such as the establishment of a workplace exercise policy
7 *Health education aimed at positive health protection,* such as the 'cover up' campaign designed to protect citizens from dangerous UV radiation in sunlight.

Ewles and Simnett (1999) recognise five approaches to health promotion:

1 *Medical approach,* which would encompass the mass immunisation of the population
2 *Behaviour change approach,* which might include, for example, information designed to help people to give up smoking
3 *Educational approach,* which might include giving people information designed to enable them to make their own choices regarding health
4 *Client-centred approach,* which might include information given by a health professional on alcohol consumption in pregnancy if the pregnant woman identifies the concern
5 *Societal change approach,* which includes the banning of cigarette smoking in public places.

The partnership approach to health promotion, including government, local communities and individuals, is much in evidence in these various strategies. Ewles and Simnett's (1999) 'societal change' approach, for example, seems to depend substantially on the efforts of government and local communities, while Tannahill's (1985) preventive health education approach depends upon local professionals giving information to groups/individuals willing to accept the information.

Activity 4.2

Design a preventive health campaign. First you will need to decide on the target audience for a health education campaign, for example children, adolescents, adults, older citizens and so on.

Research the health promotion needs of your target audience. For example, if your target audience is 'adolescents', you may elect to focus on teenage pregnancy, alcohol issues or eating disorders.

List the key messages and facts that you would put across in a campaign for a series of posters or television/radio advertisements. How could you make the different posters or advertisements interrelate to form part of a complete set?

The following section will evaluate the relative merits of the individual and societal approaches.

Individual approaches versus societal approaches

In this section, individual approaches will refer to those small-scale approaches designed to assist individuals or small groups to improve their prospects of good health, usually by lifestyle changes. Societal approaches will refer to large-scale health promotion strategies that involve the government or local community in improving the health of all its citizens.

It should be remembered that both health promotion strategies, individual and societal, have two major benefits. First, they have the potential to prevent people from succumbing to illness/disease and, second, in a time when the curative model of healthcare provision is failing to cope with the economic demands for limited resources, they offer an acceptable alternative. Most people support the philosophy that it is preferable to remain well rather than to be treated when one becomes ill. Having said this, it is equally apparent that both approaches have strengths and weaknesses.

Probably the major strength of the individual approach is that it can be tailored to meet the specific needs of an individual or small group. In this sense, it can even plug a gap in healthcare provision. The **expert patient**, for example a person suffering with a chronic long-term condition such as Parkinson's disease, can be a rich source of information as to the management of the disease to other Parkinson's sufferers. Hence the individual approach can truly offer opportunities for empowerment of the individual.

However, it can be equally argued that since these strategies usually look for a change in behaviour, the failure of the individual to comply means that the strategy is unhelpful and potentially expensive. Noncompliance can be a result of a variety of factors. There is evidence that social deprivation and low income play a role in noncompliance (Acheson 1998; DH 1999). Indeed, the government's strategies have incorporated initiatives and funding to combat inequality and assist disadvantaged clients. However, this inequality could still inhibit health promotion strategies in the foreseeable future.

Recently there has been evidence that as people become more aware of healthcare issues, an increased scepticism with regard to government and the health profession has been identified. Perhaps the best example of this is the unwillingness of parents to have their children immunised for measles, mumps and rubella (MMR), following reports that the vaccine was associated with potentially harmful side effects such as autism. The government's attempt to appease the public has not been entirely successful, possibly because the public has become equally sceptical of government statements following the previous Conservative government's handling of the BSE crisis. Whatever the ultimate reasons for individuals refusing to accept the MMR vaccine, the damage to health promotion is significant, since insufficient uptake will prevent the development of **herd immunity** to these diseases.

The blaming of individuals who fail to comply with expert advice is another disadvantage of this approach. In essence, this runs contrary to both the educational approach and the client-centred approach identified by Ewles and Simnett (1999), since citizens should be empowered to choose whether or not to take the advice given by professionals. This is unlikely to be the case because a power relationship exists between the professional and the 'patient', which may result in the noncompliant 'patient' being seen as lacking in willpower and hence open to accusations of blame (Naidoo and Wills 2001, p. 283).

The societal approach can be applied to attack health inequality, as in the White Paper *Choosing Health: Making Healthy Choices Easier* (DH 2004). In addition, there is substantial evidence that societal approaches have brought about major improvements in healthcare. Public health policy changes in the second half of the nineteenth century led to improvements in the safety of London's water supplies, for example, resulting in massive reductions in human suffering and deaths from bacterial diseases, notably typhoid and cholera, long before antibiotics were discovered to cure them. Here the interrelationship between government and private manufacturers made remarkable contributions to the public's health and it is this model of partnership that the Labour government identified as key to the societal approach. In this sense, local providers will be required to provide local solutions to their specific healthcare needs. However, it is the very 'newness' of this policy that causes one to temper enthusiasm for the immediate future at the very least and one can expect a reasonable period of time before the interactions of the various agencies gel into a cohesive health promotion package.

The Labour government itself did not escape criticism. The recent policy to introduce a ban on smoking in public places (2007) was not introduced without a degree of debate and disagreement, with many people suggesting that this was an infringement of individual liberty. This identifies one of the major difficulties for governments and societal health promotion strategies, in that such a wide-ranging approach rarely meets the approval of all citizens. This may in part explain why the decision to ban smoking in the UK lagged behind other European countries such as the Republic of Ireland.

The following sections will evaluate a number of specific health promotion areas.

Education for healthy living including the value of regular exercise

The White Paper *Saving Lives: Our Healthier Nation* (DH 1999) clearly identified government support for healthy living and regular exercise. Despite the fact that this approach essentially requires a behaviour change of individuals and hence puts the onus of health improvement on the individual, the government was keen to point out that it wanted to contribute to making 'healthier people in a healthier country' (DH 1999).

The government recognised that its citizens already knew that physical activity was a key determinant for good health and that walking, cycling and participating in sport reduced the risk of CHD as well as promoting good mental health. However, it also recognised that uptake in physical exercise depended upon individual factors such as income, work pressure and motivation. Additionally, it noted that the 'better off' were more likely to act on health information and hence recognised that the challenge was to encourage all citizens to take up physical exercise. The reasons for individuals failing to take up physical exercise include:

> lack of time
> cost
> lack of access to facilities
> embarrassment
> lack of self-belief
> lack of someone to go with/support (Morrison and Bennett 2006, p. 99).

Hence, this strategy was seen to require the partnership approach, as identified above. The intent is to encourage everyone to take 30 minutes of moderate exercise, five times per week. Failure to do this doubles the risk of suffering from CHD and trebles the risk of suffering a stroke (DH 1999). In order to support this, the government introduced a Sport Strategy in 1999 looking to introduce 'affordable' activities within local reach of citizens. It also suggested that family doctors, who would refer patients for physical activity with local providers, could give 'exercise on prescription'. The Safer Travel to School scheme required schools to support pupils walking or cycling to school. It was envisaged that this would have a positive effect on tackling childhood obesity, as well as reducing air pollution by reducing the dependence on cars. The advancement of physical education in schools was also developed through the Active Schools programme.

More recently, the Wanless Report *Securing Good Health for the Whole Population* (Wanless 2004) and the White Paper *Choosing Health: Making Healthier Choices Easier* (DH 2004) further supported the need for physical exercise, with specific requirements for tackling health inequalities. A subsequent development has been the use of lottery funding to establish over 300 healthy living centres, throughout the UK, to provide a range of activities for varied groups of people including children and older citizens.

It is now accepted that the benefits of regular exercise include reducing the risk of cardiovascular disease, reducing the risk of type 2 diabetes mellitus, reducing the risk of some cancers and obesity, and improving one's mental health (WHO 2002).

Maintaining a balanced diet

Another key area that the government supports is the maintenance of a balanced diet, in which individuals are encouraged to eat a diet low in saturated fat, sugar and salt, but high in fruit and vegetables. Diet is important, since there is overwhelming evidence that dietary factors can affect the risk of a range of diseases including CHD, stroke, cancer and diabetes mellitus. In addition, the increase in incidence of obesity in adults and children in the UK has led to a healthy diet becoming an important health promotion target.

The challenge for health promotion is to encourage all citizens to choose to eat healthy foods, but again the problem is the lack of equality between citizens. The government noted that people living in deprived neighbourhoods had difficulty reaching shops that sold affordable healthy foods and noted that local providers could be expensive. It referred to these localities as 'food deserts' and realised it needed to develop a strategy to improve access in these communities (DH 1999).

In schools, the government introduced a range of innovations to encourage children to eat more healthily and to understand the importance of a healthy diet, including:

> The School Fruit and Vegetable Scheme, part of the 5 A Day programme, which encourages everyone to eat five portions of fruit and/or vegetable every day.
> The Food in Schools programme, a joint venture between the Department of Health and the Department for Education and Skills.
> Free fruit for primary schools initiative.
> The Cooking for Kids programme, which supports the teaching of food hygiene and nutrition in the school holidays supported by high-profile celebrities such as Jamie Oliver.

These initiatives are part of a long-term strategy to reduce CHD and cancer and are supported by the Foods Standards Agency.

Recent national strategies to reduce obesity include *Tackling Child Obesity: The First Steps* (Audit Commission 2006) and *Healthy Weight, Healthy Lives* (DH 2008a). These suggest that the government is not only keen to keep 'tackling obesity' on the policy agenda but is equally willing to monitor, adapt and develop the strategy.

Looking after your heart

Coronary heart disease (CHD) is one of the biggest single causes of death

– causing approximately 115,000 deaths each year in the UK. Stroke is also a major cause of death, with 54,000 people losing their lives in 1997 (DH 1999). These conditions are major causes of increased morbidity in the UK and place extreme demands on the NHS. CHD accounts for 2.5% of NHS hospital expenditure, and strokes account for 4% of NHS expenditure and 7% of community health and social care for adults' expenditure. As they are largely preventable, it is not surprising that they represent a specific target in *Saving Lives: Our Healthier Nation* (DH 1999).

The partnership approach is key to tackling this problem and individuals are encouraged to take exercise and to eat a healthy diet. However, the government also introduced some specific initiatives pertinent to heart disease under a Health Skills agenda. This includes the Health Skills defibrillator initiative, which seeks to improve the survival rate of people who suffer a heart attack by providing **defibrillators** and trained staff in public places throughout the UK. In addition, the NSF for CHD (DH 2000) requires GPs and primary care teams to develop a register of CHD patients, so that they can receive information and prompt medication if needed. High-risk patients will receive **statins** to reduce **cholesterol** and prevent repeated attacks.

Recognising and dealing with stress and related conditions

Mental health is also a target of *Saving Lives: Our Healthier Nation* following the discovery that 4,500 deaths per year were caused by suicide and that 16% of the adult population suffered from a mental disorder such as depression, and the cost to the NHS and social services was estimated at £7.5bn per year (DH 1999).

It is recognised that **stress** can harm a person's physical health. The risk of CHD is higher in those people with more stressful occupations. The recognition of stress in an individual is, however, complex since it varies from person to person. Often there is an external event or occurrence (**stressor**) that causes the feelings of stress. These can be evidenced by an individual feeling anxious, angry or upset. It can result in difficulty in sleeping and can lead to increased headaches and high blood pressure. The range of signs and symptoms varies from person to person and the stressor can be a variety of events such as getting married, family bereavement or moving house (Morrison and Bennett 2006).

Coping with this range of problems falls within the remit of health promotion and, again, government, professionals and individuals can play a part. For example, individuals can take regular exercise, eat a balanced diet and keep physically fit. They can adopt relaxation exercises and take time away from the stressor. Local organisations and employers can offer support and guidance to employees helping them cope with stress (Morrison and Bennett 2006). Community mental health nurses play an important part in combating the effects of stress through expert counselling and support in the person's home. The government's role in reducing stress among its citizens is the same as for other areas identified above, namely that of tackling inequality, since there is:

Consistent evidence that people in lower socio-economic groups not only experience more stress than those in higher socio-economic groups, they frequently have fewer resources to help them cope. (Morrison and Bennett 2006, p. 40)

The government introduced the New Deal policy, intended to help reduce unemployment, and has introduced a range of benefits to support poorer citizens including the working family tax credit. It is hoped that these initiatives will improve the financial status of disadvantaged citizens. The improved economic status of individuals should allow them a greater opportunity to experience the benefits of the health promotion agenda.

Sexual health

Although sexual health was originally a target of the Conservative government's health promotion White Paper *The Health of the Nation* (DH 1992), it was removed as a specific target from the Labour government's *Saving Lives* (DH 1999). This may imply that the Labour government was less interested in sexual health than its predecessor; however, it would be unfair to imply that the Labour government had no interest in this area as evidenced by the publication of the *National Strategy for Sexual Health and HIV* in December 2001 (DH 2001).

This document identified the successes of previous health promotion campaigns in this area, which had, by the provision of information to individuals, led to the 'control of HIV in England'. It also praised needle exchange schemes, which had contributed to the UK having one of the lowest incidence rates of HIV in Europe, as well as free access to genitourinary medicine clinics and free contraception on the NHS. However, this document (DH 2001) identified areas in need of improvement and set out a strategy, costing £47.5m, which included:

> A target to reduce the transmission of HIV and sexually transmitted infections (STIs)
> A reduction in the prevalence of undiagnosed HIV and STIs
> A reduction in unintended pregnancies
> An improvement in health and social care for citizens living with HIV.

The role of health promotion included the provision of information, provision of contraceptive services and advice and increasing the offer of hepatitis B vaccination. The strategy identified the role of healthcare professionals and vowed to address their training and development needs across the range of sexual health services. Areas that continued to concern the government were the increase in chlamydia infections, as identified above. The programme of screening for chlamydia for targeted groups began in 2002 as part of the *National Strategy for Sexual Health and HIV* (DH 2002).

In common with other areas of health promotion discussed in this chapter, sexual health is an area that benefits from an integrated approach and is another area that will lead to decreased health inequality.

A key objective of the Labour government's health promotion agenda was tackling health inequality. How successful this strategy has been cannot yet be estimated, since the benefits of a successful health promotion strategy are likely to be long term. Indeed, most of Labour's targets were set for 2010. However, a report by the Audit Commission/Healthcare Commission (2008 p. 6) praised the government's policy on health inequality over the past 10 years. The coalition government has pledged to tackle the economic crisis, which is unlikely to result in the abandonment of the health promotion agenda. However, a 2011 White Paper on public health should clarify the situation.

The nurse's role in promoting positive public health within a social context

In 2008, the NHS celebrated its 60th anniversary. From its inception, many changes have occurred, including a complete revolution in the training and education of nurses. From the outset, doctors and clinical consultants dictated the direction of the service, with nurses being little more than handmaidens. In the early years, health education was rudimentary, the nursing curriculum being highly structured in clinical practice. Today's sophisticated health empowerment strategies, which nurses now routinely practice, took many years to develop.

Earlier in this chapter reference was made to the dynamics present in the modern service regarding the prevention and early detection of physical illness. Similar observations are made in psychiatry, where practitioners have become highly skilled in the use of therapeutic measures to help people who experience difficulties in their mental health. In learning disabilities, nurses now make wider use of their skills in health education and promotion than was ever the case in the large long-stay hospitals where their role was largely one of containment and control. Teamwork is the essence of healthcare today, and nurses work as equal partners with other disciplines to provide a seamless service to the patient or client. Examples of this can be seen in GP surgeries and health centres where practice nurses are often the first point of contact for many people who access the health service. Practice nurses run their own surgeries where patients can receive expert advice on many health-related issues such as obesity, diet, exercise, blood pressure, sexual health and keeping cholesterol in check. The raison d'être for their existence is rooted in health promotion and health education.

Activity 4.3

Organise an appointment with a local practice nurse to discuss their nursing role in maintaining the optimum health of patients. Identify the main areas of public health where the practice nurse is seen to be most effective.

Mental health nurses, through health education and health promotion, play a substantial part in supporting people in the community. Many people, who were diagnosed during the early years of the NHS, would often find themselves being treated in a large Victorian asylum. Today, many more people with mental health problems live supported lives in the community and in those instances where hospital care is indicated, it is offered in a modern, enlightened way. From a historical perspective, it was in 1982, with the advent of new curricula, that learning disability and mental health nurses found themselves at the forefront of a new ethos of care. It was here that the therapeutic age dawned and nursing in these disciplines would gradually move away from institutional measures to a delivery of care that would become more socially derived. Some new approaches inherent within these revolutionary training courses transferred to the 'general' curricula and general nurses found themselves developing health promotion, health education and counselling skills alongside the more traditional subjects.

We have mentioned government measures such as the banning of smoking in public places, promoting healthy eating in schools, and health and safety in the workplace. It is worth considering that these measures will continue to make a significant impact on the health of the nation and form a substantial part of ongoing educational programmes for nurses.

Following a review of the NHS in England (DH 2008b), a draft constitution covering health priorities for the next decade was published (see Chapter 1).

These priorities are:

> Tackling obesity
> Reducing alcohol harm
> Treating drug addiction
> Reducing smoking rates
> Improving sexual health
> Improving mental health.

This draft constitution is aimed at providing users of the health service in England with a legal right to select their GP practice and choose between different types of treatment in hospitals of their choice (Carvel 2008).

This far-reaching agenda will impact on the nursing contribution to widening and improving the access that people have to healthcare. Because people are living longer, the need for high-quality health and social care has never been greater. The continual shift of resources into early detection and prevention of disease will impact on the future direction taken by nursing education. As these measures come into force, the nursing service will be obliged to produce an even more eclectic, socially aware practitioner than we have today.

Conclusion

This chapter has focused on the development of a health promotion agenda.

It explained the meaning of health promotion and explored strategies in health education. It demonstrated the importance of both approaches in supporting the agenda to tackle health inequality, which has been fundamental to the Labour government's policy on healthcare since the publication of the Acheson Report in 1998.

The chapter also identified and evaluated the limitations of health promotion and health education, while supporting the shift of healthcare delivery from being essentially curative to one of prevention. The role of the nurse as a professional person working in this changing healthcare arena has been identified as being fundamental and the importance of nursing to the success of health promotion and health education has been emphasised.

Further reading

Naidoo, J and Wills, J (eds) (2008) *Health Studies: An Introduction* (2nd edn), Basingstoke, Palgrave Macmillan. A readable text for students who are new to the area of healthcare issues, with an excellent introductory section on health promotion as an interdisciplinary practice.

References

Acheson, D (1998) *Independent Inquiry into Inequalities in Health* (Acheson Report), London, HMSO

Audit Commission (2006) *Tackling Child Obesity: The First Steps*, London: Audit Commission

Caplan, G (1969) *An Approach to Community Mental Health*, London: Tavistock

Carvel, J (2008) NHS review: patient choice at the heart of health service revolution, *The Guardian*, 30 June

Davies, M and Macdowall, W (2006) *Health Promotion Theory: Understanding Public Health*, Maidenhead: Open University Press

DH (Department of Health) (1992) *The Health of the Nation*, London: HMSO

DH (1999) *Saving Lives: Our Healthier Nation*, London: HMSO

DH (2000) *National Service Framework: Coronary Heart Disease*, London: HMSO

DH (2001) *The National Strategy for Sexual Health and HIV*, London: HMSO

DH (2002) *The National Chlamydia Screening Programme*, London: HMSO

DH (2004) *Choosing Health: Making Healthy Choices Easier*, London: HMSO

DH (2008a) *Healthy Weight, Healthy Lives: A Cross-Government Strategy for England*, London: HMSO

DH (2008b) *High Quality Care For All: NHS Next Stage Review Final Report* (Darzi Review), London: HMSO

Ewles, L and Simnett, I (1999) *Promoting Health: A Practical Guide* (4th edn), Edinburgh: Baillière Tindall

Healthcare Commission/Audit Commission (2008) *Are We Choosing Health? The Impact of the Delivery of Health Improvement Programmes and Services*, Audit Commission, http://www.healthcarecommission.org.uk

Johnson, M and Webb, C (1995) Rediscovering unpopular patients: the concept of social judgement, *Journal of Advanced Nursing*, 21: 75–82

2

Morrison, V and Bennett, P (2006) *An Introduction to Health Psychology,* Harlow: Pearson/ Prentice Hall

Naidoo, J and Wills, J (2001) *Health Studies: An Introduction,* Basingstoke: Palgrave – now Palgrave Macmillan

Porter, S (1998) The social interpretation of deviance, in M Birchenall and P Birchenall (eds) *Sociology as Applied to Nursing and Healthcare*, London: Baillière Tindall/RCN

Stockwell, F (1972) *The Unpopular Patient*, London: RCN

Tannahill, A (1985) What is health promotion? *Health Education Journal*, **44**(4): 167–8

Wanless, D (2004) *Securing Good Health for the Whole Population,* London: HMSO

WHO (World Health Organization) (1986) *The Ottawa Charter for Health Promotion,* Geneva: WHO

WHO (2002) *The World Health Report: Reducing Risks, Promoting Healthy Life,* Copenhagan: WHO Regional Office for Europe

5 interpersonal and professional skills

Anita Maestri-Banks and Paula Pope

In this chapter we will explore:

> The code of practice and ethics
> Therapeutic communication
> Self-awareness
> Diversity
> Confidentiality
> The positive image of nursing

Introduction

This chapter introduces health professionals to the following important areas: the code of practice and **ethics**, therapeutic communication with the patient/client, family members and colleagues, diversity, and confidentiality. Finally, it reviews respect for the dying person and maintaining a positive image of nursing through personal example.

Code of practice and ethics

By now, we are sure that you have already considered what it means to be a nurse. A nurse should be an individual who enables and supports patients with their medical, physical and psychological needs. They should show understanding, care and respect to all their patients.

The British Medical Association (BMA 2009) provides a comprehensive list of health-related professions that have a regulatory body, which register practitioners in order to maintain standards and ensure protection for people using the services. The Nursing and Midwifery Council (NMC) is the regulatory body for nurses. The purpose of this organisation is to establish and improve standards of nursing care so that the wellbeing of the public is protected.

In order to practise as a competent and safe nurse, it is essential that the standards set by the NMC are adhered to. As a pre-registration student nurse, you are never professionally as accountable as you will be after you become a registered nurse; this means that you cannot be called to account for your 'actions and omissions'. However, this does not mean that you are not accountable by law for your actions and omissions as a student.

When you successfully complete your course, your higher education institution will notify the NMC that you have met the required standards and that you are eligible for entry onto the register. Once you are registered and have paid your registration fee, you will be entered onto the NMC register and will be eligible to practise as a registered practitioner.

Activity 5.1a

The Nursing and Midwifery Council is the regulatory body for nurses. Go to its website – www.nmc-uk.org – and from the information provided, write down what qualities and values a nurse needs to have to be an effective health professional.

The NMC register does not function simply as an administrative process but acts as an instrument of public protection. The NMC discusses the accountability of a nurse in its code of professional conduct (NMC 2008). It explains that accountability means that you are responsible for something or to someone. In other words, you have to recognise the consequences of your actions.

Activity 5.1b

Write down the qualities and values you have that would make you a good nurse. Compare these with the qualities and values a nurse needs to have to be an effective health professional, outlined in Chapter 1.

Other **professionals** who work with nurses also have **codes of conduct** that you may need to take into account. These professional colleagues may be social workers whose professional standards of practice are defined by the General Social Care Council (GSCC) in England, or counsellors whose values and principles appear in the ethical framework of the British Association for Counselling and Psychotherapy.

As well as distinct professional bodies, some groups set out their principles in common. See, for example, the joint statement of core interprofessional values underpinning work with children and young people that has been agreed by the General Teaching Council for England (GTC), the GSCC and the NMC, which can be found on the GTC website – www.gtce.org.uk. (Do be aware that different nations within the UK may have different councils.)

Among some of the commonly shared values are:

> treating individuals holistically and with dignity
> adopting a nonjudgmental approach that is empowering and anti-oppressive
> respecting the rights to confidentiality and choice
> acting with honesty, flexibility and integrity.

It may require taking steps to break down barriers and build common ground so that professionals can work together in response to the needs of the individual. Therefore, being a reflective practitioner is a key ingredient to providing an integrated and effective service, as it facilitates learning and development.

Therapeutic communication

The key elements of communication are:

> nonverbal communication
> verbal communication
> self-awareness
> counselling skills
> advanced communication models.

The highest form is called 'therapeutic communication' and if carried out effectively by the health professional, it can enable patients to express how they feel so that they perceive their stay in hospital more positively, thus aiding healing. When communicating, it is important to consider how the person will interpret what is being said, as experience and cultural identity can affect how a person understands the spoken message. It may lead to misinterpretation and defensive behaviour.

To avoid misunderstanding, it is important that the health professional has a good understanding of the principles of therapeutic communication. Communication is both a verbal and nonverbal dynamic interaction between individuals that is interpreted according to the individual's personal construct. Nonverbal communication is demonstrated through gestures, signs and other forms of behaviour that are used between two or more people. It gives increased meaning to the words we hear that represent our thoughts, feelings, ideas and actions.

Nonverbal communication involves taking account of:

> proximity and personal space
> orientation and posture
> paralanguage – voice tone, pacing and so on
> eye contact
> touch.

There are different cultural meanings attached to the use of touch, space, eye contact and so on, therefore it is important that these forms of communication are used appropriately and with care. The nurse needs to understand the context and adapt the style of communication in response to the needs of the patient and their relatives. For instance, physical contact may reassure, overwhelm or distress a patient depending on the individual and the context; offering emotional support also requires an awareness of your own needs and responsibilities in such situations. For example, in Europe, direct eye contact is seen to mean honesty and sincerity, whereas indirect eye contact implies dishonesty and uneasiness. However, in Southeast Asia, direct eye contact demonstrated by a woman to an unrelated man can be perceived as forward and disrespectful, while indirect eye contact shows modesty and respect.

Activity 5.2

1 Can you think of an occasion when you have felt uncomfortable or embarrassed talking to a person you were not familiar with? What happened to your eye contact in this situation?
2 Can you think of an occasion when you have felt uncomfortable or embarrassed talking a person you are very familiar with? What happened to your eye contact in this situation?

Verbal communication is demonstrated through the spoken messages that are transmitted between the sender and the receiver. These forms of communication involve using active listening skills, which include both the careful use of questions and responses:

> *Attending skills:* encourage and enable others to continue
> *Questioning:* open, closed, clarifying and probing
> *Responding:* reflection that may include paraphrasing and summarising.

Assessing a patient involves careful use of communication skills during the interview. One helpful interviewing checklist is PQRSTU, which has been devised by Gratus (2000). PQRSTU can be used when admitting patients, developing care plans or working out actions of care. PQRSTU reminds us of the stages we need to go through to attain successful interviews:

> *P: preparation* – we need to think through what we want to know or share and the appropriate way of doing this. Being self-aware of the context and patients' needs can help here.
> *Q: questions* – these may be neutral or intrusive and need to be chosen carefully.
> *R: rapport* – this is about building the relationship, and involves showing respect, honesty and understanding in our dealings with others.
> *S: skills* – those that help the interviewee to talk. Many of these are the attending and active listening skills.
> *T: termination* – this is a reminder that we need to pay attention to endings and how we complete our communication. Are we both going away with the same understanding of what has been discussed? Summarising can help here.
> *U: unfinished business* – this is when we review the outcome and check out what has been gained and what still needs to be addressed so that we can move on.

Helpful communication begins with self-awareness (Figure 5.1).

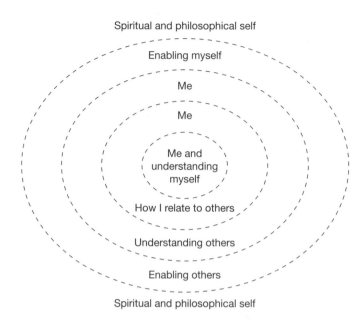

Figure 5.1 *Self-awareness model demonstrating different levels of self-awareness*

Maestri-Banks has created the above model to demonstrate the layers of self-awareness. In the small circle is 'me' as an individual and this is about understanding who I am. This person 'me' includes the roles I play, self-esteem, my cultural identity and experience, all that leads into making me the person I am.

The next circle is about how I relate to and have an effect on others through my actions and communication. The following circle is how I understand others; my ability to show empathy and see things from another's perspective and knowing who 'the other' is. The outer circle is how I enable others to move on and how I enable myself, for example through reflection, support and therapeutic communication; understanding transactions that help others to develop. You may be able to either enable yourself or others, but it takes a very insightful person to be able to do both. The outside of the circles explores a person's spiritual and philosophical self, which has an impact on each of the aspects in the circles. Interestingly, there is fluidity in this self-awareness model. You can move from one circle to another, have reached one element and not another. Depending on what is going on for you will have an impact on your own self-awareness and how you relate to others.

There are other psychological models that can help you to explore yourself. These include Johari's window (Luft and Ingham 1955), Roger's person-centred approach (1967) and Maslow's hierarchy of needs (1970).

Johari's window, developed by Luft and Ingham, represents levels of awareness of feelings and behaviour that are known to self or to others through the four states shown in Figure 5.2. These areas of awareness can be expanded when a person shares new information or receives feedback.

	Known to self	Not known to self
Known to others	Arena	Blind spot
Not known to others	Façade	Unknown

Figure 5.2 Johari's window

Roger's person-centred approach, as discussed by Mearns and Thorne (1992), is a sophisticated model that analyses the self-concept in terms of conditions of self-worth. The core conditions of a person-centred approach are:

> *unconditional positive regard*, which is a nonjudgmental respectful approach to others
> *empathy*, when you understand the situation from the other person's point of view
> *congruence*, which refers to being genuine and honest in your communication.

Maslow's (1970) hierarchy of needs is a model that shows the interrelationship from the basic physical needs of shelter and food that have to be met first, before moving on to the more complex emotional desires and self-fulfilment of potential.

Activity 5.3

Answer these questions to gain a better understanding of yourself:
• Who are you?
• What roles do you have?
• Why do you want to study nursing?

It is this insight into self that creates questions and ultimately allows us to find the answers to how we use communication with our patients and attend to process as well as outcomes. We use listening skills (or counselling skills for professional helpers) to engage with our patients. These enable social interaction and therapeutic communication; they can also facilitate greater awareness and understanding of a problem to enable the person to help him or herself.

Nurses can become counsellors with the correct training. However, counselling is a time-limited and contractual therapeutic relationship between the client or patient and the counsellor. Instead, most professionals use counselling skills rather than act as counsellors (Figure 5.3). This includes the ability to show the core conditions described in the person-centred approach. In particular, this can be achieved through empathy, where the nurse may act as the patient's advocate.

Therapeutic communication is a relationship based on respect for the individual, an ability to see things from the other's point of view. It uses the same basic listening skills as counselling and requires the same qualities and skills. It focuses on empathy, congruence and unconditional regard, which lead into advanced communication models.

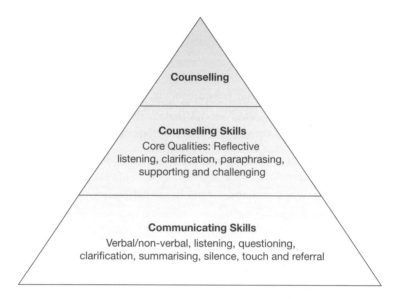

Figure 5.3 *The relationship of communication to counselling*
Source: McLeod Clark, 1981, Communication in nursing. Reproduced with the permission of the *Nursing Times*

Therapeutic communication is a different form of communication to counselling. It is a brief encounter that may be therapeutic in its nature, but it is not therapy. Not all patients are at the stage when they can help themselves. Illness and circumstances will affect the way in which a person communicates with others. Being ill also affects how people treat you, how you perceive yourself and manage everyday living.

Heron's six category analysis (1990) and Berne's transactional analysis (TA) (1961) are advanced communication models, which enable the health professional to interact with the patient and other health professionals. They offer a deep understanding of how and why individuals may react or interpret communication in the way they do. The models offer both theoretical frameworks for nursing research and practical interpersonal tools. Heron's model is explained in Table 5.1. It is helpful to draw on the range of these interventions according to your role and the needs of the patient. Also noteworthy is that more than one category can be used as part of the same intervention.

core topics

Table 5.1 *Heron's six category intervention analysis*

Authoritative category	Facilitative category
Prescriptive – being direct in what you are saying	*Cathartic* – feeling and expressing emotion
Informative – being educational	*Catalytic* – enabling and encouraging others to express feelings
Confronting – being open and honest in a nonaggressive manner	*Supportive* – being there for the person

The following practice scenario offers you the opportunity to look at how you might apply these skills in practice.

Activity 5.4

Practice scenario 1
What are some of your thoughts, feelings and sensations in these situations?

• You are a second year student on the medical ward. You approach an elderly patient to introduce yourself. The patient is hunched up and has tears in her eyes. What do you do?

Let us assume that you take steps to establish a rapport with the patient. Use Heron's six category analysis to suggest some ways in which you might do this.

• The patient discloses that she is worried about her medication.

Use Heron's six category analysis to suggest some ways in which you might respond to this anxiety.

Awareness of Berne's TA can aid communication. It focuses on the parent ego state, the adult ego state and the child ego state and is a model that can be used to move the power distribution in relationships. The most healthy power position to be in is when all individuals are in the adult state. TA is a form of therapy that is easy to understand. It uses language that is simple and accessible, employing everyday words that are familiar in describing how the person is thinking, feeling and behaving. It helps individuals to understand and make sense of their situation quickly and easily. Those who use TA have described it as potent, empowering and flexible. It derives from the positive position that each person has value and worth giving them the potential for personal growth and change. Within TA, the person becomes an active participant in their journey of self-discovery and in the process is given respect and support.

Activity 5.5

Practice scenario 2
What are some of your thoughts, feelings and sensations in these situations?

• Your first day as a student nurse entering the ward.
• Your discomfort at the ward sister's remark, 'Oh no! Not another student.'

- A month's experience on the ward, working with a supportive mentor.
- The illness of your mentor that leads you to work more closely with the ward sister.
- Your uncertainty about sharing your concerns with your course tutor.

Using Berne's theory of transactional analysis, especially with regard to the notion of growth, value and worth, explore the dynamics of these different situations and suggest some ways you might employ it towards understanding your own feelings.

Diversity

Diversity can be defined as the accepting and respecting of people's differences and the valuing of our shared humanity. Good self-awareness and effective communication skills, coupled with an understanding of diversity and respect for human rights, lead to anti-discriminatory practice. This is supported by a framework of policies and procedures on equal opportunities. The Commission for Equality and Human Rights states that individuals need to be treated with dignity, equality and respect.

As a nurse, it is important to recognise that each patient has different needs and that we appreciate and work within the boundaries of individualised care. This should not isolate the patient from the whole group as this leads to **discrimination**.

Nurses need to understand the influence of their own cultural identity and formative experiences that have shaped the person they are today. Each person has their own cultural identity that is derived from gender, race and ethnicity, sexual orientation, disability, age and class. These divisions are socially constructed, shaping personal identity, patterns of behaviour and preferred ways of being in situations.

Through reflection, nurses need to make sense of their life experiences, so that they do not prejudice how they see others and affect their relationships with other people. It involves being nonjudgmental, considering things from other points of view and enabling patients to work with their treatment in as positive way as they can. Nurses need to use all their skills when making sense of how a patient is experiencing difficulty with certain procedures or situations on the ward.

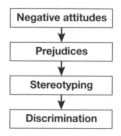

Figure 5.4 How negative attitudes can lead to discrimination

Our experiences shape our **attitudes** towards people and things. These attitudes are feelings and thoughts that may be positive or negative. They can help us to make sense of our environment and the differences between individuals. Negative attitudes are often subconscious and can have a significant impact on how we relate to others. They can create **prejudice,** which leads to **stereotyping**. This is when a person generalises or makes assumptions towards an individual or group and may lead on to discrimination.

When caring for patients who are demanding because they may be in pain or frightened, it is easy to label them as difficult and, as a result, they become 'the unpopular patient' (see Chapter 4). Your response may be to ignore that patient or talk about them negatively to other staff members. In doing this, you are treating this patient differently and therefore being discriminatory.

As health professionals, we are responsible for our own professional development. It is helpful to take stock from time to time to check out our progress as an anti-oppressive practitioner. This involves using reflection, which means looking at what you have done, why you did it and what you have learned from it. Activities 5.6 and 5.7 will help you start the process.

Activity 5.6

Diversity and personal development
Ask yourself the following questions:

- Where am I now in my anti-oppressive practice?
- Am I paying lip service, reluctant to risk, choosing and sharing, or risk taking?

Give some examples that reflect your stage of development as an anti-oppressive practitioner.

Other professional colleagues give examples of ways they have found to make a start on their anti-oppressive practice. They include learning from colleagues, undertaking training and having a personal connection. They also suggest reasons why they may struggle at times. Among them are personal safety, peer pressure, personal anger, lack of knowledge, and the situation at work, implying a lack of policy, leadership or teamwork.

Activity 5.7

Diversity and personal development
Take a moment to think about your own progress on anti-oppressive practice:

- What is helping your development?
- What is hindering your development?

Give some examples of what helps or hinders you.
Work out some action points to take you forward in the short, medium and long term.

Anti-discriminatory practice is a journey. At times we may do a course on a particular aspect of diversity and gain a certificate. However, this needs to be a stage of development rather than the final destination. We need to apply the new ideas and thinking into our everyday lives and practice, staying alert to the impact of what we say and do to others. This involves reviewing our own patterns of behaviour and points of reference that we use to make sense of situations. A systematic approach is needed to reflect and gain feedback that can enable us to move forward. (See Moon, 1999, for ideas on how to develop your own reflective practice.)

At times, nurses may find themselves resisting change. In such cases, it is important to listen to and acknowledge the anxiety, allowing time for adjustments. Health professionals have an important part to play in sharing insight from their experiences and helping to tailor new systems to best meet the practical everyday realities.

Confidentiality

As a student nurse, you are expected to understand the principles of confidentiality. An individual should have the right to have their information and story protected, so that it does not become public knowledge. Often patients will not build up trust with the health professional if they feel that their information or details have been shared unnecessarily. However, as stated by Moss (2008), confidentiality is not an absolute. There are some situations where it is paramount that you share a patient's or colleague's details. In situations like this, an individual may be at risk of harming themselves or others. It is essential that you report your concerns to your mentor or line manager, who will discuss with you the appropriate action.

With good self-awareness and effective communication skills, it is important to be able to empower patients. **Empowerment** is when you, as the health professional, support or enable the patient to achieve a goal or set of goals. It may be as simple as the patient being able to pick up their cup and drinking from it or as difficult as going shopping and counting out the correct money.

The hospital environment can protect the patient and allow them to recover physically, but it can also act as a barrier to an individual going home. Patients can become institutionalised. This is where the patient's whole existence becomes focused around the hospital routine. On entering the hospital, patients are expected to change into their nightwear, take off their jewellery and slip into the role of the patient. This can make the patient feel vulnerable. As a health professional, it is important to recognise this phenomenon, in order to support and enable the patient to adjust.

One of the roles of a nurse is to be the advocate of the patient. Advocacy is the supporting and speaking up for the patient, which may happen formally or informally. As a student nurse, it is important that advice and support is sought from your mentor. An example of advocacy may be when a patient does not want to go through any more surgery, but is unable to tell the surgeon. In this situation, the nurse may act as an intermediary, offering support in bringing the patient's views to the attention of the medical and nursing team. The nurse needs to make sure that the patient has been given all the information so that the patient is making an informed choice.

Activity 5.8

Can you think of an occasion when you spoke up for a vulnerable person. How did it make you feel?

Family members may want to be involved in the planning and decision making of the care of their relatives. Although it is important that you involve family members, the right to choose is the patient's, as long as they are physically and mentally capable to make an informed choice. Family members may react in an aggressive manner. It is important that you remember that they act like this as they are scared and out of their depth. Often families struggle to articulate their feelings and it manifests itself in different ways. If you feel out of your depth as a student nurse, it is important that you tell the relatives that you think it would be more useful if they spoke to the staff nurse in charge. As you become more experienced, you will recognise this behaviour and will learn to deal with it. Remember, you never meet aggression with aggression, but act in a calm, professional manner, reassuring the relatives and showing empathy.

Breaking bad news is always difficult and you should only do this if you feel able to. Remember that every patient is an individual and may or may not want the full facts of their diagnosis (what is wrong with them) and/or prognosis (outcome of their diagnosis). You need to be aware that every patient has a different level of understanding and therefore you need to deliver information according to the patient's understanding and need. Maestri-Banks and Gosney (1997) found that when nurses are faced with the unique and awesome task of communicating with patients and/or relatives about difficult areas such as dying, they struggled and often avoided the topic. So it is essential that health professionals have effective communication skills and good self-awareness, in order to ask for support and guidance from senior staff members when needed.

According to Kübler-Ross (1969), when a person has died, those left behind usually suffer feelings of shock, anger, denial, sadness and depression. These are normal reactions to loss and part of the natural process of grieving. As a health professional, you may also have these feelings of bereavement. It may be for a patient you have known for some time and also because the loss evokes memories of another significant person in your life. It is important that you seek support from your mentor or senior staff member. The individual needs and practices of the dying person have to be considered as these may vary between cultures and religions.

Positive image of nursing

It is important that each nurse contributes towards the operation and promotion of a professional service. This is evident in the professional image and interpersonal skills used by the nurse. Historically, nurses were known for their clean, crisp uniform, with starched aprons and perfectly shaped hats. However, due to infection control and health and safety, nurses now wear modest comfortable uniforms, which, although they do not identify nurses so clearly, act as a practical and yet smart alternative.

A uniform in nursing is essential as it acts as a barrier between the nurse and the patient. This is important for the nurse and the patient when the time comes to carry out personal treatments on the patient. The uniform allows the patient to see the nurse as a person to trust and not feel embarrassed, rather than as a young person seeing them in a vulnerable situation. The uniform also protects nurses as it allows them to act in a professional manner, recognising that they hold a lot of responsibility for the patient's wellbeing and owe the patient a duty of care.

As a student nurse, you may not be comfortable wearing a uniform and you may feel as if part of your identity has been taken away. However, this uniformity also protects you. You will have to carry out some difficult and personal care on many of your patients. The uniform allows you to recognise that you are there for the good of the patient, in a privileged position as a nurse and not just as yourself. A nurse's uniform also exists for infection control reasons. A nurse should have a clean uniform on every day and wash the uniform in a hot temperature to prevent the spread of infections.

Like all individuals, nurses have their own style and personality. It may mean that while on duty some of the ways in which this is expressed need to be moderated in order to present yourself and act appropriately as a health professional. Self-image and creative style should be saved for when you are off duty. Your dress code is important, as patients and staff will judge you from the impression you give. It is important that you keep jewellery to the minimum, again for infection control and also so you do not hurt patients when delivering care.

A professional image needs to be presented. In practice, this is about performing duties in a caring manner and in accordance with professional regulations and values. Care of the patient has to be prioritised so that the patient feels emotionally safe and secure. Nurses have to be competent, knowing what to do and when. The service nurses offer needs to change in response to the patient's need and institutional priorities.

The role requires discretion so that staffing issues and concerns do not interfere with patient care. Nursing is a flexible and responsive occupation that meets people at their most vulnerable. As such, it is a privilege and needs to be respected as such.

Conclusion

We believe that the skills and qualities expected of nurses are shared with other professionals who work in the helping professions. These interprofessional skills are increasingly important as strategic initiatives require nurses to work in multidisciplinary teams. It is about developing a dialogue and working together in the interests of the service user or patient. One example of these professional mergers is when A&E medical staff work with drug and alcohol workers who are in attendance to begin their first contact with potential clients. Another example is when school nurses find that by working with youth workers and through their relationship with young people, it can transform the take-up of sexual health services. There are many opportunities for interprofessional collaboration. Using your personal and professional skills will enable you to play your part in this process.

In summary, with good self-awareness and effective communication skills, you are likely to be able to empower your patient and fulfil what it means to be a good nurse.

Useful resources

British Medical Association www.bma.org.uk

Nursing and Midwifery Council www.nmc-uk.org

General Social Care Council www.gscc.org.uk

British Association for Counselling and Psychotherapy www.bacp.co.uk

References

Berne, E (1961) *Transactional Analysis in Psychotherapy*, New York: Grove Press

BMA (British Medical Association) (2009) Regulatory Bodies, www.bma.org.uk

Gratus, J (2000) *Sharpen Up Your Interviewing: The Systematic Approach to Effective Interviewing for Busy Managers*, London: Management Books

Heron, J (1990) *Helping the Client: A Creative Practical Guide*, London: Sage

Luft, J and Ingham, H (1955) The Johari window, a graphic model of interpersonal awareness, *Proceedings of the Western Training Laboratory in Group Development,* Los Angeles: UCLA

Kübler-Ross, E (1969) *On Death and Dying*, London: Routledge

Maslow, AH (1970) *Motivation and Personality* (2nd edn), New York: Harper & Row

Maestri-Banks, A and Gosney, M (1997) Nurses' response to terminal care in the geriatric unit, *International Journal of Palliative Nursing*, **3**(6): 345–50

Mearns, D and Thorne, B (1992) *Person-centred Counselling in Action*, London: Sage

Mcleod Clark, J (1981) Communication in nursing, *Nursing Times*, 1: 12–18.

Moon, J (1999) *Reflection in Learning and Professional Development: Theory and Practice*, London: Kogan Page

Moss B. (2008) *Communication Skills for Health and Social Care*, London: Sage

NMC (Nursing and Midwifery Council) (2008) *The NMC Code of Professional Conduct: Standards for Conduct, Performance and Ethics*, London: NMC

Rogers, C (1967) *On Becoming a Person: A Therapist's View of Psychotherapy*, London: Constable

6 user involvement and user perspectives

Tony Hostick and Elaine Margaret Hostick

In this chapter we will explore:

> What user involvement means
> Why it is important
> The political context for user involvement
> Differences between tokenism and participation
> Ways of enhancing user involvement
> Hearing the voices of service users

Introduction

This chapter aims to provide an overview of user involvement. It is written so that it can be used as both a practical guide and as a toolkit for user involvement for nursing students and anyone considering a career in nursing.

What do we mean by user involvement?

The term 'user' is commonly employed to describe someone who is currently in receipt of services, for our purposes, healthcare. Other commonly adopted terms are 'patient', 'customer', 'consumer' or 'client'. The term can also include carers. Carers are users in their own right with their own needs.

User involvement is the means for ensuring the participation of service users in the planning and delivery of healthcare. This can be as an immediate participant in treatment, care and therapy or as a distant participant at the level of planning and delivery of services (Warr and Wall 1975). The involvement of users can engage them in all aspects of their own care and gain their perspectives on healthcare-related activities, including research, education, training, recruitment, in fact everything we do at every level. Consideration can be given to involving people who have used services previously, as they will have valuable views based on their experience of healthcare. The contributions of potential users or members of the public who have an interest in health or healthcare can also be sought.

While the principles of both immediate and distant participation are the same and both require us to effectively engage with service users, the means of

core topics

engagement are different and distinct. Immediate user participation occurs as a necessity when directly using or receiving a service. As nurses providing immediate care, our contribution should be 'user centred' and the needs of users given primacy. For service users who are able to articulate their needs, the primary task is to work with them to agree what these needs are, then plan a way forward. For service users who are unable or unwilling to engage, we should ensure that our decisions are based on the best available evidence. Evidence-based practice often refers to the use of research evidence of efficacy but can also include evidence from distant user involvement. If we value the contribution that service users make and incorporate their contribution, this could be termed 'values'-based practice.

User/carer involvement within care planning

The following four case histories are taken from a student nurse's continuous assessment document and reflective diary (with permission) and are designed to demonstrate how immediate user/carer involvement may be achieved.

Activity 6.1

Read through the case studies and select one or two that interest you. Then try to develop them further. For example, what aspects of good practice stand out? Can you identify alternative approaches to increase user involvement? Discuss your ideas with other others to see how they would approach the scenarios. What similarities and differences are there?

Case study 1

Client A is a 68-year-old female with memory impairment and limited mobility, whose husband and main carer had experienced difficulty assisting his wife in maintaining her personal hygiene and a balanced diet.

Prior to care planning with this lady, I gained knowledge of her past hygiene routines and dietary preferences by initially engaging with her carer (husband). He provided essential basic information that guided my approach to discussing these issues with the lady. Client A had valued her privacy in the past when washing and dressing and now objected to her husband's interventions to assist her. Her short-term memory impairment impacted upon her understanding of what was requested of her. Visual clues, simple language and directions all enabled the lady to be involved with her care. This approach also provided the carer with basic management techniques of his wife's experienced difficulties.

Ensuring user involvement within care planning to maintain a balanced diet for this lady was influenced by many factors. The environment of a hospital ward enforces restrictions upon choice and flexibility with established ward routines, menus and mealtimes. The lady was able to identify food and drink preferences visually if not verbally and due to short-term memory impairment, she required reassurance and support with maintaining a balanced, individualised diet.

Case study 2

These same principles were applied when caring for children (aged between 2 and 12 years). The child that is informed and included in decision making will feel safer, valued and potentially more motivated to be active in managing their health.

A six-year-old child with breathing difficulties requires care planning to maintain prescribed oxygen therapy. The child had been noncompliant in the past and his parents have experienced difficulties assisting him.

The child and parents responded positively to inclusion and negotiation in addressing this problem. The child had become fearful and mistrustful of the hospital environment following his repeated admissions and need of medical interventions. The parents voiced concern and frustrations regarding their inability to actively help their son. I explained to the child the importance of his treatment and the role of oxygen therapy within it. The use of appropriate language and providing simple choices resulted in the identification of and care planning for his individual care needs. The child talked of his fear of having an oxygen mask secured to his face. We discussed this and agreed that the elastic strap be removed and he was supported to hold the mask to his face for increasing periods of time. Providing the child with physical control of the equipment reduced his fear and the prescribed oxygen therapy was achieved through reward and positive feedback. In collaboration with the child and his parents, a plan of care was agreed. The parents and nurses encouraged the child to fill in a simple tick chart to record the times/duration of the self-administration of his oxygen. The child was then encouraged to present these documents to his consultant at the ward round.

Case study 3

A 12-year-old female was admitted for abdominal surgery with no previous experience of surgical intervention. The child had limited knowledge of her diagnosis, treatment and care needs following surgery.

The child's parents were engaged in conversation to establish both parental and client norms and values within managing health. The parents had limited the information given to their daughter regarding planned surgery in an effort to reduce her anxieties. By providing the child with basic knowledge of the sequence of events prior to and following her surgery, she was able to ask questions and share her anxieties. Her expressed fear of needles and injections was alleviated to some extent by informing her of skin anesthetising patches used prior to injection if needed. The child was enabled to make choices regarding these issues through discussion with her anaesthetist. Direct inclusion of the child, her parents and other healthcare practitioners in the care planning process and implementation contributed to a positive healthcare experience for this anxious child.

Case study 4

A 24-year-old male client was admitted to a mental health unit via the crisis resolution service. This gentleman was experiencing acute psychosis, currently homeless and unable to identify his next of kin.

Initial care planning with this gentleman was governed by his experienced symptoms and altered perceptions of time, place and person. He was able to make simple choices within meeting his basic needs and able to communicate these to staff. Due to homelessness, his routines had been changed and become erratic. He related sleeping during daylight hours as safer, as sleeping in the open at night made him feel vulnerable to attack from others. Obtaining a regular and balanced diet was governed by many factors such as finances, whereabouts and the charity of others. The gentleman was unable or unwilling to identify his next of kin to staff. He identified his wish that his parents not be informed of his admission or whereabouts. His right to refuse this course of action was acknowledged and he was encouraged to think of any trusted person/significant other who he wished to contact. His care plan clearly identified his wishes and he stated that being listened to and respected by others was something he valued greatly. This gentleman's circumstances and lifestyle choices differed greatly from ward routines and social norms but were broadly accommodated within his planned care. Care planning to ensure his basic needs required adaptation and compromise. To ensure he obtained rest and a balanced diet, he agreed to decrease the time he slept during the day and be respectful of others sleeping at night, keeping his activities to a minimum. He was encouraged to prepare himself simple foods/drinks in the ward kitchen if not able to eat at routine ward times initially; this was an agreed temporary measure to be reviewed after five days. An adaptive and inclusive approach to care planning with this gentleman provided the foundations for building a therapeutic and trusting relationship between a service user and care providers.

User/carer involvement in service planning and delivery

By definition, distant user participation usually occurs 'away' from direct care or treatment and is concerned with engaging service users to:

> help improve the quality of services
> make services more sensitive and responsive to the needs of service users
> contribute to the design of services
> help manage services
> monitor services.

These are some examples of general activities in which service users can be involved:

> Participation in the development of service strategies and frameworks
> Identifying and prioritising needs and allocating resources
> Planning and commissioning services
> Developing care pathways or care packages
> Monitoring, reviewing and evaluating services and taking part in inspections
> Staff selection, training and development
> Training of service users, frontline staff, senior managers and directors
> As representatives of a group with a particular interest, for example use of a

particular service, living in a particular area, having a specific condition such as diabetes or asthma

> Advocacy for other service users and carers.

Why is user involvement important?

User involvement is not an end in itself but a way of achieving three fundamental objectives:

1 strengthened accountability to local communities
2 a health service that genuinely responds to patients and carers
3 a sense of ownership and trust (DH 2003, p. 4).

Since the late 1960s, there has been pressure for greater involvement of both patients and the public in health and social care (Walsh and Hostick 2004). Arnstein's (1969) ladder of citizen participation was aimed at involving the public in community planning and this model of involvement can be applied to involvement in healthcare and service planning. Published a little later, Wolfensberger's (1972) normalisation theory was aimed at helping learning disabled people become more socially included in 'normal' life and remains influential. (Chapter 14 discusses normalisation in detail.)

In 1978, responding to international crises in health, the *Declaration of Alma-Ata* at the International Conference on Primary Health Care stated:

The people have the right and duty to participate individually and collectively in the planning and implementation of their health care. (WHO 1978)

The 'consumer' of health services came to be recognised as the main judge of quality (Gregory and Walsh 1993) and risk is also seen as possibly best managed with broader involvement of service users (Hood et al. 1992). Therefore the involvement of service user and carer is seen to have many benefits (CCNAP 2001):

> Increased trust and confidence in open, accountable and respectful services
> Services that are more responsive to public needs and views
> Local ownership of and commitment to health and social services
> Local understanding of changes to services
> Constructive working relationships
> Sensitivity to the voices of users and carers as experts on their own needs and desires
> Identifying where standards are not being met
> Praise for excellence in performance
> More well-informed public making more appropriate use of services
> Promotes creativity and new ideas
> Increased understanding of patient and carer experience of services
> Reduces the risk of abuse of service users

> Protects patient and carer rights

> Increases control over decisions that are important to patients.

The political context

There is a long tradition of national policy approaches to public involvement in healthcare from the establishment of community health councils in 1974 as local bodies to mediate between local people and the NHS. Pressure for broader participation led to a number of policies being produced (James 1992; DH 1992, 1995, 1996), and the modernisation of the NHS in England through *The NHS Plan* (DH 2000) re-emphasised the need to put the patient at the centre of everything the NHS does. In health services, clinical governance is a system through which NHS organisations are accountable for continuously improving the quality of their services and safeguarding high standards of care, by creating an environment in which clinical excellence will flourish (DH 1997; NHS Executive 1998, 1999). A key dimension of clinical governance is the user experience and the involvement of service users, carers and the public in all aspects of healthcare delivery. These developments culminated in the publication of guidance (DH 2003) to support Section 11 of the Health and Social Care Act 2001, which identifies the need for partnerships between the public, patients and health providers within whole communities.

The NHS Reform and Healthcare Professionals Act 2002 abolished community health councils and established patient and public involvement (PPI) forums in each trust, a Commission for Patient and Public Involvement in Health and the NHS Centre for Involvement. More recent policy changes have replaced PPI forums with Local Involvement Networks through the Local Government and Public Involvement in Health Act 2007, which emphasised involvement in the commissioning of services and sought to increase patient choice.

While it could be argued that these changes have been generally structural, it is clear that public services have a duty to demonstrate that public involvement has occurred, how involvement has impacted and how participants have been informed of outcomes. Indeed, involving service users and the public is seen as a vital way of forcing health and social services to think about how to improve their purpose, culture and activities (Smithies and Webster 1998).

The difference between tokenism and participation

Arnstein (1969) provides a ladder of citizen participation (Figure 6.1), with each rung representing the degree of power a citizen holds from the lowest rung of manipulation through a number of levels of nonparticipation, tokenism and citizen power to citizen control as the top rung. Arnstein (1969, p. 218) states:

> the fundamental point [is] that participation without redistribution of power is an empty and frustrating process for the powerless. It allows the

power holders to claim that all sides were considered, but makes it possible for only some of those sides to benefit. It maintains the status quo.

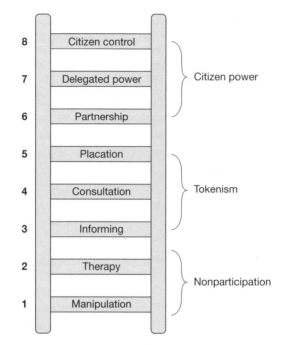

Figure 6.1 Arnstein's ladder of citizen participation
Source: Arnstein (1969) A ladder of participation, *Journal of the American Institute of Planners*, 35: 216–24. Reproduced with permission

Arnstein describes the type of 'nonparticipation' represented by the lower two rungs on the ladder as attempts to 'educate' participants. Levels 3 and 4 allow participants to hear and have a voice, but they have no power to ensure that their voice has influence. At level 5 participants can offer advice, but the right to decide is retained by the agency. True participation begins where 'partnerships' enable negotiation and shared decision-making responsibility. Arnstein considers that partnership working is most effective when participants have an organised and resourced base from which to work, and to which they are accountable. At levels 7 and 8, participants form the majority in decision-making arenas, or hold managerial power.

Activity 6.2

Apply Arnstein's model to your own experience or to examples of user involvement in decision making in the settings you have worked in:

- Where would you place yourself or the service users on the ladder?
- Did you or the service users have clear, genuine reasons for being there?
- What did you think and feel about your involvement?
- What did you learn from the experience?

core topics

Arnstein's model has subsequently been adapted, for example by Wilcox (1994), who suggests that our intent (purpose) when involving people might be:

> information giving
> consultation
> deciding together
> acting together
> supporting independent community interests.

1 *Information giving*: Good quality, appropriate, accessible information underpins all involvement, but does not in itself constitute involvement. Giving information alone is a one-way process. It suggests that there are no alternative options and that no contribution is required from the public/service users. Just giving information may be appropriate when:
   ▶ there is no possibility of negotiation, for example you are following a legal requirement
   ▶ you want to get a message across but don't require feedback or comment
   ▶ you are initiating a process, and people need information to become involved at a later stage.

2 *Consultation:* Allows choice between limited, predetermined options, but not an opportunity to propose alternatives or take part in putting plans into action. Consultation (only) may be appropriate when the range of options is genuinely limited.

3 *Deciding together:* Views are shared, options are generated jointly, and a course of action decided upon. Deciding together will be appropriate when:
   ▶ there is a possibility of negotiation
   ▶ an agreed agenda needs to be reached among different interests
   ▶ implementation requires the cooperation of other people.

4 *Acting together:* Working with others to make decisions and carry through the action agreed. This may be appropriate when:
   ▶ there is a shared agenda
   ▶ there is an ongoing process of development of trust and cooperation between the parties
   ▶ the imbalance of power or resources has been addressed.

5 *Supporting independent community interests:* Supporting independent groups to develop and implement their own solutions. This may be appropriate when:
   ▶ there are adequate resources and support for the group
   ▶ a longer timescale is possible
   ▶ participation is currently on one level.

These models illustrate levels or degrees of participation that are appropriate for a particular purpose. On another level, they illustrate the progression that takes place as service users become more involved, and their power and responsibility develops and extends.

Ways of enhancing user involvement

There is no single 'right way' or 'best method' for involving people. The approaches you choose depend on what you want from the process. There are ways that are better or worse for particular ends, in particular circumstances, or for working with particular people. You will need to use a variety of approaches; however, if we adopt user involvement as a core value, it offers the means to engage staff from different professions, disciplines and services in meaningful discussion that is often made difficult by professional boundaries and beliefs (Nolan and Grant 1993; Pendleton and King 2002; Fulford and Williams 2003).

Before you ask how, you may ask some other questions about commitment, resources and support (CCNAP 2001):

> How committed are you?
> Are you clear about your reasons for involving people?
> Do you have an adequate budget?
> Is there a strong lead within your organisation or workplace?
> Are members of staff on board?
> Have you considered the impact on the people you are asking to participate, and their information and support needs?
> Are you prepared to act on what they tell you?
> How will you deal with the change in the balance of power that meaningful involvement brings?

It is especially important that involvement initiatives are seen to be both genuine and practical. Failure in this will at best simply waste a lot of time and at worst may lead to disillusionment and resentment (Wilcox 1994), which may affect staff, patients and carers who have not been directly involved.

Consider this checklist, adapted from Wilcox (1994), for involving people in service settings:

> In planning to involve service users, are you responding to what service users want, or are you initiating the process?
> If you are planning an initiative, how will service users view what you are doing?
> What do you want to achieve?
> Who can help?
> What might restrict you?
> Are other staff members committed?
> Have staff members been offered opportunities to work through their fears?
> Do you have the skills and resources you need?

> Have you thought through the consequences of your actions in changing the balance of power between staff and service users?

> What might the service look like as a consequence of what you are doing?

> Who will have the final say over decisions? Can you deliver the service that users want?

This list looks daunting, and you will only be able to answer some of the questions as you develop your plan. There is plenty of evidence that considering these things, and getting everyone on board before you start, goes a long way towards ensuring that your initiative will be successful.

Hearing the voices of users

While there are many ways of enhancing user involvement, listening, understanding and action are core activities within each. Within the Trent Quality Initiative, Gregory et al. (1994) identified two key ways in which involvement can be improved generally:

1 Providing the opportunity to clarify what has been said or written in terms of:
  ▶ intelligibility (of words, ideas)
  ▶ acceptability (legal, moral, social)
  ▶ sincerity (of the speaker)
  ▶ evidence (facts or opinions or feelings).
  A request for clarification needs only to be as simple as being able to say 'please clarify X'.

2 Being willing to respond to requests for clarification.

By listening to people who use our services, we can start to identify ways in which those services need to be improved. By including them in the planning of services, they can help to put things right or ensure they are right from the start. Time to listen is often pressurised, so create time for yourself and the service user, check out your understanding of what is being said, reflect on what has been said and act upon it. Every healthcare organisation will have systems for involving service users. For example, these will include forums, PPI strategies, user member meetings in foundation trusts, clinical governance, customer care or patient experience teams, and policies for dealing with complaints and suggestions. As with the examples used for involving users and carers in care planning, there will be opportunities to involve different groups of users and carers in service planning and delivery. Groups include children, older people, people with learning disabilities, people with short-term acute needs and people with longer term needs. All will require different approaches to involvement.

Conclusion

User involvement is fundamental to all that we do. You can make it real and meaningful by valuing the contribution that service users can make and by putting the needs of the service user at the centre of decision making. User involvement is not easy; it needs commitment, planning, time and resources. However, it is evident that the benefits are many. As a nurse, you are ideally placed to facilitate user involvement and the activities outlined in this chapter can help. How would you want to be involved? How can you make sure users are involved? How can you make sure that others involve users?

Useful resources

NHS Centre for User Involvement http://www.nhscentreforinvolvement.nhs.uk/

Joseph Rowntree Foundation http://www.jrf.org.uk/publications/user-involvement-and-seriously-ill

Acknowledgement

Thanks to Dr Mike Walsh for his comments on the draft versions of this chapter.

References

Arnstein, S. (1969) A ladder of participation, *Journal of the American Institute of Planners*, 35: 216–24

CCNAP (Community Care Needs Assessment Project) (2001) *'Asking the Experts': A Guide to Involving People in Shaping Health and Social Care Services*, available at http://www.library.nhs.uk/PPI/ViewResource.aspx?resID=289379

DH (Department of Health) (1992) *Local Voices: The Views of Local People in Purchasing for Health*, Leeds: DH

DH (1995) *Consumers and Research in the NHS: An R&D Contribution to Consumer Involvement in the NHS*, Leeds: DH

DH (1996) *Patient Partnership Strategy*, Leeds: DH

DH (1997) *The New NHS, Modern and Dependable*, Cm 3807, London: TSO

DH (2000) *The NHS Plan: A Plan for Investment, A Plan for Reform*, London: DH

DH (2003) *Strengthening Accountability: Involving Patients and the Public*, Policy Guidance Section 11 of the Health and Social Care Act 2001, London: DH

Fulford, KW and Williams, R (2003) Values-based child and adolescent mental health services? *Current Opinion in Psychiatry*, **16**(4): 369–76

Gregory, W and Walsh, M (1993) Quality, ideology and consumer choice, in M Malek, P Vacani, J Rasquinha and P Davey (eds) *Managerial Issues in the Reformed NHS*, Chichester: Wiley

Gregory, WJ, Romm, NR and Walsh, MP (1994) *The Trent Quality Initiative: A Multi-agency Evaluation of Quality Standards in the National Health Service*, Hull: Centre for Systems Studies

Hood, C, Jones, D, Pidgeon, NF et al. (1992) Risk management, in *Risk Analysis, Perception and Management: Report of a Royal Society Study Group*, London: Royal Society

James, A (1992) *Committed to Quality: Quality Assurance in Social Services Departments*, London: HMSO

NHS Executive (1998) *A First Class Service: Quality in the New NHS*, London: DH

NHS Executive (1999) *Clinical Governance: Quality in the New NHS*, London: DH

Nolan, M and Grant, G (1993) Action research and quality of care: a mechanism for agreeing basic values as a precursor for change, *Journal of Advanced Nursing*, 18: 305–11

Pendleton, D and King, J (2002) Values and leadership, *British Medical Journal*, **325**(7376): 1352–5

Smithies, J and Webster, G (1998) *Community Involvement in Health*, Aldershot: Ashgate

Walsh, M and Hostick, T (2005) Improving health care through community OR, *Journal of the Operational Research Society*, **56**(2): 193–201

Warr, P and Wall, T (1975) *Work and Well-being*, Harmondsworth: Penguin

WHO (World Health Organization) (1978) *Declaration of Alma-Ata*, The International Conference on Primary Health Care, available online at http://www.who.int/hpr/NPH/docs/declaration_almaata.pdf, accessed 1/1/2010

Wilcox, D (1994) *Participation Guide*, Brighton: Partnership Books

Wolfensberger, W (1972) *The Principle of Normalization in Human Services*, National Institute on Mental Retardation, Toronto

7 understanding the social context of healthcare

Peter Morrall

In this chapter we will explore:

> Imagination
> Globalisation
> Medicalisation
> Madness
> Sexuality

Introduction

What has the academic study of society got to do with the practical occupation of nursing? In this chapter I argue that a sociological understanding of health is fundamental to nursing care. (Connections can be made between some aspects of the social context of healthcare as argued in this chapter with those presented in Chapter 4.)

Undoubtedly, students of nursing should concentrate more on learning skills, attributes and knowledge, such as compassion, kindliness, empathy, anatomy/physiology/pathology, drug administration, wound care and hand washing, rather than the often abstract and frequently complex notions emanating from sociology. Despite being an ardent advocate for a sociology of and in nursing – and all other health/medical disciplines (Morrall 2001, 2009) – I accept unreservedly that the basic premise of nursing must encompass caring, competency and cleanliness. Without first empathising with the patient's plight, executing treatments effectively and doing them no harm, there is little point in realising that people's lives are shaped substantially by society – the basic premise of **sociology**.

At a macro-level, sociologists point out how social factors, situations and trends can undermine, shape and ameliorate health dramatically. For example, the 2008 crisis in the global banking system, the ongoing inequities of global food production and distribution, along with global ecological mismanagement, can be connected to the higher infant mortality, lower life span, increase in life-threatening diseases and environmental disasters found in such countries as Ethiopia, Bangladesh and Haiti. At a micro-level, sociologists points out that labelling a patient as 'bad' or 'good', cooperative or uncooperative, likely to live or die can have a profound effect (positive or negative) on that individual. Indeed, the very diagnosis of a disease may alter substantially how the patient thinks, feels and acts, leading to a 'patient career' related to that diagnosis.

So, in this chapter, I first set out to explain the **sociological imagination** in order to provide the essential 'tools' of sociology, that is, the subject's intellectual heritage which underpins its theories and research. This is followed by sections on globalisation, medicalisation, madness and sexuality. The first section I have chosen because of a desire to demonstrate how we live now in a global society and that the nature of this global society has direct relevance to nursing. The other sections have been chosen to reveal the expansiveness and appeal of the sociological imagination. Inevitably, this means other, perhaps more expected, sections, for example on social class, poverty and social exclusion, have been omitted. However, overall, the chapter contains explicit or implicit reference to a much wider range of sociological interests than the section headings imply. Moreover, some of the points made here may seem provocative to the reader. This is deliberate. While not wanting to offend gratuitously, I have attempted to stimulate those new to sociology into thinking and thinking differently (Morrall 2010).

The 'sociological imagination' provides nurses with broader awareness and deeper insights regarding their work. Research and theorising derived from the sociological imagination help to educate rather than just train nurses. The results from research and the ideas from theories contextualise healthcare. This may lead indirectly or directly to adjustments in how nurses think and therefore how they carry out their practice, where in the world they want to practise, and possibly to personal or collective 'moral action', whereby nurses campaign for a better world and, in particular, improved healthcare (Morrall 2009).

Imagination

Humans have, since the first collections of hominids in the African rainforests millions of years ago, existed in what could loosely be described as 'societies'. That is, the evolutionary precursors to humans and subsequently *Homo sapiens* virtually always belonged to a social grouping of one type or another. Initially, these were in the form of clusters of intimate relationships, which became what we now refer to as 'families', and small bands, whose members collaborated for their mutual protection and to obtain food more efficiently than could a few operating together or lone individuals.

It is the belonging to social groupings and how that inevitably alters how people 'perform' (think, feel and behave) that is of interest to the sociologist. Today, human social groupings are varied and multilayered. People usually belong to a family. But there are many different sorts of families. For example:

> married or cohabiting couples
> single parent (female or male)

> nuclear (two adults and their children)
> polygamous (men having more that one wife)
> polyandrous (women having more than one husband)
> extended (many different generations)
> step (two adults with children from this and previous relationships)
> homosexual/lesbian (with or without legal status).

Apart from families, people can belong to an assortment of associations, **cultures**, subcultures and communities, based on, for example, work, ethnicity, religion, volunteering, hobbies or criminality (Giddens 2009). They will also belong to a society, for example British, French, South African, or Irish, and possibly a supranation (such as the European Union). Moreover, because of advanced communication systems (especially the internet and television) and travel (for holidays, adventure and business), a **global society** is developing. This is either 'real' (people come together face to face) or 'virtual' (people connect with each other via the internet and telephone). The exceptions might be hermits, castaways, new age subcultures, although even they will have come from, and may go back to, social groupings of one sort or another.

So, how does belonging to these social groupings influence health and therefore nursing? Health is affected by the beliefs, values and customs (called 'norms' by sociologists) of the associations, cultures, subcultures, communities and global society, the decisions made by governments (particularly those of the industrialised West and the rapidly industrialising countries of China, India and Brazil) and employers (above all the executives and major shareholders of global corporations).

Health is also influenced by the way in which individuals choose to live their lives. For example, having lung cancer, liver cirrhosis, diabetes, obesity, or/and anxiety and depression is related to a number of social factors:

> how fervently tobacco companies push their products, whether or not a government decides to regulate the selling of cigarettes, and the age group, gender, social class or culture we belong to
> the price per unit of alcohol, acceptability of a binge-drinking culture, and the availability of alcohol
> whether or not the food industries stop adding so much sugar and fat to their products, the amount of advice about diet being disseminated by health agencies, and how ideas in the media of femininity and masculinity relate to weight
> how much the 'stress' to earn more and more to buy more and more is stimulated by the values of our particular social class or lifestyle.

Furthermore, high alcohol intake, smoking, ingesting sugary and fat-laden snacks and drinks, and being a workaholic and a rampant consumer are also to do with our personal preferences. There are pressures from global corporations to drink and eat their unhealthy if not lethal products and demands by governments and employers for people to accept their responsibilities to work. However, consumers demand these products and want to be employed.

Not only is the contracting of such diseases related to social factors, but so is their diagnosis and treatment. The amount of health resources allocated and health research conducted will depend on the priorities of governments and their health agencies, as well as on public opinion. The finances of a society can be ploughed into treating and researching cancer, cirrhosis, diabetes, obesity and stress, rather than, for example, procuring armaments, the laying of more roads, or building more fast-food outlets, bars and nightclubs.

Moreover, sociology is not merely common sense. At times, sociology coincides with conventional wisdom, but only after the veracity of the relevant assumptions has been investigated thoroughly. At other times, what is commonly taken as an obvious fact is contradicted by sociological analysis. It was, for example, accepted as common sense for hundreds of years that nursing was 'women's work', medicine was 'men's work', and patients should do as they are told by both. Sociologists have contributed to the successful undoing of those particular stereotypes.

George Ritzer (2006) suggests that what he calls 'social thinking' is very different to ordinary thinking. It is more disciplined, broader, orderly and deliberate, and makes reference to thoughts of previous social thinkers. Essentially, the basis of social thinking, or the 'sociological imagination' (Mills 1959), is to look beyond the obvious and minutiae, and to challenge preconceived ideas (including those of sociologists). Above all, it is to provoke thinking by asking the question 'why', and to keep on asking the question 'why', scrutinising systematically all possible answers.

There are various ways of thinking sociologically, but most emanate from one of three:

1 The *structuralist* sociologist views much, if not all, of **human performance** as being 'determined' by society. Specifically, the institutions of society (including those of education, criminal justice, the family, industry and commerce, media, psychotherapy and health), and the ways in which society is divided (principally by social class, gender, ethnicity, religion, age, and geography) set out the boundaries for human performance. Moreover, the structuralist argues that these social institutions and divisions produce a hierarchy in society founded on status, power and wealth. The notable contribution from structuralist sociology is that people at the bottom of the social hierarchy are likely to suffer from far more chronic diseases and die far younger than those at the top.

2 The *interactionist* sociologist takes a modified stance to understanding society to that of the structuralist. Human performance for the interactionist is definitely linked to social circumstances. But humans have much more choice than the structuralist accepts, and they constantly and consciously elect to make life meaningful for themselves even though their choices are

to some degree restricted by, or indeed opened up by, society. Importantly, the interactionist points out that social groups, for example nursing, can campaign to improve their standing in society. That is, within this model of society, the social hierarchy is far more fluid than the structuralists suggest. Furthermore, for the interactionist, contracting cancer, diabetes, obesity, or depression has different meanings for different people. To understand health and disease, nurses (and medical practitioners and other healthcare workers) have to appreciate what meanings are attached to these states by specific individuals and groups. Interactionists also describe how some people have 'spoiled identities' because of the stigma from the physical, psychological or social labels they attract. Through regular negative feedback, individuals can come to perceive themselves as in some way not quite 'normal' or 'whole'. They may feel 'damaged' or 'contaminated', and self-worth becomes undermined. A diagnosis of schizophrenia or HIV/AIDS, having a stutter, facial disfigurement or a disabled limb, or even just being described by nurses as an 'awkward patient' may attract stigma and therefore furnish a spoiled identity.

3 The *constructionists* take much further the notion that individuals give 'meaning' to their lives. For the constructionist, the social world does not have an unadulterated objective existence. All social phenomena are to a greater or lesser extent 'constructed'. Things become 'real' only because humans and their societies attach particular meanings to them. From this point of view, diseases and states of mind are human fabrications. They do not exist without someone recognising and defining them. Whereas the medical scientist believes that cancer, diabetes and depression actually exist and can be identified and described as 'facts', the constructionist argues that they only have the appearance of having a reality because of the coming together of certain historical and social processes. At other times, and in other places, they would either not be construed as real at all or they would be interpreted as different entities.

Activity 7.1

Do you dare to think differently? Buy a magazine/newspaper/book that you have not read before but which may provoke you into understanding a topic or the world in an alternative way.

Globalisation

From a structuralist perspective, the creation of a global society is fundamentally about the worldwide transmission of a Western (capitalist) way of life rather than a pooling of cultures from all parts of the globe. Together with more freedoms for businesses to sell their goods and consumers to buy more commodities, an increase in respect for human rights, an unrestricted press and freedom of speech, what has also been transmitted globally are widespread inequalities. Wealth is not shared equally between the three economic segments of the world: developed (Western) countries; developing countries, principally, Brazil, Russia, India and China; and underdeveloped countries (many African and South American nations). Furthermore, the wealth divide has grown substantially within most countries, no matter what stage of economic emergence they are in.

Indeed, the divide globally between the wealthy minority and impoverished majority is growing rapidly. The ecological and material self-interest of the corporate and governmental stratums in developed and developing countries, along with corruption among the elites of the underdeveloped countries, has created a polarised world population:

> 10% of the richest adults in the world own 85% of global household wealth
> the richest 2% own more than 50% of global wealth
> the richest 1% own 40% of global wealth
> half of the world's adult population own less than 1% (Davies, 2008).

In Britain, the National Enquiry Panel (2010) reported that the gap between the rich and the poor in Britain had become wider that ever before, with the richest 10% more than 100 times as wealthy as those in the poorest 10%. The report also commented that it is 'obvious' this wealth divide is connected to 'startling' differences in life expectancy (p. 23).

Moreover, environmental pollution, brought on by the spread of industrialisation, may be tipping the earth into a spiral of ecological collapse characterised by droughts, famines, floods, tsunamis and earthquakes (Gore 2006; Lovelock 2006; Monbiot 2007). Violence is endemic, and the global murder rate per annum is rising towards one million (Morrall 2006). One billion people in the world are impoverished, hungry, diseased or have no access to the basic amenities of life such as safe water (Sachs 2007; Collier 2007).

Children's life expectancy is also dependent on the socioeconomic status of their country. As with life expectancy overall, there has been significant improvement in child survival globally. However, the divergence is immense. Whereas there are six deaths before the age of five per live 1,000 births in most developed countries (with only three in Sweden, Singapore, San Marino, Liechtenstein, Iceland and Andorra), Sierra Leone has 270 deaths before the age of five per 1,000 live births, Angola 260, Afghanistan 257, Niger 253, and Liberia 235. Every day, 26,000 children under five die mostly from diseases that can be prevented through vaccination, better nutrition, safe water, better sanitation and hygiene, or basic medical input. That is, approximately 10 million children under the age of five die every year from easily preventable diseases (WHO 2008; United Nations Children's Fund 2008).

Life spans vary widely. People born in Japan, Iceland, Israel, Norway and Sweden reach around 80 years of age, with people born in the UK, Italy,

Germany, France, Canada, Australia and Singapore not far behind. Notwithstanding the 2008 'credit crunch', the USA remains the wealthiest and most powerful country on earth, with a life expectancy rate of 77.5 years. But in many sub-Saharan African countries, far from life expectancy rising, there has been a huge lowering due to the interrelated factors of HIV, destitution, famine, war, environmental disaster and unbalanced Western-orchestrated trading arrangements. Tens of millions of people in sub-Saharan countries have lower life expectancies than the working classes of England in the 1840s. People from Rwanda will probably only live for the first few years of their fourth decade, those from Malawi and Angola will maybe just to get to 40, and those from Zambia will be extremely lucky if they reach 40 years, while being born in Swaziland means that you will probably die at just over 30 years, and in Sierra Leone at about 29 years (UN 2006; ESRC 2008; Jones et al. 2008).

Furthermore, some subregions and substrata of countries, which overall have respectable life span and infant mortality profiles, contain populations that on average die at significantly younger ages; for example shanty town dwellers in Brazil, blacks in the southern states of the USA, peasants in Indo-China, the Aborigines of Australia, industrial workers in the special economic zones of the People's Republic of China, and the millions of people being exploited as 'modern slaves' throughout the world. Similarly, within developed countries, wide disparities in longevity mean that the executive, management and white-collar classes in countries such as Britain die up to 10 years older than those with menial jobs and those in the underclass – the long-term unemployed, homeless, and chronically and severely ill. Infant mortality difference between the classes is evident, but not as marked as those of life span.

This is what is going on in the world. Nurses, I argue, should be aware of not just how to deal with the health issues of the patients in their locality, but of how other people in a global society, a society to which they belong, deal with health issues not usually experienced in the UK.

Activity 7.2

List five improvements you would like to make in one of the clinical areas you have experienced. Make suggestions as to how these improvements could be brought about.

What steps would you take to promote better health in the world?

Medicalisation

The sociological theory of **medicalisation** proposes that medical intervention, and by implication that of nursing and other healthcare disciplines, in everyday life is out of control (Morrall 2009). That is, more and more of our thoughts, emotions and behaviours are becoming susceptible to medical interference, and new syndromes and diseases are being discovered (or, from the constructionist sociologist viewpoint, 'invented') regularly. This, according to Peter Conrad (2007), has led to the 'medicalisation of society'.

Some members of the profession of medicine have actually adopted this critical sociological approach and use it for the purpose of self-criticism. For example, Michael Fitzpatrick (2000) is a GP. His experience of working in a British inner-city practice confirms for him that the 'health propaganda' contained in the plethora of government policies is having an unhealthy effect on society. Fitzpatrick argues that patients are made to feel unnecessarily anxious because of the constant health scares in the media, which are reinforced by government health agencies. The risks, he suggests, of normal activities such as eating, sunbathing and having sex are being hugely exaggerated. Medical practitioners, he continues, don't merely try to cure disease, but are encouraged by the government's 'health police', for example GPs and primary care nurses/health visitors, to tell people how to live their lives in great detail.

Many specific examples of this medicalisation are offered by those who propose the medicalisation thesis. Menstruation is no longer a natural if unwelcome curse, but a medical condition that can be regulated. Premenstrual tension is not a period of unavoidable hormonal imbalance, but an unhealthy symptom to be remedied. A large body size, which at one time would have been viewed as the result of a 'healthy appetite', and in some cultures may still signify wealth and high social status, has been reclassified as 'obesity'. Feeling tired, disinterested and miserable is rescheduled as 'chronic fatigue syndrome'. If repeating the same physical movement causes pain, no longer is a sensible and quick way of stopping the pain to stop the movement, but instead a diagnosis of 'repetitive strain injury' is given, with special repetitive strain injury pain-relieving medications prescribed. Binge drinking is no longer a personal lifestyle choice or cultural habit of certain social groups (all be it a self-destructive one) but 'alcoholism'. Bodily blemishes, wobbly bits, small bits, large bits and fat bits can all be cosmetically reconfigured. Naughty school children become sufferers of 'hyperactivity' or 'attention deficit syndrome'. Difficulties in writing (dyslexia) are traced to specific abnormalities in the brain, rather than being accepted as an issue to do with learning. Having bombs drop on you, your family and your neighbours while under siege from some rampaging and merciless army (and thereby collectively becoming scared witless) is not explained as perfectly understandable, given the terrible circumstances. It is given the medical epithet of 'complete mass conflict disorder'. Sex offending is not only a reprehensible criminal offence, but is treatable with medication and/or psychotherapy. Being a grumpy man is not a regrettable gender trait, but 'irritable male syndrome'.

For Ivan Illich (1977), the profession of medicine (and increasingly nursing) has put both the health of individuals and society in jeopardy as a consequence of medicalisation. Illich uses the term 'iatrogenesis' (meaning doctor-induced disease) to describe the negative consequences of medicalisation. Illich argues that there are three types of iatrogenesis:

1 *Clinical iatrogenesis*, the straightforward and relatively immediate

complications and side effects of surgical operations (either conducted unnecessarily, or which cause unintended damage) and medicines. For example, the British Medical Association has reported that over 250,000 people suffer from adverse reactions from medicines prescribed for them, and about 5,000 die (Boseley 2006). This is aside from the number of errors made in medical prescribing, reckoned by the NHS Healthcare Commission (2006) to be approximately 40,000 in English and Welsh hospitals alone, and by the World Health Organization (WHO 2005) to affect 1 in 10 patients globally.

2 *Social iatrogenesis*, whereby the whole of society, as a consequence of medicalisation, becomes dependent on the medical profession. People become addicted not just to medicines but to the medical profession. Such dependency is what, for Illich, has made the medical profession extremely and worryingly powerful.

3 *Cultural iatrogenesis* is the end product of the medical destruction of personal autonomy. Illich argues that clinical and social iatrogenesis lead to such entrenchment of medical authority in all areas of human life that individuals lose their ability to make decisions for themselves. Whether it is about how to bring up our children, how to care for each other, whether or not we should work, how to grow old, how to procreate or have sex, or how to die, doctors are consulted. Moreover, for Illich, cultural iatrogenesis has incapacitated individuals to the point that they are unable to accept pain, suffering or death as an inescapable element of human existence. Being pain free is to be less than fully human. Humans, suggests Illich, need discomfort and grief to be in touch with the natural world of which they are part.

Obviously, medical intervention has a function in the diagnosis and treatment of such serious diseases as breast cancer and coronary heart failure. To argue otherwise would be absurd. It is also unfair to blame medicalisation totally on doctors and nurses. Such a perspective considers people as passively entering what structuralist sociologist Talcott Parsons (1951) describes as 'the sick role' and accepting what they are told is good for their health, whereas the demand for pills, potions and operations can (and often does) come from the consumer. From an interactionist viewpoint, the massive rise in alternative complementary healthcare is indicative of people actively wanting more and more remedies for an ever increasing range of self-identified health problems (Morrall 2008a). Moreover, the overmedicalisation of the developed world should be contrasted with the undermedicalisation of the underdeveloped world. Millions of children and adults die in sub-Saharan Africa, South America and Southeast Asia because there is a lack of medical provision, although the root of their diseases may well be socio-environmental.

Madness

Nurses come across madness frequently. They do so of course in the dedicated mental health units, but also in A&E departments, elderly care facilities, and when working in the community.

In the West (and increasingly globally) the overriding explanation of madness comes from the profession of medicine. That is, madness is construed explicitly as an 'illness' akin to physical ailments, and is treated by doctors specialising in psychiatry. The psychiatric account of madness suggests that 450 million people worldwide are affected by mental health problems at any time, and roughly 850,000 people commit suicide every year. These mental health problems are common to all countries, cause immense suffering and have staggering economic and social costs (Morrall and Hazelton 2004).

The structural sociologist accepts the existence of mental disorder, but acknowledges that the poor suffer far more than the wealthy. For example, there is a strong connection between (lower) social class and alcohol and drug addiction, schizophrenia, depression, Alzheimer's disease and personality disorder. However, some mental illnesses do occur more frequently among those further up the social scale, for example eating disorders, manic depression and the anxiety states (Rogers and Pilgrim 2005).

A structuralist position is taken by Andrew Scull (1979, 1984). He refers to the specific role of psychiatry as an agency of social control, which serves the state by keeping 'the mad', who may disrupt the order of society, under control. Erich Fromm (1963) argues that it is (capitalist) society that is insane rather than individuals. Capitalism, for Fromm, is a form of social disease. It contains major contradictions and irrationalities that have immense social and economic consequences. For example, wars are fought regularly to protect markets. Periods of high unemployment alternate with periods of worker shortages. Mass entertainment, such as daytime television, 'dumbs down' humanity, rendering life meaningless and devoid of interpersonal intimacy. An ethic of materialism, whereby commodities are valued above everything else, has replaced any semblance of spiritual or human-oriented regard of life.

Using labelling theory, a branch of interactionist sociology, Thomas Scheff (1966) proposes that mental disorder is 'residual' rule breaking, not an illness as such. That is, the label of 'madness' will be put to use by the agencies of social control, for example the police, psychiatrists and judges, because no other label (such as criminality) seems to fit. Thomas Szasz (1972) argues that mental illness is a myth. Psychiatry, for Szasz, deals not with disease but with ordinary 'problems with living'. Therefore, for Szasz (as with Scull), psychiatry, and by implication psychiatric nursing, is acting inappropriately as an agency of social control, and people should be liberated from the influence of psychiatry and deal with their own problems, perhaps with the help of friends, family and paid helpers such as psychotherapists.

However, some sociologists – such as me – suggest that 'madness', although difficult to understand because what it is and how it should be treated changes over time and place, is not a myth (Morrall 2008b, 2009). People suffering from severe madness – no matter what a culture or discipline decides to describe it as – often do need help. This help may be that of medication or some form of talking therapy, notwithstanding the dangers of both. But accepting that some people with madness need help of this sort does not dismiss the sociological realisation that there is a link between the 'mental health' of a society and the healthiness of that society, and today that means the healthiness of global society.

Activity 7.4

In what clinical and social situations have you come across 'madness'?
How might society influence positively or negatively the mental health of individuals?

Sexuality

Society is drenched in sex. Sex impinges on health. Hence, nurses should be interested (professionally) in sex. The drenching of society in sex is obvious:

> the selling of cars, boats, clothes, alcohol, films, magazines and books frequently involves bottoms, breasts and 'six-pack' bellies to seduce the consumer
> the display and trading of 'adult' imagery and services permeate the internet
> pornography is a multibillion dollar industry in the USA alone
> 'cyberdating' and 'cybermating' – contacting and flirting with potential sexual partners, and maintaining sexual relationships via the internet – are becoming normalised
> mainstream literature and cinema encompass a flourishing 'erotic' division
> not just the middle aged but also the elderly are accepted as having sexual needs
> hardcore sexual wares are sold in high-street shops
> Viagra, and similar drugs, allows sex to be performed at length and on demand
> email 'spam' is usually offering ways of heightening sexual potency, increasing penis size, or rejuvenating vaginas

> prostitution has been legalised in many countries, or tolerated within set areas of cities (Morrall 2009).

Overall, the effect on society of this emersion has been the shifting of sexuality from procreation (having sex to have babies) to recreation (enjoying the pleasures of sex for their own sake). Moreover, there are now a multitude of sexualities (heterosexuality, bisexuality, homosexuality/lesbianism, metrosexuality, transsexuality), while the sanctification of sexual abstinence and virginity is making a comeback. While the debate about how much 'gender' (the attributing by society of appropriate male or female thoughts, feelings and behaviours) is determined by 'nature' or 'nurture', sexuality appears to cross the boundaries of role-specific styles. That is, particular sexual patterns are not necessarily confined to one gender or another.

Such a soaking in sex brings with it major social problems:

> the trafficking and exploitation of women and children through prostitution
> the sexualisation of childhood by the fashion industries
> unplanned/underage pregnancies.

Furthermore, there are huge inconsistencies about sexuality within global society. Emerging in Western society are new sexualities, deviances and exploitations. In other parts of the world, especially in theocratic, fundamentalist and totalitarian countries, as well as areas of the West that are influenced by right-wing religious groups, there has been an increase in sexual repression and oppression.

Nurses should be concerned about sex because:

> supposed 'holistic' care promoted in nursing by definition should include attending to sexual needs; for example, in parts of Australia, as part of their care for people with learning disabilities, nurses take their patients to prostitutes (Aylott 2001)
> nurses are part of providing advice and treatments relating to sexual health
> nurses may be specifically involved in treating sex and pornography addiction, sexual dysfunction, and the physical and psychological effects of sexual abuse and rape
> nurses can be at the forefront of reducing continued prejudice about certain sexual identities and practices.

Activity 7.5

Observe and record how many and the type of sexual images and products there are in the public domain – perhaps do this when you go shopping in a city centre.

In what way do you think sexuality may affect your practice?

Conclusion

The heart of nursing, I argue, is care, competence and cleanliness. However, to appreciate fully the health needs of humans, consideration must be given to wider issues than nurse–patient communication, proficiency in a series of nursing skills based on robust knowledge, and creating sanitary conditions in which to carry out nursing. Applying the sociological imagination demonstrates that the social grouping people belong to has dramatic effects on health. The above discussion about health inequalities in global society, the untoward impact of the profession of medicine on health, alternative perceptions about madness, and transformations in human sexuality is an introduction to some of those effects aimed at provoking further thinking.

References

Aylott, J (2001) Developing a positive sexual identity, *Nursing and Residential Care*, **3**(6): 257–4

Boseley, S (2006) Doctors urged to be more vigilant over drugs' side-effects, *The Guardian*, 12 May, p. 12

Collier, P (2007) *The Bottom Billion: Why the Poorest Countries are Failing and What Can be Done About It*, Oxford: Oxford University Press

Conrad, P (2007) *The Medicalization of Society*, Baltimore, MA: Johns Hopkins University Press

Davies, J (ed.) (2008) *Personal Wealth From a Global Perspective*, Oxford: Oxford University Press

ESRC (Economic and Social Research Council) (2008) *Global Life Expectancy 2008*, London: ESRC

Fitzpatrick, M (2000) *The Tyranny of Health: Doctors and the Regulation of Lifestyle*, London: Routledge

Fromm, E (1963) *The Sane Society*, London: Routledge & Kegan Paul

Giddens, A (2009) *Sociology* (6th edn), Cambridge: Polity Press

Goffman, E (1959) *The Presentation of Self in Everyday Life*, Garden City, NY: Doubleday Anchor

Gore, E (2006) *An Inconvenient Truth: The Planetary Emergency of Global Warming and What We Can Do About It*, London: Bloomsbury

Healthcare Commission (2006) *Medicines Management Review*, London: Healthcare Commission

Illich, I (1977) *Limits to Medicine: Medical Nemesis and the Expropriation of Health*, Harmondsworth: Penguin

Jones, K, Patel, N, Levy, M et al. (2008) Global trends in emerging infectious diseases, *Nature*, 451: 990–3

Lovelock, J (2006) *The Revenge of Gaia: Why the Earth is Fighting Back – and How We Can Still Save Humanity*, London: Allen Lane

Mills, CW (1959) *The Sociological Imagination*, Oxford: Oxford University Press

Monbiot, G (2007) *Heat: How We Can Stop the Planet Burning*, London: Penguin

Morrall, P (2001) *Sociology and Nursing*, London: Routledge

core topics

Morrall, P (2006) *Murder and Society*, Chichester: Wiley

Morrall, P (2008a) Snake-oil peddling: nurses and complementary and alternative medicine, in J Adams and P Tovey (eds) *Complementary and Alternative Medicine in Nursing and Midwifery: Towards a Critical Social Science*, London: Routledge

Morrall, P (2008b) *The Trouble with Therapy: Sociology and Psychotherapy*, Maidenhead: Open University Press/McGraw-Hill

Morrall, P (2009) *Sociology and Health: An Introduction*, London: Routledge

Morrall, P (2010) Provocation: reviving thinking in universities, in T Warne and S McAndrew (eds) *Creative Approaches in Health and Social Care Education and Practice: Knowing Me, Understanding You*, Basingstoke: Palgrave Macmillan

Morrall, P and Hazelton, M (2004) *Mental Health: Global Policies and Human Rights*, London: Whurr

National Equality Panel (2010) *An Anatomy of Economic Inequality in the UK*: Report of the National Equality Panel, London: Government Equalities Office

Parsons, T (1951) *The Social System*, New York: Free Press of Glencoe

Ritzer, G (2006) *Contemporary Sociological Theory and its Classical Roots: The Basics* (2nd edn), New York: McGraw-Hill

Rogers, A and Pilgrim, D (2005) *Sociology of Mental Health and Illness* (3rd edn), Maidenhead: Open University Press

Sachs, J (2007) Bursting at the Seams, BBC Reith Lectures, Lecture 1, available online at http://www.bbc.co.uk/radio4/reith2007/lecture1.shtml, accessed 12/3/2010

Scheff, TJ (1966) *Being Mentally Ill: A Sociological Theory*, Chicago: Aldine

Scull, AT (1979) *Museums of Madness: The Social Organisation of Insanity in Nineteenth Century England*, Harmondsworth: Penguin

Scull, AT (1984) *Decarceration: Community Treatment and the Deviant – a Radical View* (2nd edn), Cambridge: Polity Press

Szasz, TS (1972) *The Myth of Mental Illness*, St Albans: Paladin

UN (United Nations) (2006) *Social Indicators*, United Nations Statistical Division, available online at http://unstats.un.org/unsd/demographic/products/socind/health.htm, accessed 12/3/2010

United Nations Children's Fund (2008) *The State of the World's Children 2008*, New York: UN

WHO (World Health Organization) (2005) World Health Organization Partners with Joint Commission and Joint Commission International to Eliminate Medical Errors Worldwide, News Release, available online at http://www.who.int/patientsafety/newsalert/WHO_final.pdf, accessed 26/7/2010

WHO (2008) *10 Facts on the Global Burden of Disease*, available online at http://www.who.int/features/factfiles/global_burden/en/index.html, accessed 12/3/2010

8 the psychological context of healthcare settings

Rebecca Jayne Stack

In this chapter we will explore:

> Various approaches to the study of psychology
> Health-related thoughts and behaviours
> Memory
> Stress and coping with stress
> Child development in healthcare settings

Introduction

Psychology is the study of **behaviour**, thought and **emotion**. One of psychology's aims is to understand people's behaviour, and the driving forces behind behaviour. Actives such as communicating with patients, observations and decision making all involve an understanding of the mind and behaviour. Therefore, many aspects of nursing practice can be improved by understanding and applying the principles of psychology.

This chapter provides an overview of psychology and discusses how psychology can be applied to daily activities of nurses. By the end of this chapter you should have an understanding of how psychological principles can be applied to nursing practice and the ways that psychology can be used to improve the experiences of both patients and nursing colleagues.

Approaches to the study of psychology

Over the years different theories about the mind and behaviour have been developed by psychologists. These approaches are not necessarily competing theories, but are different perspectives on the factors that drive behaviour. Some examples of these psychological theories and their application to nursing are outlined below.

Psychodynamic theories

One of the earliest approaches to psychology came from **psychodynamic theories**, which focused on the unconscious motivations that drive behaviour; essentially, factors beyond our awareness. These theories suggest that, during

core topics

childhood, interactions and conflicts between unconscious mental forces shape the way we think and can create problems in adulthood.

Sigmund Freud (1856–1936) developed the psychoanalytic approach, the most widely known theory that derived from psychodynamic approaches to psychology. According to Freud, the mind is divided into three parts, which represent different levels of **consciousness** (awareness):

> *Conscious:* the part of the mind we are aware of, which consists of the mental processes that actively occupy our current thoughts.
> *Preconscious:* contains thoughts, memories and knowledge not currently available to the conscious mind but can be accessed easily, typically through memory.
> *Unconscious (or subconscious):* the part of the mind beyond our awareness containing thoughts, urges and impulses associated with pain or anxiety.

Freud also suggested that the personality is divided into three parts, which are the source of the mental conflict that takes place during childhood. The conflict between the different parts of the personality is the cause of distress and behavioural problems in later life:

> *Id:* The first part of the personality, called the id, is an innate drive that seeks out instant gratification, such as desiring to be fed instantly to satisfy hunger.
> *Superego:* As the child develops, a second part of the personality, called the superego, emerges, which embodies the values, morals and rules of society. The presence of the newly formed superego clashes and begins to conflict with the pleasure-seeking desires of the id.
> *Ego:* To regulate this conflict, the final part of the personality, called the ego, develops. The ego uses a number of defence mechanisms to regulate the conflicting goals of the id and superego; these include denial and repression.

Defence mechanisms can also be used to protect the individual from threatening or dangerous feelings, thoughts and fantasies. An example of a defence mechanism is denial, where a person convinces themselves that the problem they are experiencing does not exist, which helps to prevent threatening thoughts from entering the conscious.

Psychoanalytic therapy aims to relieve tension and distress by uncovering the unconscious content of a person's mind. Nurses who speak to people experiencing a high level of anxiety or panic may notice defensive overtones and a psychoanalytical approach may be used to understand why a person is behaving in a defensive manner. Fredric et al. (2008) suggested that panic disorders create ego defence mechanisms, which included denial. A psychodynamic psychotherapist uses psychodynamic principles to help a person to recognise and reappraise their frightening thoughts, emotions and fantasies.

Behaviourism is a scientific approach to psychology that focuses on observable behaviour, not the internal processes of the mind (unlike psychodynamic approaches). This approach argues that behaviour occurs through **learning**. Behaviourism is divided into two core theories, operant conditioning theory and classical conditioning theory.

Ivan Pavlov (1849–1936) developed the theory of **classical conditioning** through his observation of dogs. He observed that when food and the sound of a bell continually occurred at the same time, the dogs would learn to associate the sound of the bell with food and eventually salivate at the sound of the bell alone (see Walker and Payne 2003).

Pavlov called this process 'learning through association'. This happens when two or more stimuli (for example people, object or events), which occur at the same time, are mentally linked together. For example, if a child finds medical procedures at a hospital painful, they will associate hospital with pain and unpleasant experiences, which may result in a high level of distress being displayed during hospital visits.

Classical conditioning can be applied to any reflex or automatic behaviour such as salivating or flinching. For example, imagine the light in a room flashes and then you are hit by a wet sponge. At first, you may conclude that this is an unfortunate coincidence. If the same thing happened again and again, you would begin to pair the flashing light with being hit by the sponge and you would learn to flinch or duck on seeing the light flashed to avoid the unpleasant experience. Essentially your response to the light flashing would become conditioned and this would become your automatic response (beyond your control), which would continue to occur even if the sponges stopped being thrown. The association between flashing lights and a horrible event may become generalised to other situations, for example you may flinch at a flashing traffic light for fear of a negative consequence.

Classical conditioning can explain how fear and phobias are developed, and would explain why some people develop needle phobias.

Activity 8.1

Below are the key features in classical conditioning. Using the wet sponge example, work out which of the following objects matches with the definitions provided:

1 Flinching because of the light
2 Flinching or ducking
3 Flinching because of any light
4 A wet sponge being thrown

Features in a classical conditioning experiment	Definitions	Object
Unconditioned response	This is a naturally occurring response, that is, not learned (hint – in our example, what you may expect to see happen naturally if you threw a wet sponge at someone)	
Unconditioned stimuli	A naturally occurring stimulus (hint – in our scenario, this will be the object that elicits the natural response of flinching	
Conditioned response	A learned response that has been paired with a stimulus (hint – in our scenario, this is a person's reaction to a flashing light once the flashing light has been paired with the wet sponge)	
Generalised conditioned response	A response that occurs when learning is transferred to other similar stimuli (hint – this is a response that has been generalised to other similar circumstances)	

Classical conditioning has been used to help people overcome behaviours that have negative health consequences. In **aversion therapy**, a pleasurable behaviour is associated with an unpleasurable effect. For example, disulfiram is an emetic drug often prescribed to support the treatment of chronic alcohol abuse. This drug disrupts the way that the body breaks down alcohol, making the body extremely sensitive to the presence of alcohol. This process causes severe vomiting when alcohol is ingested, leading to alcohol consumption being paired with the negative event of vomiting, which should lead to a decrease in alcohol consumption (Suh et al. 2006).

An alternative approach to behaviourism, called **operant conditioning**, was proposed by BF Skinner (1904–90) (see Walker and Payne 2003). Skinner observed that behaviour was influenced by reinforcement or the consequences of behaviour. Reinforcement is a consequence that causes a behaviour to occur with greater frequency, punishment is a consequence that causes a behaviour to occur with less frequency, and extinction is the lack of any consequence following a behaviour. The main difference between operant conditioning and classical conditioning is that operant conditioning affects voluntary behaviour (not reflexes).

As an example, a high proportion of people in methadone treatment programmes smoke cigarettes, which can result in adverse health effects. Dunn et al. (2008) examined the effectiveness of vouchers as a positive form of reinforcement for people who initiated and maintained smoking cessation. Voucher-based reinforcement was found to significantly enhance the number of people who ceased smoking. This research shows the positive effect reinforcement can have on improving healthy behaviours and eliminating unhealthy behaviours.

Social learning theory

Albert Bandura (1925–) suggested that direct reinforcement could not account for all types of learning and that rewards were not always extrinsic (given externally, such as money or vouchers), but could be produced internally and include sensations such as pride or happiness. Bandura proposed the **social learning theory,** which views learning as a social process of observing, imitating and modelling the behaviour, emotions and attitudes of other people (see Bahn 2001). Social learning theory suggests that four psychological processes also help learning to occur:

> **attention** – for example, focusing concentration on the learning experience
> *retention* – storing or memorising the information for later use
> *reproduction* – the ability to reproduce the behaviour
> *motivation* – the desire to reproduce the learning experience.

Without these four psychological processes, social learning is unable to occur.

Let us take an example. Compliance to hand hygiene regulations in hospitals is vital for reducing hospital-acquired infections. However, research has found that it can be difficult to motivate people to maintain good hand hygiene. Barrett and Randle (2008) examined nursing students' perceptions of hand hygiene practice in hospitals. A number of factors such as busyness, hand condition and lack of knowledge were identified, but, interestingly, students' perceptions of what other healthcare workers did was very important. Many felt that they should fit in to their surroundings; essentially, students modelled their behaviour on those around them and would not participate in hand washing if others had not.

Activity 8.2

When a local hospital wants to improve hand washing, a psychologist recommends the following strategies based on social learning theory, but the hospital wants to know which part of modelling each recommendation will be affecting. Can you help them by giving one of the following labels to each recommendation?

A Attention   C Production
B Retention   D Motivation

1 The hospital should keep records of how each nurse has improved in hand washing, and records of improvements in hospital-acquired infections. These records are then shown to the nurses regularly to show how they have progressed and the improvements their actions have caused.
2 The correct hand washing procedure is shown to all staff for the first time very slowly, allowing staff to concentrate on all the key tasks involved in the activity, with the aim of staff retaining this information for use later on.

3 Place catchy posters in the wards to remind staff to wash their hands. These posters may contain memorable phrases or rhymes to help staff to remember to wash their hands.

4 Spend an hour on the ward with each member of staff to highlight hand washing opportunities, which should show staff that they have the ability to reproduce hand washing behaviour in their busy schedules.

Cognitive psychology

Cognitive psychology focuses on mental processes such as memory, perception, attention and information processing. This approach views people as information processors; attending to information, formatting information so it can be held in memory, then memorising it and finally recalling information.

As people grow older, subtle changes in cognitive abilities occur. Generally, researchers suggest that the speed of abilities such as memory recall, attention and perception reduces and declines as we get older. This is an important issue for nurses to consider (Vance 2009). Reductions in the speed of communication and the performance of everyday tasks may be noted. Also, nurses may find that patients wish to discuss changes in their cognitive abilities, and may require referrals to specialist practitioners. However, nurses may find that they are able to offer patients advice or simple solutions to managing cognitive difficulties. For example, as people grow older, they may find that they are prescribed multiple medicines for multiple conditions; these medicines may become increasingly difficult to manage. Older people prescribed multiple medicines often report that they forget to take their medicines (Stack et al. 2008). A simple strategy to help people overcome forgetting to take their medicines is giving people dosette boxes to help organise their medicines (usually by the time and day that particular doses are required).

Our cognitive processes are used to monitor and control our behaviour. Cognitive approaches focus on addressing/changing irrational thoughts and improving the monitoring of cognitive processes. Therapeutic applications of **cognitive therapy** help people to identify distorted thinking and change maladaptive thoughts, emotions and behaviour.

Cognitive behavioural therapy (CBT) was developed by merging **behaviour therapy** with cognitive therapy. CBT examines **cognitions**, behaviours and emotions and physical responses in combination. For example, a CBT programme for pain management may address thoughts and beliefs about pain, mood and emotion management, relaxation training to reduce stress, education about the processes of pain, and an assessment of behavioural responses to stress.

CBT is considered to be effective for treating mild levels of psychological distress in a range of physical and mental health conditions. Nurses in some areas may find that the waiting lists for referral for psychological therapy are long. One approach to meeting demand is through the use of self-help CBT materials and computerised CBT. Warrilow and Beech (2009) described how CBT could be transformed into self-help material for people with depression. Furthermore, the National Institute for Health and Clinical Excellence recommends two computerised packages for CBT for use by the NHS in England and Wales (NICE 2006). Nurses should consider the different therapeutic options available for people experiencing mild levels of psychological distress.

Humanistic approaches to psychology

Humanistic psychologists suggested that approaches such as psychoanalysis and behaviorism were negative, pessimistic and deterministic (not accounting for human free will and choice). Humanistic psychology encourages people to think in the here and now instead of examining past experiences (unlike psychodynamic therapy, which typically examines past experiences) or attempting to predict future events. The **humanistic perspective** focuses on the personal nature of the human experience, the uniqueness of individuals and the potential for personal growth and self-actualisation (the ability to realise one's full potential).

This approach emphasises individual control over health and the ability to determine the course of one's health. Humanistic psychology often looks beyond the concepts of mental illness and psychological distress as being negative and maladaptive states. Instead, people are viewed as good. It is suggested that mental illness and social difficulties result from environmental influences (as opposed to focusing on internal thoughts and desires). Self-improvement, personal reflection and self-understanding lead to happiness; these are often the aims of humanistic therapy. It is becoming increasing recognised that nurses should provide person-centred care, which emphasises humanistic principles.

Activity 8.3

Consider how using humanistic principles or taking a humanistic approach may enhance patients' experiences of the following nursing activities:

- While assisting a patient with oral hygiene
- When meeting and greeting patients
- Supporting patients to make appropriate diet choices
- Supporting and advising carers who are experiencing feeding difficulties with the cared-for person
- During a pressure sore risk assessment
- While communicating with patients/clients during and after an multidisciplinary team meeting

Health-related thoughts and behaviours

The way we think about the world can take the form of beliefs, perceptions, attitudes and preferences, all of which are thought to influence our behaviour.

Beliefs and attitudes about health and illness can influence the way people behave in nursing settings. Beliefs and attitudes also influence the behaviour people undertake when ill and the behaviours people partake in to protect their health. The way a person thinks about the world can determine their judgements, decision making and behaviour.

Making decisions about health behaviours involves deliberate and systematic processing of information. Some suggest that the key to decision making is a cost–benefit analysis, where the decision maker aims to minimise the costs and maximise the benefits of their choice. The health belief model (proposed by Rosenstock in 1966) describes four types of thoughts and the way they predict future health behaviours. The four thoughts are perceived severity, perceived susceptibility, perceived barriers and perceived benefits (see Activity 8.4 for a description of each term). A person would use these beliefs to evaluate a health threat and weigh up the costs and benefits of a particular course of action.

Activity 8.4

Below are examples of how the health belief model can be applied to understanding sexually transmitted infections (STIs) and condom use. Consider what you may say to a person to try and encourage them to think more favourably about condom use. How would what you say change if you were trying to address each of the beliefs within the health belief model?

1 *Perceived susceptibility* would relate to whether a person believes they are at risk of acquiring an STI from unprotected sex.
2 *Perceived severity* would relate to a person's assessment of the seriousness of contracting an STI and the consequences.
3 *Perceived benefits* of condom use would not only include avoiding STIs, but would also include avoiding unwanted pregnancy or being viewed as a socially responsible individual.
4 *Perceived barriers* to condom use would include factors that make the behaviour harder to perform, such as the cost of condoms, or being afraid to ask a partner to use condoms.

The self-regulation model (SRM) proposed by Leventhal (Leventhal and Cameron 1987) suggests that when a person becomes ill, they attempt to make sense of their illness. The SRM suggests that people develop emotional and cognitive representations of illness. Emotional representations of illness may include distress, anger, sadness, surprise or fear. In healthcare settings, emotions become a concern when they develop into anxiety or depression. According to the SRM, cognitive representations centre on five components:

> *identity beliefs* concern the labels attached to an illness and the symptoms associated with that illness
> *cause beliefs* include lifestyle, environment or genetic factors
> *timeline beliefs* relate to the perceived duration of the illness – whether it is acute or time limited, chronic or cyclical

> *consequence beliefs* reflect the range of potential costs an illness may have – physical, psychological, social or financial
> *cure/control beliefs* relate to perceived curability, perceived treatment control and perceived individual control.

These illness cognitions influence the behaviour a person undertakes in response to illness.

Illness beliefs also have an effect on the way that people respond to a suspected illness, behaviours such as attending screening appointments and seeking help for a suspected illness have all been linked to illness perceptions. O'Mahony and Hegarty (2009), for example, investigated women's reasons for delays in seeking help after finding an adverse breast symptom (such as a lump). One of the main reasons women gave for putting off contacting a professional was the beliefs they held in relation to the breast symptom they had found. Nurses need to be aware that the beliefs that people hold about potential illnesses relate to their clinic attendance and decisions to seek help.

Activity 8.5

Think about the last time you were ill. Try to remember the types of beliefs you had, did they fit into the five constructs of the SRM presented below? Did these beliefs about illness influence the way you behaved, that is, did you seek help, did you take medicines, did you carry on as before, did you rest? If your cognitions were different, how would your behaviour have changed?

Cognitive illness construct	The type of thought originating from that construct
Cause	What caused it?
Identity	What is the condition?
Consequences	How will or how has it affected me?
Timeline	How long will it last? Will it be constant or variable?
Cure/control	Can it be controlled or cured?

Memory

Memory is vital for learning, receiving information, holding conversations and problem solving. A good understanding of memory processes may maximise communication, facilitate patient self-management and ensure that health-related information has been received and retained, so it can be acted upon at a later date.

A large amount of the information available to our senses (through vision, touch, sound, smell and taste) is coded by our brains so that it can be retained in memory for use at a later point in time. Therefore, **memory** can be defined as the ability to store, retain and recall information.

A widely held view of memory is that it is an ability that occurs in stages. The first stage is **sensory memory,** where information from our surroundings is attended to, a process referred to as 'attention'. Relevant information is then passed on to the next store called **short-term memory** (STM). STM holds a limited amount of information. STM is also a temporary store, so if information is not rehearsed or transferred into a more permanent store, that is, **long-term memory** (LTM), it will begin to degrade and will be lost.

Miller (1956) conducted digit span experiments, where he gave people ever increasing series of numbers and asked them to recall them. Miller found that most often people could hold about seven digits in STM, which could then be recalled accurately. Based on this experiment, Miller believed that the 'span' or capacity of STM was 7 +or− 2 digits – meaning that 7 is the average, with 5 being the minimum capacity and 9 being the maximum capacity of STM. Miller's 7 +or− 2 indicates that STM is only able to hold a limited amount of information. Therefore, when giving information to patients, it may be best to limit it to seven core pieces of information.

Activity 8.6

Read the dialogue below. Think about how you would organise this information. What potential problems can you recognise? What are the most important pieces of information? If you had to shorten this conversation to seven key pieces of information, which key terms/phrases would you choose?

Nurse–patient consultation dialogue

Well, you know the recommended dietary allowance is no more than two units of alcohol per day for women and it sounds like you're drinking more than a safe amount of alcohol. One unit is about one glass of wine, so if you work it out, it's too much. And because you're a woman, you're vulnerable. Women just don't process alcohol well, it stays in your system longer and can cause things like liver cirrhosis, which is really irreversible scarring on the liver. You also have to think about your weight, you know that a large glass of wine is about 200 calories. Women's bodies have 10% more fat than men's and they have less fluid to dilute the alcohol, so the concentration of alcohol in the body is higher. I can make you an appointment to see an adviser.

Memory experiments on our ability to store information showed that people remember the first thing and last thing they are told, and the information in the middle tends to be lost. This is because it cannot be rehearsed and transferred into LTM and it cannot be stored within STM because now information is competing for STM storage. This is known as the **primacy effect** and the **recency effect**.

Activity 8.7

Read each of the words below. Then cover the words over and write down all the words you can remember.

1	Lymph	6	Dislocate	11	Pulse	16	Anxiety
2	Fever	7	Retina	12	Seizure	17	Chronic
3	Mucus	8	Bacteria	13	Kidney	18	Tendons
4	Allergy	9	Alcohol	14	Vaccine	19	Insulin
5	Nausea	10	Artery	15	Biopsy	20	Hormone

Having done Activity 8.7, you may have found that you remembered the words at the start of the list as these were easily transferred to your long-term memory. You may also have found that it was easy to remember words towards the end of the list, as they were still available in your STM and had not been pushed out by the presentation of new words when you began to recall the list. This suggests that to enhance memory, the most important pieces of information should be presented at the beginning and the end of a conversation.

Finally, you may also find that you have remembered words that are meaningful to you, known as 'association'; this involves your mind linking familiar information (such as experiences, people or event) to a piece of unfamiliar information (such as the information presented in the word list).

Go back to Activity 8.6 and think about how you would rearrange the conversation between the nurse and patient to ensure that the most important messages are placed at the beginning or end of the conversation. Also, think about how you could use association to ensure that a conversation is accurately recalled.

It is in STM that information is processed in greater depth before select information is transferred to the LTM store. Each store differs in the length of time information is held. LTM stores information over long periods of time, in three distinct categories – **episodic memory**, semantic and **procedural memory**:

> *Episodic memory* represents moments in our personal history and experience. It can be thought of as autobiographical memory, as all the information stored is of a personal nature. This type of memory is explicit because we can declare that we know the answer to questions of episodic memory; this type of information is available to our consciousness.

> *Semantic memory* is memory not tied to a specific event, which can be thought of as general world knowledge, for example vocabulary and grammar. Again this type of information is explicit because you can describe what you know about a topic. You don't have to go to the Sahara desert to know that it's sandy, but knowing the Sahara's environmental features may be a form of semantic memory (not tied to an event or episode when you visited the Sahara).

> *Procedural memory* is memory storage of skills and procedures that are difficult to verbalise. Procedural memory can be thought of as the 'know-how' memory and is responsible for the performance of automatic tasks such as driving a car or riding a bike. Procedural memory is related to the

knowledge of rules of action and procedures, which can become automatic with learning and repetition.

Understanding the difference between these different types of memory can be used to enhance patient health behaviour. For example, simple health-related tasks can be taught to people in many different ways so that they are stored in different parts of memory, hence being less likely to be forgotten. For example, a person with diabetes may see a TV programme describing how to monitor their blood glucose; this type of information may be entered into event memory (episodic memory). However, a person may also be physically taken through the procedure to monitor blood glucose again and again until it becomes part of procedural memory.

Stress and coping with stress

Stress is seen as a person's response to the characteristics of the environment, and can cause changes in a person's emotional, physical, cognitive and behaviour reactions. Therefore, a person experiencing stress may find that it impacts on many aspects of their life. Situations that cause stress (known as a stressor) are also highly varied and personal, but all will require the person experiencing the stress to make an adjustment or an adaptation to the stressful situation. Therefore, stressful situations require people to change in some way or find a way of getting used to the presence of the stressor.

Physical response to stress

When an individual experiences a stressful event, a number of physical reactions can occur. These reactions have evolved to enable one to flee the danger or fight the stressor; a concept referred to as 'fight or flight'. The physiological changes that occur because of a stressor include increases in heart rate, adrenaline, blood pressure and an increase in the metabolism of fatty acids, cholesterol and triglycerides. These changes provide a large amount of energy that allows the individual to flee or fight the threat. Furthermore, platelet adhesiveness and aggregation also increases, which facilitates rapid healing, should the person choose to stay and fight. Other physical changes include a decrease in blood flow to non-vital systems such as the kidneys, skin and gut; this helps to conserve energy.

Stress in the workplace

All these changes help to ensure the survival of a person facing an immediate threat or danger. However, this reaction can cause a large amount of damage to the body if it persists for a long time; essentially, the aroused state causes the body to become exhausted. Stress in the workplace is usually a type of stress that one cannot escape from or physically battle. However, the high state of physiological arousal caused by a continued workplace stressor can cause long-term physical and psychological damage.

Stress is a common reaction to workplace pressures and demands for nurses. The Royal College of Nursing recognises that stress in the workplace can adversely affect the delivery of patient care and can be a distressing experience, resulting in a negative impact on health (see Murray 2005). Managing workplace stress is an important aspect of nursing practice.

The ways that people react when stressed can include increasing the amount of alcohol consumed, smoking, poor diet, drinking more caffeinated drinks and inattentiveness. Inattentiveness can be a particularly dangerous effect of stress for nurses who are under stress and pressure, while the other negative behavioural effects of stress can be detrimental to nursing staff personal health and wellbeing.

Activity 8.8

Below is a visual analogue scale which can be used to measure stress. Consider using it from time to time to monitor your own levels of stress and be aware of the situations that cause higher scores. In these circumstances, it may help to consider strategies that help you to reduce your stress levels.

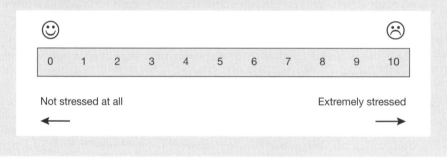

The negative physical consequences of stress

Stress and physical illness have a complex relationship; as the prospect of illness can be highly stressful and conversely stress can have a direct effect on health. It is well known that stressful situations can adversely affect the immune system. Research has shown, for example, that people who are stressed out are more likely to develop colds. Cohen et al. (1991) asked people to complete a stress questionnaire and then exposed them to respiratory viruses. They found that people who were the most stressed were more likely to develop colds. Stress can also interact with a pre-existing vulnerability towards an illness and is linked to physical illness, such as cardiovascular disease, infections (such as flu), diabetes, asthma and headaches, to name a few.

Stress can also lead to behavioural changes that can be damaging to health, for example undereating, overeating, drinking alcohol, drug taking and smoking. These behaviours may help a person to manage their stress levels and cope with the stressful situation, but may ultimately make the individual's stress worse because of the negative health consequences these behaviours cause. The next section describes some of the ways people may choose to cope with the presence of a stressor.

Coping with stressful situations

Coping is a term used to describe the process of managing stressful situations. Coping behaviours can be positive or negative responses to a stressful situation. A coping behaviour may be directed at overcoming the source of stress, minimising or reducing the stressful situation or helping the individual to tolerate a stressor. Lazarus and Folkman (1984) suggested that coping is a multidimensional process of cognitive and behavioural efforts to manage external or internal demands that tax or exceed resources during stressful situations. Two categories of coping are described; problem-focused coping and emotion-focused coping:

> *Problem-focused coping* involves activities focused on the challenge of addressing the problem; stress is reduced through behavioural and environmental challenges being addressed.
> *Emotion-focused coping* involves activities that modify the emotional impact of stress and make the situation more tolerable. These activities would focus on reducing emotional distress through emotional expression, avoidance, distance, detachment and withdrawal.

A therapeutic approach to coping involves strategies such as active problem solving and information gathering, which focus on the sources of stress and reactions to it. Avoidance coping involves a strategy that places the focus of attention and resources away from the sources of stress and reactions to stress; these strategies may include withdrawal and denial.

Summary

Psychology can view stress from a number of perspectives. The first is to explore the type of events, or environmental factors, that cause stress, known as stressors. The second way psychology can contribute to our understanding of stress is to consider the relationship between the person and the stressor by looking at the different ways that people cope with stress. Finally, psychology often investigates the way people respond to the presence of stress; these responses can be behavioural, such as inattentiveness, and physical, such as developing an illness.

Child development in healthcare settings

Children are not just mini-adults – their bodies and their minds work in very different ways to the minds of adults. Understanding the way that children develop is vital for nurses who have contact with young people. This understanding is vital for understanding distress, effective communication and the role of carers. This section will explore how a child develops and describe the ways that nurses may minimise the impact of illness or hospital visits for children.

Intellectual development

Intelligence involves a variety of mental abilities, which include understanding, acquiring knowledge and learning from previous experiences. Children's understanding of the world changes as they get older. Nurses who work with children need to understand the way that children interpret the world around them; particularly being aware of the many ways that children of different ages understand information about their health. Theories in the area of child development outline the way children's intelligence and knowledge of the world develops.

Jean Piaget (1896–1980) describes the development of intelligence in sequential stages. Essentially, Piaget's theory of cognitive development suggests that children's intelligence develops in stages that build upon one another. Piaget suggested that information about previous experiences is stored in **schemas**, which can then be used to evaluate future experiences. Intelligence involves a variety of mental abilities, which include understanding, acquiring knowledge and learning from previous experiences. Schemas are units of information that represent some aspect of the world. For example, the way that a child understands an illness may be made up of lots of different schemas, which may represent different aspects of a child's illness experiences such as discomfort, fatigue or treatment. New information is either assimilated to fit into existing schemas or schemas are changed to accommodate new information. So, providing a child with new information about an illness will either result in the information being made to fit into the child's existing understanding, or the child's understanding of their illness having to change to accommodate the new information.

The developmental stages are as follows:

> *Sensorimotor stage – 0–2 years of age:* Piaget suggested that newborns have no self-concept – the ability to differentiate self from the environment and think of oneself as an agent of action who can intentionally manipulate their environment. During the sensorimotor stage, the infant will begin to differentiate themselves from their environment. Other characteristics that Piaget suggested represent the sensorimotor stage include 'object permanence': the knowledge that objects still exist even when out of sight or reach of other senses. To begin with, a child believes that if an object is out of their visual range, it ceases to exist; gradually they come to understand object permanence. Also, thought is reliant on action and intelligence is based on a practical knowledge of the world, for example the word 'drink' may be used to represent a cup. During this stage, children can become frustrated when these communication attempts are not understood.

> *Preoperational stage – 2–7 years of age:* During this stage, a child learns to

represent objects with symbols, images or words. This allows the child to move beyond an understanding of the world through actions. During this stage, the child can only use one feature at a time to classify an object. For example, a child may group objects based on their texture, regardless of their shape or colour; secondary features are not comprehended. Therefore a child may be unable to categorise their medicines into subgroup according to colour, size, shape or texture. Also, during this stage, a child has difficulty understanding other people's point of view; Piaget described children at this stage as being 'egocentric', meaning that they perceive, understand and interpret the world in terms of the self. This can result in a child being unable to take the perspective of another person; they may be incapable of empathising with another person's distress or may find it difficult to understand why a person experiencing an illness is in need of rest. Nurses working with children may need to spend extra time explaining the perspective of other people. One way that an egocentric perspective can be challenged is to relate the experiences of other people to the child's own experiences, for example encouraging empathy with a parent's illness by asking the child to think about a time when they were ill and how this situation felt to them.

> *Concrete operational period – 7–11 years of age:* During this stage, the concept of 'conversion' is tackled. Children often have difficulty imagining that the same volume of water can be poured from a tall thin container to a shorter wider container. The same amount of water in a tall thin jar is often concluded to be different from the same amount of water in a small wide jar.

> *Formal operational period – 11–15 years of age:* At this stage, abstract and logical thinking is achieved. The ability to generate hypotheses appears and during this stage the child may be an active partner in decisions about their health, as their ability to contemplate the consequences of a medical intervention may have developed.

Nurses must develop an understanding of what a child perceives and thinks, as this will influence the way that nurses communicate with children. This process is vital for keeping children informed about their health or the health of family members and friends, and also to avoid unnecessary distress to children who have contact with nursing services.

Early relationships and childhood attachments

John Bowlby (1907–90) suggested that children are born with the drive to form a secure attachment with an adult. Bowlby's attachment theory considered that human babies, like other species, are born with behaviours that help to keep them close to a parent or carer. A good and secure attachment is suggested to be a deep emotional bond between the infant and primary carer. When this bond is formed, the infant will aim to be close to their carer, particularly during times of stress and uncertainty.

Newborn babies have a variety of capabilities that facilitate attachment. An example is facial expression imitation; if you stick your tongue out at a newborn baby, they will also stick their tongue out. This is an unusual skill because newborns have not learned the connection between expressions, movement and their facial muscles. It is thought that imitation skills allow babies to form attachments with adults. It is in the interests of the newborn to form attachments to ensure that parents or carers will bond with them and protect them.

In the early months of a child's life, developing the attachment bond is an important task for parents and child. Nurses and midwives can support the process of becoming a new mother and helping parents to form strong long-term attachments, for example skin-to-skin contact through mothers massaging their babies can help to facilitate parent–child bonding.

Psychologist Mary Ainsworth (1913–99) conducted an experiment called the Strange Situation, in which the behaviour of a child and carer were observed during a series of events (Box 8.1).

Box 8.1

Event 1   The carer and infant are alone
Event 2   A stranger joins the carer and infant
Event 3   The carer leaves the infant and stranger alone
Event 4   The carer returns and the stranger leaves
Event 5   The carer leaves and the infant is left completely alone
Event 6   The stranger returns
Event 7   Finally, the carer returns and the stranger leaves

During the experiment, the child's reaction to each of these scenarios was monitored and used to categorise the type of attachment the child has with the carer. Three types of attachment were recognized by Ainsworth; children who are securely attached, those categorized as having an anxious-resistant insecure attachment and those who have anxious-avoidant insecure attachments.

Children with a secure attachment will typically use the carer as a safe base to explore their environment; the child is calm and continues to play when the stranger enters the room. However, when the mother leaves, the child becomes distressed and will avoid contact with the stranger. Upon the carer's return, the child returns to a calm state and will be willing to play with the stranger as long as the mother remains present. Ainsworth suggested that 65% of children–carer relationships are securely attached.

Fewer children were classified as having an anxious-resistant insecure attachment with their carer. During the experiment, these children typically avoided contact with the stranger, and when the carer left, the child showed intense distress upon separation. When the mother returned to the room, the child typically approached the carer but was difficult to comfort, resisted contact, and even attempted to push the carer away.

The final type of attachment identified by Ainsworth was anxious-avoidant insecure attachments. Children with this type of attachment showed no sign of distress when mother left the room; the child played normally in the stranger's company. Furthermore, the child showed little interest in the mother when she returned to the room and if the child did become distressed, both the carer and stranger were equally able to comfort the child.

Ainsworth's experiment highlights the different types of attachment styles that can occur between child and carer, as well as the different reactions separation from a carer can cause, and what can happen when a child is left alone with a stranger. Nurses caring for children should be aware that separation from a carer can be distressing for some children; however, the level of distress is often a reflection of the type of carer–child attachment. Nurses should also consider the impact prolonged hospitalisation may have on a child. John Bowlby suggested that hospitalized children were often emotionally damaged by their experiences. He suggested that children may endure extreme emotional trauma during hospital stays due to being separated from a carer for a prolonged period of time.

Conclusion

This chapter has provided a brief overview of psychological principles that relate to nursing practice. Nurses regularly interact with patients, provide health advice and work with other healthcare professionals; psychology is a core part of all these activities. This chapter explored examples of how understanding thought processes, emotions and behaviours through the study of psychology can contribute towards nursing practice. However, there are many more ways that psychology can affect nursing practice, and time should be taken to reflect on how psychology can be introduced into other aspects of nursing.

References

Bahn, D (2001) Social learning theory: its application in the context of nurse education, *Nurse Education Today*, **21**(2): 110–17

Barrett, R and Randle J (2008) Hand hygiene practices: nursing students' perceptions, *Journal of Clinical Nursing*, **17**(14): 1851–7

Cohen, S, Tyrrell, DA and Smith, AP (1991) Psychological stress and susceptibility to the common cold, *New England Journal of Medicine*, **325**(9): 606–12

Dunn, KE, Sigmon, SC, Thomas, CS et al. (2008) Voucher-based contingent reinforcement of smoking abstinence among methadone-maintained patients: a pilot study, *Journal of Applied Behaviour Analysis*, **41**(4): 527–38

Fredric, N, Busch, MD, Barbara L and Milrod, MD (2008) Panic-focused psychodynamic psychotherapy, *Psychiatric Times*, **25**(2): 1–2

Lazarus, RS and Folkman, S (1984) *Stress, Appraisal and Coping*, New York: Springer

Leventhal, H and Cameron, L (1987) Behavioral theories and the problem of compliance, *Patient Education and Counseling*, 10: 117–38

Miller, GA (1956) The magical number seven, plus or minus two: some limits on our capacity for processing information, *Psychological Review*, 63: 81–7

Murray, R (2005) *Managing your Stress: A Guide for Nurses*, London: Royal College of Nursing

NICE (National Institute for Health and Clinical Excellence) (2006) Depression and Anxiety: Computerised Cognitive Behavioural Therapy, available online at http://guidance.nice.org.uk/TA97, accessed 26/7/2010

O'Mahony, M and Hegarty, J (2009) Help seeking for cancer symptoms: a review of the literature, *Oncology Nursing Forum*, **36**(4): 178–84

Rosenstock, IM (1966) Why people use health services, *Milbank Memorial Fund Quarterly*, 44: 94–124

Stack, R, Elliott, R, Noyce, P and Bundy, C (2008) A qualitative exploration of multiple medicines beliefs in co-morbid diabetes and cardiovascular disease, *Diabetic Medicine*, 25: 1204–10

Suh, JJ, Pettinati, HM, Kampman, KM and O'Brien, CP (2006) The status of disulfiram: a half of a century later, *Journal of Clinical Psychopharmacology*, **26**(3): 290–302

Vance, DE (2009) The emerging role of cognitive remediation therapy, *Activities, Adaptation and Aging*, 33: 17–30

Walker, J and Payne, S (2003) *Psychology for Nurses and the Caring Professions*, Maidenhead: Open University Press

Warrilow, AE and Beech, B (2009) Self-help CBT for depression: opportunities for primary care mental health nurses?, *Journal of Psychiatric & Mental Health Nursing*, **16**(9): 792–803

9 helping people to manage pain

Emma Briggs

In this chapter we will explore:

> What pain is
> Nurses' role in pain management
> Pain assessment
> Pharmacological management of pain
> Non-drug approaches to pain management

Introduction

All human beings experience pain yet it is a unique experience, no one else can tell you how intense your pain is or what it feels like. For the most part, pain has a protective function; it stops us hurting ourselves such as dropping a hot plate, or if tissue damage has occurred, it stops us causing more harm such as resting a twisted ankle. Some people experience long-term, persistent pain that does not seem to serve any function. Whatever the cause or type of pain, it can have a detrimental effect on people's recovery, mobility, sleeping patterns, eating, mood, social and family activities and their working lives. This chapter examines the different causes of pain and nurses' role in assessing and managing pain through medication and non-drug techniques.

Before we can care for others and manage their pain effectively, we need to examine our own reactions, beliefs and attitudes towards pain. Complete Activity 9.1 before starting this chapter.

Activity 9.1

Think about a recent experience of short- or long-term pain and write down the answers to the following questions:

- How did the pain make you feel, for example upset, frustrated, depressed?
- How did you behave, for example winced, cried, rested, took painkillers?
- How do react when you see someone else in pain – sympathy, not sure what to do?

This chapter will help you to understand why our reactions to pain are all individual; even if we experienced the same surgery, our levels of pain and our reactions to it would be different. Understanding this helps us to care for other people by accepting that they will not necessarily react to pain in the way that we do.

What is pain?

Describing pain in words that we can all agree on is difficult but the International Association for the Study of Pain (IASP 1994) offered this definition of pain:

> An unpleasant sensory and emotional experience associated with actual or potential tissue damage, or described in terms of such damage. Note: The inability to communicate verbally does not negate the possibility that an individual is experiencing pain and is in need of appropriate pain-relieving treatment.

This definition emphasises the physiology of pain, the emotional experience and that sometimes we experience pain even though we cannot communicate it to others. Nurses care for many people who may not be able to communicate their needs. Complete Activity 9.2, which thinks about this in more detail.

Activity 9.2

Under the four branches of nursing – adult, child, learning disability, mental health – identify people who may have difficulty communicating their pain. Think about particular age groups, conditions that may affect speech or procedures in hospital that may hinder verbal communication.

What clues could you look for when caring for people that might indicate they were in pain?

The IASP (1994) also highlights that pain is always subjective, a sentiment echoed by a well-known nursing definition of pain: 'Pain is whatever the experiencing person says it is, existing whenever the person says it does' (McCaffery 1979, cited by McCaffery and Pasero 1999).

There are three main types of pain:

> Acute pain is short term, usually less than three months, and disappears when an injury heals or a condition resolves.
> Persistent or chronic non-malignant pain (sometimes called 'neuropathic' pain) lasts for longer than three months and may not have a foreseeable end, such as osteoarthritis or persistent back pain.
> Finally, pain may also be caused by cancer.

The physiology and therefore the treatment of these types of pain often differ.

In acute pain, the normal physiological process of pain (called 'nociception') can be described as a series of stages (based on McCaffery and Pasero 1999), as shown in Table 9.1.

Table 9.1 Basic principles of nociception

Stage 1	Stage 2	Stage 3	Stage 4
Damage and the detecting of noxious stimuli	Transmission of the signal to the spinal cord and brain	Pain becomes a conscious experience, once the signals have reached the brain	Modulating the painful stimulus

Stage 1: damage and detecting noxious stimuli

During this stage, the tissues (skin, muscle and so on) are damaged and nerve endings pick up this information, converting it into an electrical stimulus. Depending on the injury, this damage could be caused by overstretching the tissues, laceration, shearing, extremes of temperature, compression, infection and inflammation. The damaged cells release a number of chemicals that make the nerve endings very sensitive. This is why touching and moving an injured area is painful when it was not previously.

Stage 2: transmitting the signal to the spinal cord and brain

The electrical stimulus now travels up to the spinal cord via two different types of nerve fibre, A delta and C fibres:

> A delta fibres are covered with a fatty myelin sheath (myelinated) that insulates the fibres, ensuring that the signals travel extremely quickly (6–30 metres per second). These nerves are responsible for the sharp, stabbing pain that initially happens with injuries.
> C fibres are not insulated (unmyelinated) and the signals travel more slowly (0.5–2 metres per second). C fibres are responsible for the dull, throbbing pain that continues after an injury to try to prevent further damage (Melzack and Wall 1996).

Different areas of the body have different proportions of A fibres and C fibres, which helps to explain why pain from the abdomen differs from a painful joint.

Once the signal has reached the spinal cord, neurotransmitters (chemicals that transmit impulses to another nerve or muscle fibre) pass the signal across to a nerve that extends into the brainstem and brain. Several factors influence whether neurotransmitters are released in the spinal cord and the number of signals that reach the brain. In response to pain, the body produces natural opioids (painkillers or analgesics) such as endorphins. These may alter the sensation of pain by preventing the release of neurotransmitters and therefore stop some signals reaching the brain. Medication also works in this way.

Nerve fibres responsible for touch (A beta) can also stop the signals reaching the brain. The touch signals travel much faster than A delta or C fibres and because the brain can only receive so many signals, the sensation of touch is sensed. This is essentially like an engaged telephone, the pain signals from the other fibres cannot get through. This is why 'rubbing it better' works when you have a minor injury.

Stage 3: pain becomes a conscious experience

Once the signals have reached the brain, pain becomes a conscious experience. Although it is not known which part of the brain interprets pain, several areas are involved, including those responsible for emotion and memory. Research studies have suggested that, as infants, we can become sensitised to painful experiences such as taking repeated blood samples and have an increased physiological and behavioural response to pain. Then, as children, our memories of painful events can influence how we react as adults (von Bayer et al. 2004). These two aspects begin to explain the individuality of pain and responses to it; our nervous system is subjected to different painful experiences throughout our life that may cause sensitisation and evoke negative emotions. This also highlights the importance of pain management in children.

Stage 4: modulating the painful stimulus

As well as the strength of the signal being altered at the spinal cord, the brain can influence the information it receives by sending signals back down the spinal cord to prevent or increase neurotransmitter release. A sports person may not notice a minor injury until they have finished playing, because they are distracted and because of emotion and adrenaline (epinephrine in the USA), pain is not felt until much later. Having the opposite effect, fear, anxiety and depression all increase the pain people feel.

Chronic or neuropathic pain is sometimes difficult to understand especially when the original damage has healed or there has been no injury at all. The physiology is still not completely understood but is thought to be due to changes in the nervous system such as the peripheral or spinal cord nerves becoming hypersensitive and hyperactive (McCaffery and Pasero 1999). This means that touch or movement that used to be correctly sent to the brain is now being passed on as pain messages. Chronic pain can also occur when nerves are damaged such as limb amputation.

Effects of pain

Pain is more than a symptom; it can have a devastating effect on people's physical, psychological and social wellbeing (Table 9.2). Acute pain stimulates a complex physiological reaction that is similar to the 'fight or flight' or stress response. This may not harm someone if they are generally well but it can cause complications for people with existing medical conditions. For example, tachycardia (increased pulse rate above 100) and hypertension (high blood pressure) can increase the risk of abnormal heart rhythms or a myocardial infarction (blockage to blood vessels in the heart) (NHMRC 1999). Pain also prevents people from mobilising or coughing, leading to respiratory infections, blood clots (deep vein thrombosis and pulmonary emboli) or pressure ulcers.

People experiencing chronic pain may not have the stress response as the body physiologically adapts over a period of time. However, chronic pain is a major cause of disability and can affect people's daily activities such as eating, sleeping, getting dressed, shopping, as well as their mental health, social and family roles, working lives and financial income. Pain relief is necessary for humanitarian reasons and some argue that it is a basic human right (Leibeskind and Melzack 1987), but preventing the harmful consequences of pain and promoting recovery is one of the key roles of a nurse.

Table 9.2 *Effects of pain*

Physiological effects (acute pain only)	Psychological and social effects	Behaviours
Increased heart rate Increased blood pressure Increased respiration rate Elevated blood sugar levels Decreased gut motility Nausea and vomiting Increased sodium and water retention	Fear Anxiety Negative moods Irritability/aggression Agitation Depression Reduced sleep Loss of appetite Loss of the will to live Change in family role Changes in working lives and possibly reduced income	Verbal reports Grimacing Limping Rubbing the painful area Guarding the painful area Withdrawal Immobilising the painful area Seeking medical advice Seeking methods of relief

Nurses' role in pain management

Pain is the most common reason that people visit their health centre or attend hospital, and during their treatment, several healthcare professionals may be involved in their care. Every member of the multidisciplinary team has a role in helping people to manage their pain (see Table 9.3), but nurses usually spend the most time with people and therefore have the closest relationship with them. Nurses are in a unique position to help and the International Council of Nurses (ICN 2000) recognises the alleviation of suffering as one of our fundamental responsibilities. Nurses alleviate suffering by detecting when people are in pain, assessing pain regularly, administering medication and pain management techniques (such as cold packs), manage specialist procedures such as epidurals, document and evaluate pain relief. They also refer patients to GPs, hospital doctors or pain management specialists when pain is unrelieved or particularly complex. The following sections describe how nurses can assess and help to manage pain using medication and non-drug approaches.

Table 9.3 The role of other healthcare professionals in pain management

Healthcare professional	Role
Healthcare assistants	Conduct pain assessments, document and communicate findings to registered nurses (RNs)
Student nurses	Conduct pain assessments, document and communicate findings to RNs Administer prescribed analgesics under supervision of RNs Evaluate pain relief measures
Physiotherapist	Assess and document pain Promote pain management to ensure physical rehabilitation Use pain relief measures such as heat or cold packs, massage, manipulation and acupuncture
Occupational therapist Speech and language therapist Dietician	Assess pain and promote relief to ensure that daily activities can be continued
General practitioner Hospital doctor	Assess and document pain Prescribe appropriate analgesics Evaluate pain relief measures
Anaesthetist	Assess and manage pain during hospital procedures involving sedation or general anaesthetics Initiate and manage specialist pain management techniques such as epidurals
Pain management specialists: Clinical nurse specialist Consultant nurse Consultant anaesthetist	Manage groups of patients experiencing severe, unrelieved or complicated pain. This may be people undergoing major surgery, receiving palliative care or long-term pain

Pain assessment

Pain is such an individual, subjective experience that we need to help people to communicate their pain in order to treat it effectively. Pain assessment may help to diagnose the cause of pain, to describe the effect of pain, to choose pain relief strategies and evaluate whether they are working. Through sensitive questions, nurses can explore people's experiences and negotiate goals such 'treating pain so that Mrs Phillipe is comfortable undertaking her physiotherapy and walking to the toilet independently'. During pain assessment, a number of key areas need to be assessed:

1 *Location:* Finding out where the pain is helps the diagnosis of pain. If someone has a number of painful areas, it may be helpful to use a body chart to document each area.

2 *Intensity:* The level of pain should be assessed using an assessment tool so that people are using the same words or numbers to describe their pain each time. Figure 9.1 describes some pain assessment tools.

3 *Quality:* The type of pain is important, for example cardiac pain can be quite crushing, squeezing, but there are other causes of chest pain that will feel different. Ask the person to describe the pain and give a few words if it helps (for example sharp, dull, throbbing).

4 *Onset and duration:* Asking the person when the pain started and how long it lasts can give clues as to its cause.

5 *Factors affecting the pain:* Ask people to describe what makes the pain worse and what makes it better. People often have their own pain relief strategies or know which drugs have been effective.

6 *Effect of the pain:* Ask the person to describe how pain affects their daily activities, such as eating, sleeping and mobilising, their mood and personal and social wellbeing.

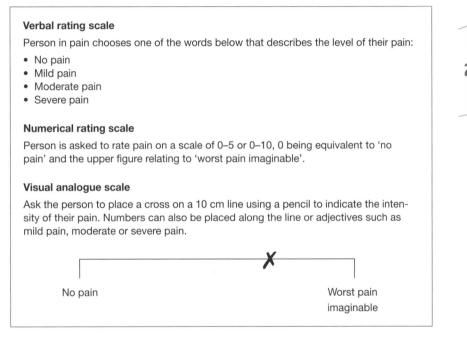

Verbal rating scale

Person in pain chooses one of the words below that describes the level of their pain:

- No pain
- Mild pain
- Moderate pain
- Severe pain

Numerical rating scale

Person is asked to rate pain on a scale of 0–5 or 0–10, 0 being equivalent to 'no pain' and the upper figure relating to 'worst pain imaginable'.

Visual analogue scale

Ask the person to place a cross on a 10 cm line using a pencil to indicate the intensity of their pain. Numbers can also be placed along the line or adjectives such as mild pain, moderate or severe pain.

No pain   Worst pain
                                           imaginable

Figure 9.1 Pain assessment tools

The frequency of assessment depends on the clinical situation. In acute hospital settings, pain assessment is now considered the fifth vital sign (British Pain Society/Royal College of Anaesthetists 2003). Following the four patient observations of blood pressure, pulse, respiration and temperature, pain should always be assessed (see Box 9.1). The amount of information gathered may differ in different scenarios. When experiencing severe pain, location, quality and intensity may be all that is required and more in-depth assessment may be conducted when pain relief has been given. Activity 9.3 presents three case studies to help you think about the sort of questions you could ask as part of a pain assessment.

Box 9.1 Observations

Taking and accurately recording regular measurement of a patient's temperature, pulse, respiration and blood pressure is referred to as 'observations'. Initially, they are taken as baseline measurements on admission. These observations, when recorded together on a graph, will give a profile of the patient's general condition. The doctor will determine how often during a 24-hour cycle the observations will be taken. In circumstances of intensive care, they are monitored constantly.

Observations are useful in charting recovery from infection, the effectiveness of certain treatments and recovery from surgery. A fluctuation in one or more of these measurements can alert the nurse or doctor to changes in the patient's general condition. For example, a raised temperature and a quickening of the pulse could indicate infection. A rise or fall in blood pressure will alert the nurse to physiological changes that may require treatment, and severe pain can bring about fluctuations in temperature, pulse rate and respiration. A skilled nurse is able to interpret these fluctuations and take the necessary action.

Activity 9.3

Case study 1

Patricia is a 35-year-old woman who has recently had surgery to remove her gall bladder (**cholecystectomy**). She appears restless and cannot concentrate on reading a magazine or the television and refuses to drink any fluids. Eight hours after returning to the ward, her observations are as follows:

- Blood pressure: 130/82
- Pulse rate: 88
- Respiration rate: 16
- Temperature: 36.7 °C

Her pain and levels of nausea need to be assessed:

- What questions would you ask Patricia about her pain and nausea?
- What pain assessment tools could you use?
- As a student nurse, what would you do with this information?

Case study 2

Ali is an 8-year-old boy with mild cerebral palsy who attends the local junior school. He has one-to-one help in the classroom as he can have jerky, unpredictable movements of his arms and his speech is slightly slurred. You have been working with him and his classroom assistant and notice a change in his behaviour after he had a fall at playtime, landing on his hip and elbow:

- What questions could you ask Ali to assess whether he is in pain?

- Which pain assessment tools would be useful?
- Who needs to be informed about your concerns and assessment of Ali?

Case study 3

Jacob is a 37-year-old man who is being visited regularly by his community psychiatric nurse due to a history of depression and suicide attempts. Two years ago, Jacob experimented with illegal intravenous drugs, the injection site on his arm became infected and he had to be admitted to hospital for surgery. Since then, the site of the infection has been a source of constant pain, which has contributed to his depression, lack of sleep and reduced food intake. Part of the treatment plan for Jacob is to help him manage his pain but first his experiences need to be assessed:

- What questions could you ask Jacob as part of his pain assessment?
- What pain assessment tools would be useful?

Jacob is experiencing long-term, persistent pain that is not controlled and may need to be referred to his GP or a specialist pain outpatients' clinic.

Pain assessment can be more difficult with neonates, very young children or when people are unable to communicate, such as when being assisted to breathe via a ventilator in intensive care. Specialist pain assessment tools have been designed for these situations based on observations by nurses. Older adults or people with mild-to-moderate intellectual impairment can successfully use the pain assessment tools in Figure 9.1, and observational skills and involving carers can help to assess people with severe impairment.

Pain assessment results should always be documented in the nursing notes, on a pain assessment chart or a routine observation chart. This can be used when evaluating pain relief methods and aids communication between professionals caring for the individual over a period of time. Some people with persistent pain find it useful to write a pain diary so that they can track the changes in their pain or monitor the effectiveness of pain management strategies.

Pharmacological management of pain

A wide range of pain relief medication is available over the counter at pharmacies and prescription only medicines. Some of the most commonly used drugs are highlighted in Table 9.4.

They can be broadly classified into three types; non-opioids, combination drugs and opioids:

> *Non-opioids* (for example paracetamol, anti-inflammatory drugs) are used for mild-to-moderate pain and work by preventing the production of chemicals (usually prostaglandins) that are released and cause pain after an injury or during inflammation.

Table 9.4 *Commonly used drugs in pain management*

Mild-to-moderate pain	Moderate-to-severe pain	Severe pain
Paracetamol Aspirin Co-codamol (each tablet 8 mg codeine, 500 mg paracetamol)	*Non-steroidal anti-inflammatory drugs* Ibuprofen Diclofenac *Combination drugs* Co-codamol (30 mg codeine, 500 mg paracetamol) *Weak opioids* Tramadol Codeine Dihydrocodeine	*Strong opioids* Morphine Diamorphine Pethidine Fentanyl

> *Combination drugs* contain two drugs that are more effective together than they are separately. Used for moderate-to-severe pain, co-codamol is an example containing paracetamol and codeine, a weak opioid.

> *Opioid drugs* mimic the natural endorphins produced by the body by attaching to special opioid receptors on the nerves in the brain and spinal cord. Once attached, opioids prevent the release of neurotransmitters that are required to pass pain information from one nerve to another. Therefore the brain does not receive signals about pain. Opioid drugs can be described as weak or strong depending on their affinity with the opioid receptors. Staff and patients can often hold misconceptions about opioids because of their potential side effects, such as respiratory depression or because they relate opioids to illegal drug use. Opioids are extremely effective for pain relief and can be used safely; the risk of respiratory depression or addiction is estimated at less than 1% (McCaffery and Pasero 1999; Carr and Mann 2000).

The analgesic ladder is a commonly used guide for pain management and different levels of pain. The World Health Organization (WHO 1996) originally designed the ladder for cancer pain and to promote the use of stronger drugs as pain levels increase. Also, the ladder suggests the safe use of drugs combinations, which are more effective than individual doses of one drug. Figure 9.2 illustrates the WHO (1996) analgesic ladder along with an acute analgesic ladder (*Bandolier Extra* 2003) where pain is severe and will subside with healing. Therefore we work down the ladder, starting with the strongest pain relief.

Analgesics can be given through a number of routes, although oral medication is the most common (see Box 9.2). There are also a number of specialist pain management techniques such as nerve blocks, intravenous patient-controlled analgesia or epidurals. The details of these are covered in the pain management textbooks in the Further reading list at the end of this chapter.

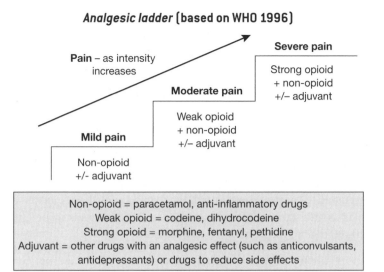

Analgesic ladder (based on WHO 1996)

Pain – as intensity increases

Severe pain
Strong opioid
+ non-opioid
+/– adjuvant

Moderate pain
Weak opioid
+ non-opioid
+/– adjuvant

Mild pain
Non-opioid
+/- adjuvant

Non-opioid = paracetamol, anti-inflammatory drugs
Weak opioid = codeine, dihydrocodeine
Strong opioid = morphine, fentanyl, pethidine
Adjuvant = other drugs with an analgesic effect (such as anticonvulsants, antidepressants) or drugs to reduce side effects

Acute pain analgesic ladder (based on *Bandolier Extra* 2003)

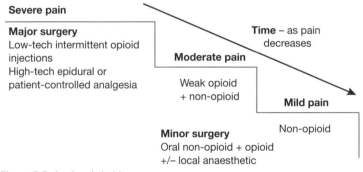

Severe pain

Major surgery
Low-tech intermittent opioid injections
High-tech epidural or patient-controlled analgesia

Time – as pain decreases

Moderate pain
Weak opioid
+ non-opioid

Mild pain
Non-opioid

Minor surgery
Oral non-opioid + opioid
+/– local anaesthetic

Figure 9.2 Analgesic ladders

Box 9.2 Main analgesic routes

> Oral – tablet, suspension
> Subcutaneous injection – under the skin
> Intramuscular injection – into the muscle
> Intravenous injection – into a vein
> Rectal – via the rectum
> Transdermal – absorbed through the skin
> Transmucosal – absorbed through the oral membranes
> Patient-controlled analgesia – an infusion pump attached to a handset controlled by the patient. Depressing the button delivers a dose of analgesic usually via an intravenous infusion
> Epidural – drugs are delivered through a tube into the epidural space in the spinal cord

It is important to note that the same drug can be given through different routes although the dose and frequency rate would vary because absorption would differ. Compare the adult doses of morphine below according to route:

> *Intravenous injection delivered into a vein* where it then circulates round the vascular system and to the brain and spinal cord nerves. Ordinarily, 1–2 mg morphine is needed and the drug takes minutes to work.
> *Intramuscular injection delivered into the muscle* and then absorbed slowly into the vascular system. Takes 5–15 minutes to work and the dose is usually 10–15 mg.
> *Oral* dose is absorbed through the gastrointestinal system but some is metabolised as it passes through the liver. Liquids have quicker absorption than coated tablets but both can take 30–60 minutes to be effective and 20–30 mg of morphine is the usual dose.

Learning about pharmacological pain management can be complicated. Always use the generic names for drugs rather than brand names to prevent confusion. Using analgesic ladders and learning which group of drugs are suitable for mild, moderate and severe pain can help the process of assessing pain.

Work with your patient and mentor to decide which prescribed analgesics will help to manage pain and always refer to a pharmacological publication such as the *British National Formulary* (British Medical Association/Royal Pharmaceutical Society of Great Britain 2010). This contains details of all medication including side effects and contraindications and is updated twice a year.

Non-drug approaches to pain management

Although medication is usually the first line of defence, non-drug approaches can play an important role in pain management. The Nursing and Midwifery Council (NMC 2006) offers guidance on the use of alternative therapies by nurses, emphasising obtaining informed consent, safe practice, promoting the interests of patients or clients and the need for discussion with the multidisciplinary team. Techniques such as acupuncture, massage and aromatherapy need additional qualifications to be practised. However, there are simple techniques that can provide additional relief and relaxation for mild-to-moderate pain.

Psychological techniques

Relaxation through slow breathing, relaxing and tensing different muscle groups and music therapy can all contribute to the reduction in muscle tension and promote the release of the body's own opiates, the endorphins. Simple distraction such as carrying out favourite activities can help pain and children often use play as a distraction technique. Guided imagery helps people to imagine a scene or journey to induce relaxation and is a form of distraction.

This can be done on a one-to-one basis or through using commercially available tapes and CDs.

Cutaneous stimulation

As described earlier, the use of touch or 'rubbing it better' can promote pain relief and there are several non-drug methods that stimulate the skin and deeper tissues. Heat packs are useful for joint and muscle pain but are not recommended in any situation where there is inflammation, bleeding or loss of sensation (neuropathy). Cold packs provide very quick pain relief, reducing inflammation, muscle and joint pain and are good for acute injuries. These should not be used where there is bleeding, neuropathy or when the individual is confused or has a cognitive impairment.

A trans-electrical nerve stimulation (TENS) machine uses electrodes placed on the skin and connected to a battery-operated device that generates electrical impulses. This creates a tingling sensation across the skin, giving the electrical equivalent of 'rubbing it better' and longer use is thought to stimulate endorphin release (King 2001). TENS machines can be useful for persistent pain or during childbirth.

Non-drug approaches can be extremely useful, providing relief and relaxation and encouraging people to play an active role in their pain management. A careful assessment of the individual needs to be done and their consent gained before using these techniques. This will help to ensure that the technique is appropriate and assess their understanding and willingness.

Conclusion

Pain is a subjective experience that is influenced by several factors that can increase and decrease the sensation of pain. Also, our emotional and behavioural response to pain is as individual as we are because our experiences to date have been different. The potential physical, psychological, social and economic effects of pain illustrate why its management is fundamental and often called a basic human right. In every area of nursing, nurses play a key role in the multidisciplinary team by detecting and assessing pain and helping people communicate their personal experience in order to provide appropriate treatment. A wide variety of analgesic drugs are available and before administration, nurses need to be aware of their indications, contraindications and side effects. Non-drug approaches also play a key role in helping people to manage pain by providing relaxation, distraction and increasing their coping strategies.

Further reading and resources

Carr, EC and Mann, EM (2000) *Pain: Creative Approaches to Effective Management*, Basingstoke: Palgrave Macmillan

McMahon, S and Koltzenberg, M (2005) *Melzack and Wall's Textbook of Pain* (5th edn), Edinburgh: Churchill Livingstone

Schofield, P (ed.) (2005) *Beyond Pain*, London: Whurr

British National Formulary www.bnf.org

British Pain Society www.britishpainsociety.org

Nursing and Midwifery Council www.nmc-uk.org.uk

Oxford Pain Internet Site www.jr2.ox.ac.uk/bandolier/booth/painpag/

Pain Relief Foundation www.painrelieffoundation.org.uk

Pain Talk www.pain-talk.co.uk

Pain Support www.painsupport.co.uk

Pain Association Scotland www.chronicpaininfo.org

References

Bandolier Extra (2003) *Evidence-based Health Care: Acute Pain*, special issue, February, available online at http://www.msdforphysicians.co.uk/bandolier/apain.pdf, accessed 15/2/2010

British Medical Association/Royal Pharmaceutical Society of Great Britain (2010) *British National Formulary*, London: BMA/RPSGB

Carr, EC and Mann, EM (2000) *Pain: Creative Approaches to Effective Management*, Basingstoke: Palgrave Macmillan

IASP (International Association for the Study of Pain) (1994) IASP Terminology, available online at http://www.iasp-pain.org/AM/Template.cfm?Section=Pain_Defi...isplay.cfm&ContentID=1728, accessed 3/5/2010

ICN (International Council of Nurses) (2000) *The ICN Code of Ethics for Nurses*, Geneva: ICN

King, A (2001) *King's Guide to TENS* (2nd edn), Glossop: Physiomed

Leibeskind, JC and Melzack, R (1987) The International Pain Foundation: meeting a need for education in pain (editorial), *Pain*, 30: 1–2.

Melzack, R and Wall, PD (1996) *The Challenge of Pain* (2nd edn), London: Penguin

McCaffery, M and Pasero, CL (1999) *Pain: Clinical Manual* (2nd edn), St Louis, MO: Mosby

NHMRC (National Health and Medical Research Council) (1999) *Acute Pain Management: Scientific Evidence*, Canberra, Australia: NHMRC

NMC (Nursing and Midwifery Council) (2006) *Complementary Alternative Therapies and Homeopathy*, London: NMC

Pain Society/Royal College of Anaesthetists (2003) *Pain Management Services: Good Practice*, London: Pain Society

Von Baeyer, CL, Marche, TA, Rocha, EM and Salmon, K (2004) Children's memory for pain: overview and implications for practice, *Journal of Pain*, **5**(5): 241–9

WHO (World Health Organization) (1996) *Cancer Pain Relief* (2nd edn), Geneva: WHO

10 contemporary preoperative and postoperative care

Mark Mitchell

In this chapter we will explore:

> Day and short-stay surgical nursing
> Contemporary physical aspects of care
> Management of postoperative nausea and vomiting
> Patient psychoeducational experiences

Introduction

During the past few years, there have been major changes in surgical practice to the point where many operations that once required a stay in hospital are now routinely performed as day surgery. It has been reported that:

> Minimally invasive surgery will continue to improve. In the next ten years, endoluminal surgery – entering the body through its natural 'holes', such as the throat – will become the standard method of treating many complex cases. Better diagnosis will also help most surgery to become non-invasive.
> (Darzi 2007, p. 7)

In 1999, the British Association for Day Surgery recommended that 50% of cholecystectomies (surgical removal of the gallbladder) should be undertaken in day surgery facilities (Cahill 1999). Moreover, an increasing range of surgery able to be undertaken on a day-case basis is continuously emerging – **thyroidectomy, genitourinary surgery, gastrointestinal surgery, orthopaedic surgery** and **neurosurgery**. As a result of such surgical advances, together with improvements in anaesthesia and pharmacology, much of the physical nursing interventions once associated with care following inpatient surgery are becoming obsolete for the vast majority of patients undergoing elective surgery. This is an escalating and irreversible trend. Minimal access surgery (keyhole surgery), advances in anaesthesia, innovation in **postoperative** recovery practices, increasing healthcare costs and public demand have all contributed to this surgical revolution.

Five central strategies to assist the continued development of day surgery are being pursued:

1 Encouragement to increase capacity

2 Building of new treatment centres (formally diagnostic and treatment centres)

3 Introduction of national tariffs

4 NHS Elect programme

5 Darzi Review (DH 2008).

1 Wide variations in day surgery activity exist throughout the UK. If all day surgery units were as efficient as the best performers, an extra 120,000 day-case procedures could be undertaken annually. More recently, the British Association of Day Surgery (BADS 2007) has added its weight to this claim by stating that if all appropriate procedures were to be undertaken on a day-case basis, an overall day-case rate of 75% could be achieved. Efforts are therefore being made to encourage NHS trusts to enhance their potential and undertake more day surgery.

2 The government commissioned the building of new treatment centres in the NHS and the independent sector as the lack of facilities delayed day surgery expansion. Treatment centres are new dedicated day surgery units, generally built a short distance away from acute hospital services. Approximately 60–80 treatment centres were planned for England by the end of 2005 and a further 100 by 2006.

3 Alongside such expansion, a programme of national tariffs or 'payment by results' for surgery undertaken was commenced:

> It will mean that NHS organisations are paid more fairly for the treatment they provide. Money will be linked directly to patients and patient choice so the more productive and efficient an NHS Trust, the more it will benefit from extra resources. (Cook et al. 2004, p. 61)

The more efficient NHS trusts who undertake more day surgery will thereby be better rewarded, financially. The Department of Health, with the NHS, will work to develop incentives that help to reduce unnecessary hospitalisation. The payment by results scheme has been gradually phased in and is now fully operational.

4 New centres of innovation and training in short-stay elective care are being developed and built (referred to as the NHS Elect programme). The purpose of such centres is to help teach 'early career' surgeons the new skills necessary in order to undertake laparoscopic (keyhole) surgery. These short-stay units will employ many of the practices pioneered in day surgery and undertake surgery, which according to the Department of Health, will 'push the boundaries of day surgery' (DH 2005, p. 12).

5 An increase in the amount and variety of elective surgery possible in day surgery facilities and a reduction in hospital stay following elective surgery is an implicit part of the Darzi Review. Lord Darzi states:

> Ten years ago, my patients would sometimes wait over a year for treatment, and now they wait just a few weeks – and even less if cancer is

suspected. My patients are treated using keyhole surgery enabling them to leave hospital in days rather than weeks. (DH 2008, p. 1)

It is therefore inevitable that both the amount and variety of surgical procedures undertaken on a day or short-stay basis will continue to rise over the coming years.

The impact on nursing practice resulting from these innovative developments in surgical healthcare is considerable. This chapter will focus on **preoperative** and postoperative nursing interventions required by patients who experience a brief hospital stay for intermediate, elective day surgery, which is defined here as planned uncomplicated surgery under general anaesthesia, which can be undertaken in an operating theatre in approximately one hour. This is because it is suggested that in the future *all* elective surgery in the UK will become day or 23-hour-stay surgery (Baskerville 2007), and to examine more traditional aspects of surgical nursing intervention would be a retrograde step. The discussion in this chapter will therefore be more relevant to your future practice.

Day and short-stay surgical nursing

Minimal access surgery offers many considerable advantages over previous methods of surgical approach (Cuschieri 1991). For example:

> reduction in trauma of access
> virtual abolition of surgical wounds
> ability to undertake complex surgical procedures within a closed physiological environment
> avoidance of abdominal wall retraction
> drastic reduction of contact with the patient's blood
> accelerated recovery
> rapid convalescence
> virtual eradication of wound infections and other wound-related complications.

Surgical robotics systems currently under development will result in further radical changes (Darzi and Mackay 2002). However, such innovation in surgical techniques has not occurred in isolation. Advances in anaesthesia have witnessed the introduction of total intravenous anaesthesia – TIVA, general anaesthesia controlled totally by intravenous drugs administration – where patients can now wake rapidly from general anaesthesia and return to the ward fully alert. Additionally, more surgical procedures are being undertaken utilising local and regional anaesthesia. Therefore, from an anaesthetic viewpoint, the surgical patient of the future will also increasingly require considerably less physical care. Currently, some patients require so little physical care that they are ready to be discharged within one or two hours of their surgery; and such procedures are not minor surgical procedures – quite the contrary.

With the more traditional physical aspects of care becoming redundant, nursing responsibilities are increasingly moving in a more multiskilled direction. For example, pre-assessment nursing, anaesthetic nursing skills, nurse surgeons and endoscopy nurses are all relatively 'new' nursing roles. Moreover, with the expansion of modern surgery, this multiskilled day surgery role of the future may be based more on a competency rating scale, that is, the ability to perform tasks such as venipuncture, cannulation, electrocardiograph (ECG) reading and so on. Additionally, many of the responsibilities within these multiskilled roles are undertaken within a very brief time frame, for example prompt admission, crucial perioperative interventions, recovery and discharge planning. Many such roles have evolved to help augment safe and efficient day surgery practices. It is suggested that nurses should welcome such change as new opportunities will become available such as convenient working hours, scope for extended roles, improved continuity of patient care, new well-equipped clinical environments and the possible introduction of new 'school term' contracts.

Such a decline in the extensive physical nursing interventions provides the ideal opportunity for this steady move towards the incorporation of quasi-medical practices into mainstream surgical nursing. Before the 2010 general election, the Labour government had projected a clear vision for the future of elective surgery and under the new coalition government, we can expect this vision to remain in place and nursing practices to continue moving into areas of devolved medical skills. While the adoption of such diverse medical tasks may be vital to ensure the safe and efficient throughput of day surgery patients, it may detract somewhat from the creation, development and utilisation of contemporary nursing-based knowledge fit for this modern surgical era (Weinberg 2003). Indeed, there appears to have been little innovation and change in nursing practices in day surgery since Gilbert (1989) described the day surgery nurses' role, advocating pre-assessment utilising a medically derived pro forma, and ensuring patients' progress through the day surgery unit.

It has been recognised that the whole day-case surgery process is treatment centred and the environment/organisation of care might limit patient/staff interaction (Suhonen et al. 2007). Given that both nursing knowledge and nurse education in modern day surgery are a little impoverished, what will the future hold for surgical nursing if this trend for the indiscriminate inheritance of unwanted medical tasks continues? Much nursing evidence is available to help fill the void left by the demise of physical nursing care and must be pursued in the interests of high-quality surgical nursing intervention fit for the twenty-first century. Such innovative nursing evidence can be broadly divided into two main aspects of intervention – contemporary physical aspects of care (pre-assessment, pain management and management of postoperative nausea and vomiting) and patient psychoeducational experiences (information provision, anxiety and satisfaction) (Gilmartin and Wright 2007; Mitchell 2007).

Contemporary physical aspects of care

Ambulatory surgery nursing unit

First, in order to avoid cancellation and delay on the day of surgery, 58% of current day surgery units in the UK utilise a pre-assessment clinic (Healthcare Commission 2005). Pre-assessment clinics help to confirm fitness for surgery and are an extremely valuable source of information for patients and can greatly assist in the management of patient anxiety. However, this pre-assessment visit is primarily concerned with ensuring medical fitness for surgery, that is, a medical assessment using a medical pro forma prior to the day of surgery to avoid delays and cancellations. As a result of this formal medical focus, psychological considerations can become informal and somewhat marginalised. In a day surgery survey, it was stated that:

> even with those who attend a pre-assessment clinic, they are often seen by the most junior members of the surgical team, in many cases pre-registration house officers, whose main task is to assess the patient's fitness for surgery, rather than to ensure the adequacy of information given. (Pai and Nicholl 2005, p. 512)

Therefore, alongside such medical assessment, there must in future be a more formal nursing assessment so that the psychoeducational aspect of care can gain greater prominence (Mitchell 2005). As day surgery numbers grow, together with the amount of patients undergoing more complex surgery, greater patient insight will be essential to help aid recovery once home.

In future, it is hoped that following the medical pre-assessment phase, a nursing assessment will be undertaken to encompass the essential clinical management and psychoeducational interventions (Box 10.1). Such an assessment would involve the structured provision of information to patients and relatives, together with information regarding pain management, dealing with anxiety and recovering at home (Mitchell 2005). This should then be more accurately named as the 'medical and nursing pre-assessment' and take place in a designated area termed the 'ambulatory surgery nursing unit' and not merely the pre-assessment clinic. Once well established, ambulatory surgery nursing units could also help to plan the discharge of patients and arrange the level of community support required (NHS Scotland 2005). This is the hope for future practice.

Box 10.1 Ambulatory surgery nursing unit assessment

Nursing assessment

> Provision and documentation of desired level of information, that is, standard, intermediate or full

> Discussion of information with patients and relatives

> Discussion and documentation of pain management, including patients' attitudes to the experience of pain
> Discussion and documentation of the management of postoperative nausea and vomiting, including patients' attitudes to its effective management
> Discussion and documentation of anxiety management
> Discussion and documentation of post-discharge contact
> Discussion regarding physical and psychological aspects of home recovery
> Communication with primary healthcare team

Management of postoperative pain

Adequate pain management is a considerable issue for day-case surgery especially one to three days following surgery (Coll et al. 2004). However, it should be noted that not all patients experience pain, many (approximately 33% and above) may experience very little pain (Hein et al. 2001; McHugh and Thoms 2002). Nevertheless, liaison with a hospital pain team or nurse specialist is an essential first step together with good pain assessment.

Following the medical assessment, any nursing assessment should include accurate and realistic pain management information (Jakobsen et al. 2003; McGrath et al. 2004). The lack of information concerning analgesia is a considerable issue and a number of studies have demonstrated improved pain control when information provision is enhanced (Skilton 2003; Prewett et al. 2008). During such discussions, patients' attitudes towards pain management can be explored (Dewar et al. 2004; Coll 2006). In the study by Dewar et al. (2004), it was discovered that patients held many misconceptions regarding pain management, for example the need to experience pain in order to monitor healing, and concerns about addiction, side effects and constipation. In addition, patients do not always follow their analgesia regime once home (Older et al. 2010).

Pain assessment, relief and management

Patients should have their pain assessed at regular intervals prior to discharge, as this can be essential in avoiding poor pain management during recovery at home. For example, an increase in pain experience prior to discharge can be a strong indicator of increased pain during the first 24–48 hours, so the timely administration of medicines, regular formal assessment of pain by the hospital staff prior to discharge, and continuing support for patients following discharge are important. Prepacked analgesia has also been recommended to avoid delayed discharge and to ensure the correct level of medication is provided for the surgery undertaken, that is, analgesia pack composition prescribed according to the type of operation undertaken (Mitchell 2004).

Recovery at home with little or no professional advice can be detrimental to swift recovery. For example, research has found that childcare, climbing stairs, cooking, cleaning and shopping were all resumed on the same day as surgery (Jakobsen et al. 2003). Patients should therefore be given realistic recovery advice and informed that pursuing demanding activities too early in the recovery period may result in an increase in pain experience. It is highly likely that patients will have forgotten much information once home and require additional postoperative information to aid their recovery. In an experimental study by Moran et al. (1998), it was established that patients who received a postoperative telephone call were significantly less likely to seek help from their primary healthcare team. Therefore all patients should ideally be contacted by telephone 24–48 hours following surgery.

Activity 10.1

If you were a patient, what information would you want to know before and after surgery? How would you like this information conveyed to you, for example by a leaflet, a one-to-one chat, or on a website?

Box 10.2 Essential pain management

Nursing intervention

> Consultation with hospital pain management team or nurse specialist regarding protocol
> Discussion and documentation of pain management including patients' attitudes to the experience of pain
> Adequate pain assessment and monitoring
> Explicit communication of expectations, that is, the extent of pain, duration and appropriate physical activity
> Detailed verbal and written information provision specifically concerning pain management
> Graded prepacked analgesia given on discharge
> Nurse-initiated telephone service

Management of postoperative nausea and vomiting

Postoperative nausea and vomiting (PONV) is a common problem following day surgery. It has been suggested that PONV has multiple causes and thereby requires a combination of actions to treat it, such as good pain relief, adequate information provision, avoidance of opioids, use of local anaesthesia to infiltrate the wound during surgery and use of non-steroidal anti-inflammatory drugs (NSAIDs). The Royal College of Anaesthetists (2006) also recommends advising patients to avoid sitting up too quickly, avoid drinking and eating immediately following surgery and to take slow deep breaths to help reduce the sensation of nausea.

> **Box 10.3 Essential PONV management**

Nursing intervention

> ❯ Discussion, assessment and documentation of the management of PONV, including patients' attitudes to its effective management
> ❯ Ensure good pain relief and adequate information provision
> ❯ Enquire regarding the possible use of opioids, local anaesthesia infiltration of wounds during surgery and beneficial effects of NSAIDs
> ❯ Advise patients to avoid sitting up too quickly, avoid drinking and eating immediately following surgery, and to take slow deep breaths to help reduce the sensation of nausea

Once the patient has arrived home, post-discharge nausea and vomiting (PDNV) can occur. According to Wu et al. (2002, p. 997): 'Approximately 36% of patients who experienced post-discharge nausea and vomiting do not experience any nausea and vomiting before discharge from hospital.' Fetzer et al. (2005) interviewed 190 day surgery patients regarding the cause of their PDNV and discovered that 36% was caused by their analgesia, 13% their pain, 24% the anaesthesia and 18% movement while travelling home or movement after arrival home.

Assessing each patient prior to surgery regarding their potential to develop PONV is a vital first step. Apfel et al. (1999) constructed one of the most widely utilised preoperative risk assessment scores to gauge the potential for development of PONV.

This calculator summarises individual susceptibility to postoperative nausea and vomiting. It employs a simple yes/no tick box system to record responses to the following relevant questions:

> ❯ What is the patient's gender?
> ❯ Does the patient have a history of motion sickness?
> ❯ Is the patient a nonsmoker?
> ❯ Are postoperative opioids to be used?

The incidence of PONV can be predicted from the overall score. For example, a score of zero = the lowest incidence, while a score of 4 = the highest incidence. If two or more of these factors are present, a change to anaesthetic technique is suggested.

Using this scale, it is clear that the most susceptible patients are adult females, with a history of motion sickness, non-smoker and exacerbated by the planned use of opioids. When all such factors are present, such a person would have a 79% risk of developing PONV. However, a criticism of Apfel et al. (1999) is its lack of anaesthesia-related factors (drugs employed during anaesthesia, for example) (Sinclair et al. 1999).

To aid the assessment and treatment of PONV, the British Association of Day Surgery has provided an online risk and treatment calculator, based on the extensive study by Sinclair et al. (1999), and a poster that provides treatment options (both can be accessed from the BADS website at www.daysurgeryuk.org).

More recently, van den Bosch et al. (2005) suggested slightly differing criteria, that is, females from puberty onwards, age (younger people more susceptible), non-smoker, a history of motion sickness or PONV, lower abdominal surgery or middle ear surgery, use of Isoflurane anaesthesia (a clear colourless liquid, pungent smell, principal effect general anaesthesia but with little analgesic effect), use of postoperative opioids and a patient with increased anxiety. Gan (2006) suggested that these risk measures are quite accurate, although they could be improved somewhat as other factors may also impact (history of migraine, history of PONV or motion sickness in a child's parent or sibling, intense preoperative anxiety, surgery type, decreased perioperative fluids and increasing duration of anaesthesia). However, such assessment measures may be unreliable when a patient is having regional anaesthesia (Williams et al. 2003). Conversely, the use of regional anaesthesia may significantly reduce a patient's length of stay on the day of surgery (Weltz et al. 2003).

Patient psychoeducational experiences

Information provision

The provision of patient information within the sphere of modern surgery is a national and international challenge and has been the case for many years:

> Fundamental to the success of day surgery is adequate patient preparation and support. Although every member of the multi-disciplinary team can play a part by conveying a positive mental attitude, day surgery nurses have a pivotal role in this respect. (Smith 2006, p. 247)

The main challenges concern the differing levels of information required by individual patients and the inclusion of suitable information for home recovery (Figure 10.1). Patients can be classified in one of the following three groups:

1 *Blunters/avoidant copers:* some patients require less information than others to help manage their anxiety when experiencing an event such as day surgery, as too much information has the potential to increase their anxiety. Such patients have been termed 'blunters' or 'avoidant copers'.
2 *Monitors/vigilant copers:* some patients require more information to help manage their anxiety as too little information has the potential to increase their anxiety. Such patients have been termed 'monitors' or 'vigilant copers'.
3 *Fluctuating copers:* as the first two are extreme coping methods, a third group of patients, who may require a variable level of information, have been termed 'fluctuating copers' (Krohne 1978). Fluctuating copers have been viewed as the most difficult to care for in respect of their anxiety

(Rosenbaum and Piamenta 1998). Unlike vigilant and avoidant copers, fluctuating copers' informational requirements cannot be as readily determined. For example, such patients may require an intermediate level of information in one area, such as information regarding their operation, but little in another area, such as general anaesthesia.

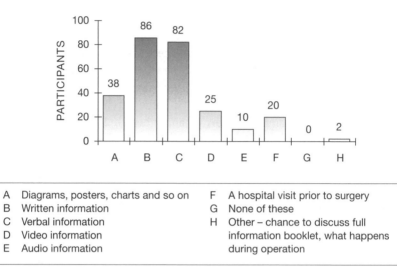

Figure 10.1 *Most preferred prior method of receiving information*
Source: Mitchell 2000b. Reproduced with permission

Activity 10.2

Visit the nearest hospital that offers a day surgery facility and pick up a patient information leaflet. Place yourself in the position of someone who is to be admitted for day surgery and assess how informative the leaflet is. For example, would you feel reassured from reading the leaflet that your operation will be carried out effectively and that you would receive all the care necessary for your recovery? Does the leaflet provide sufficient information regarding:

• Time to arrive
• What to bring with you
• Driving
• Hospital smoking policy
• All activities of daily living
• Visitors during the time you are in the unit
• A map of the hospital with the unit clearly marked.

Having read the leaflet, is there anything missing that you feel should be there? How can a nurse ensure that information incorporated in the leaflet is understood by the patient on admission? How do 'coping identifiers' assist in the general preparation of day patients?

core topics

Patients can be given a choice of full, intermediate or standard information disclosure. Such a choice also provides the opportunity to discuss the information with a member of staff and be exposed to various modes of information presentation (Figure 10.1). This chosen level of information provision should continue throughout the day of surgery experience.

Some studies have concluded that the discharge information is not always realistic or adapted sufficiently for home recovery. For example, Bradshaw et al. (1999) determined that improved information provision was required concerning postoperative pain management, wound healing, bathing, exercise, return to work, driving and sexual relations. More extensive information (where requested) may also help to prevent issues of 'trial-and-error' recovery (Kleinbeck and Hoffart 1994). A number of day surgery studies have also uncovered patients' desire to be informed of the possible complications that can occur postoperatively together with how such complications can be recognised and managed (de Jesus et al. 1996; Ruuth-Setala et al. 2000). Finally, the use of a nurse-initiated telephone service together with an additional 'helpline' service represents a way of providing patients with information once they have been discharged from hospital (see Box 10.4). Perez et al. (2006) point out that the use of mobile telephones, video imaging and the internet add further to the possibilities for developing new and innovative methods of postoperative monitoring.

Activity 10.3

1 Go to the internet and Google 'patient information leaflets'.
2 Download a selection of these and compare them for clarity.
3 Identify at least three points from two leaflets that can be incorporated into a nurse's practice leading to patient discharge.

Box 10.4 Essential patient information

Nursing intervention

> Nursing assessment to ascertain the level of information required, that is, standard, intermediate or detailed
> Provision of chosen level of information throughout whole day surgery experience (verbal and written)
> Explicit identification of patients' informational requirements on the day of surgery
> Provision of identified level of written information at discharge pertaining to a home recovery and to help inform carers
> Nurse-initiated telephone call 24–48 hours postoperatively
> Provision of patients' helpline telephone support

Anxiety management

Increased patient anxiety prior to general anaesthesia and surgery has, for a number of years, been recognised as a pertinent issue. Patient anxiety has not diminished with the advent of modern day surgery (Figure 10.2); indeed, it has evolved alongside such innovative healthcare practice (Mitchell 2005, 2008). For example, for many years, patient anxiety arose from the apprehension concerning the anaesthesia, operation, pain and being unconscious. This remained constant for many decades until the rise in day surgery. Modern day surgery studies have revealed that the waiting period prior to surgery is an additional anxiety-provoking aspect (Mitchell 1997, 2000a) (Figure 10.3).

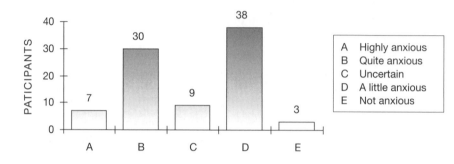

Figure 10.2 Anxiety prior to day surgery
Source: Mitchell 2000b. Reproduced with permission

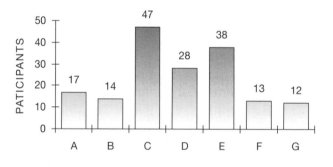

A Operation	G Other – possibility of reduced health,
B Unconsciousness	hunger, possibility of nausea and
C General anaesthetic	vomiting, IV line being resited, needles,
D Possible pain and discomfort	discharged too early, parking, ward
E Wait	layout, lack of warmth, operation being
F Social arrangements, such as child-	cancelled again, separation from
minding, work and so on	husband

Figure 10.3 Aspects increasing anxiety prior to day surgery
Source: Mitchell 2000b. Reproduced with permission

core topics

Despite the vast majority of patients experiencing anxiety over many decades, its management has remained informal, marginalised and largely pharmacological in nature (Mitchell 2005). Early pioneering nursing studies all recommended information provision as a central factor in preoperative anxiety management (Volicer 1973; Hayward 1975; Wilson-Barnett 1976; Boore 1978) and this approach remains true today (Royal College of Surgeons of England 2007; Demir et al. 2008). However, today, additional intervention is required to compensate for the limited time patients now spend in the acute hospital setting (Crockett et al. 2007; Gilmartin and Wright 2008). Primarily, anxiety management should involve assessment, adequate information provision, enhancing personal control and self-efficacy, the therapeutic use of self and managing the environment. First, therefore, patients' anxiety regarding their planned surgery and anaesthesia must be assessed, perhaps during their visit to the ambulatory surgery nursing unit (as discussed above). Rosenberger et al. (2006) suggested that key questions to be asked were:

> Knowledge of planned surgical procedure
> Anticipation of a difficult recovery
> Possible or current depression
> Positive expectations about the surgery and recovery
> Realistic expectations about the surgery and recovery
> Confidence regarding managing postoperative pain and discomfort
> Planning to be an active participant in the recovery process.

Crucial to effective anxiety management is the provision of the desired level of preoperative information. (In the section Patient psychoeducational experience, you will find more about information provision.) With the ever decreasing contact with healthcare professionals and increasing self-recovery inherent in modern day surgery, good information provision is vital (Mitchell 2005). Once the desired information provision has been established, further aspects of formal psychological intervention can be implemented.

Raising patients' experience of personal control can help to reduce anxiety. Studies have suggested that the experience of control can be strongly influenced by the environment (Shiloh et al. 2003; Lorenz 2007). Patients entering a day surgery unit can quickly feel events to be largely determined by powerful others (doctors and nurses) (Fox 1999), leaving them feeling somewhat less in control. The modern surgical environment provides a strong example of how such a shift in self-control evaluation can occur, that is, brief hospital admission, environment dominated by rigid schedules, consent signing, undressing, administration of powerful drugs and all maintained by uniformed doctors and nurses (powerful others) (Douglas and Douglas 2004). The level of control required by patients may only need to be minor, real or perceived. For example, in an older study, an increase in self-control was demonstrated merely by permitting blood donor patients a simple choice of which arm to be used during the procedure (Mills and Krantz 1979). Obviously, which arm used mattered little to the hospital personnel but for the patient it bestowed the perception of choice. If, therefore, patients are provided with a perception of choice, their experience of health control may greatly increase (Ward et al. 2007). Conversely, according to Mauleon et al. (2007, p. 897): 'When patients felt they were ordered about and they could not resist or argue, this led to distrust and a sense of anger and disappointment.'

As the ability to exercise some control in an acute day surgery setting is highly limited and the perceived ability to retain some aspects of healthcare control is reduced for some patients (Mitchell 2000a), a deliberate planned attempt on your part, as a member of the nursing staff, is required. Doctors and nurses must identify simple aspects of intervention that have the ability to bestow a perception of control; for example the choice to remain dressed if their surgery is later in the operating schedule, choice of relatives to remain with the patient, staggered admission times and so on. Such interventions need only be minor, but if each member of the clinical team behaved in such a manner and provided such minor or inconsequential options, the overall perception of personal control would be considerable.

Second, self-efficacy enhancement can have a positive influence on recovery. Self-efficacy or the confidence in one's ability to behave in such a way as to produce a desirable outcome can give rise to considerable distress if these abilities are reduced (Bandura 1982). As a patient's stay in day surgery is so brief and preparation and recovery at home the greater part of the surgical experience, patients require buoyant self-efficacy beliefs in order to assist recovery. Dental day surgery studies have demonstrated that recovery is enhanced when patients experience an increase in self-efficacy appraisal (Litt et al. 1995, 1999). Again, the modern surgical environment may negate personal attempts to establish an increased level of self-efficacy, for example brief hospital admission, unfamiliar environment, rigid schedules and powerful uniformed others determining complex medical events.

As the perceived ability to cope with day surgery is reduced in some patients (Mitchell 2000a) and much recovery occurs at home, a deliberate planned effort on the part of the medical and nursing staff to enhance self-efficacy appraisal is required. Healthcare professionals must again identify simple interventions that can aid the enhancement of self-efficacy, for example explaining all events and providing the desired level of information, the guarantee of a nurse-initiated telephone call during the postoperative period, and the desired level of information provided at discharge. If each member of the clinical team were to behave in such a manner and such interventions become commonplace, the overall perception of self-efficacy attainment would be considerable.

Third, the therapeutic use of self has demonstrated a positive influence on recovery from surgery (Costa 2001; Dewar et al. 2003; Krohne and Slangen 2005). Therapeutic use of self has been defined as:

Supportive intervention characterized by the physical and emotional presence bestowed when a nurse, doctor or relative is in close proximity to a patient. However, it is not merely the physical presence but also the interactions and statements of reassurance that are important. (Mitchell 2005, p. 202)

Here therapeutic use of self will be divided into three aspects:

> *Social support*: Social support on the day of surgery is clearly limited in modern surgery, as the surgical environment may preclude the presence of relatives or other supportive members for good clinical reasons. In such circumstances, the presence of a doctor or nurse as an agent of social support has been viewed as highly beneficial (Leino-Kilpi and Vuoren-heimo 1993; Krohne and Slangen 2005). Their presence has been compared with the assuring attendance that a parent or guardian bestows upon an infant, that is, the infant feels safer when the parent is in sight (Teasdale 1995). Therefore, merely being close to and communicating with the patient may provide a considerable element of safety (Figure 10.4).

> *Optimism enhancement:* Positive expectations or an optimistic outlook concerning a stressful medical event have been observed to have a considerable impact on postoperative outcomes (Mahler and Kulik 2000; McCarthy et al. 2003). However, such studies have mainly investigated patients undergoing major inpatient surgery and the impact this can have on short/long-term recovery and wound healing (Flood et al. 1993; Schroder and Schwarzer 1998). A more recent study examining patients' experiences of a brief hospital stay for hernia repair demonstrated the negative effects of increased preoperative stress on wound healing (Broadbent et al. 2003, p. 867): 'This study found that higher reported psychological stress before surgery predicted lower cellular wound repair processes in the early post-operative period.'

> *Provision of cognitive coping strategies:* The final aspect associated with therapeutic use of self concerns patients' cognitive coping strategies. Cognitive coping strategies are defined as the purposeful emotional attempts to prompt less negative or catastrophising thoughts concerning a given situation, for example when undergoing general anaesthesia. Optimising patients' cognitive coping strategies can help to dispel false or unfounded fears. For example, patients could be advised that the hospital performs much surgery safely every day or that the anaesthetists, surgeons and nurses are all highly trained. When concerned about their general anaesthetic, Lack et al. (2003, p. 67) recommend informing the patient that: 'Anaesthesia is ... a state of carefully controlled and supervised unconsciousness which allows surgery to be performed painlessly.'

The implementation of such care will inevitably overlap with self-efficacy enhancement and the encouragement of a more optimistic stance. However, the central importance of such intervention has been established in many studies (Leinonen et al. 1996; Costa 2001; Moon and Cho 2001). Despite this evidence, no studies to date have uncovered the most appropriate words or phases of assurance during such interactions. Doctors and nurses merely employ phrases and utterances they personally deem to be the most appropriate. Information regarding the most appropriate expressions is vital for a comprehensive preoperative psychoeducational plan of care. Research is ongoing to uncover the most effective cognitive coping strategies for use in these situations, such as most helpful words, phases and encouraging statements.

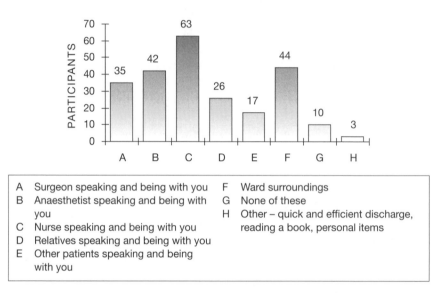

A   Surgeon speaking and being with you
B   Anaesthetist speaking and being with you
C   Nurse speaking and being with you
D   Relatives speaking and being with you
E   Other patients speaking and being with you
F   Ward surroundings
G   None of these
H   Other – quick and efficient discharge, reading a book, personal items

Figure 10.4 Anxiety reduction in day surgery

The final aspect of anxiety management concerns the environment. The environment will be divided here into the behaviours of the medical and nursing staff and the physical environment. Few studies have examined these aspects within the day surgery environment, although the impact of the environment has been clearly identified (Box 10.5). In a study by Parsons et al. (1993), the nursing behaviours deemed by patients to be caring behaviours were examined. Various categories emerged, although the three most effective caring behaviours were viewed to be:

> Nurses' reassuring presence
> Verbal reassurance
> Attention to physical comfort.

Therefore, the nurse just being in close proximity to the patient while they were in the day surgery facility and expressing concern was very helpful. In a survey by Mitchell (2000a), the aspects of care that helped to reduce anxiety the most were the presence of the nurse, closely followed by the ward environment. In this study, the ward surroundings could be described as quiet, calm and professional with music playing quietly in the background. However, the precise elements that contributed to the environmental perception of safety are unclear. The implicit and explicit messages of safety present within the day surgery environment therefore require further examination so that future action can be taken to enhance the positive influences and diminish the more negative experiences.

In a survey of 214 day surgery patients undergoing surgery and local anaesthesia (Mitchell 2008), 77% stated that they were anxious. The main cause of their anxiety was the thought of being awake during surgery, feeling the surgeon, seeing the body cut open, the surgery being more painful because of the local anaesthetic and numbness possibly wearing off too quickly. Other studies have also uncovered similar findings, that is, raised anxiety because of possibly feeling the surgery (de Andres et al. 1995), seeing the surgery, hearing intraoperative conversation (Gajraj et al. 1995) or experiencing pain (Gajraj and Sidawi 1993; Koscielniak-Nielsen et al. 2002). Clearly, such anxiety is largely completely unfounded, although these patients had not been informed about their intraoperative experience or had forgotten such information (Box 10.5).

Box 10.5 Essential anxiety management

Nursing intervention

> Assessment of level of anxiety with regard to both surgery and anaesthesia
> Provision of chosen level of information throughout whole day surgery experience (verbal and written)
> Enhancement of patient self-control and self-efficacy
> Therapeutic use of self in the form of:
>> Social support
>> Optimism enhancement
>> Optimising cognitive coping strategies
> Reducing the negative impact of the clinical environment and encouraging implicit and explicit messages of safety

---

Patient satisfaction

Finally, many of the fundamental influences on patient satisfaction have been previously discussed. However, it is beneficial to conclude with the main features by which patients measure satisfaction with day and short stay surgery. First, pain, nausea and vomiting are highly influential factors. In an international study of patients undergoing general anaesthesia for a variety of surgical procedures (Pfisterer et al. 2001), postoperative nausea and vomiting were most problematic in patients undergoing gastrointestinal (32%), gynaecological (15%) and general surgery (17%). Additionally, some patients experienced nausea and vomiting for up to five days postoperatively – 17% upon waking, 14% travelling home and 3% by the fifth day. It was concluded that postoperative nausea and vomiting remained a problem for patients many days following discharge. Immediate postoperative assessment and intervention has been viewed as vital to overcome this issue, as a strong correlation exists between immediate and more prolonged postoperative nausea and vomiting (Parlow et al. 1999; Fetzer et al. 2004, 2005).

Information provision has also been strongly linked with satisfaction and must be suited to help inform patients recovering at home (Williams et al. 2003; Yellen and Ricard 2005; Royal College of Surgeons of England 2007; Freeman and Denham 2008). Furthermore, although the specific ward environment has been discussed, a number of studies have highlighted problematic areas concerning the general hospital environment such as car parking, privacy and information (Royal College of Surgeons of England/East Anglia Regional Health Authority 1995; Georgalas et al. 2002; Hazelgrove and Robins 2002; Hammond and Smith 2004). Finally, social support and anxiety have both been highlighted as influential factors in patient satisfaction and require careful consideration (Costa 2001; Stevens et al. 2001) (see the section on anxiety management) (Box 10.6).

Box 10.6 Essential management for patient satisfaction

Nursing intervention
> Effective and responsive pain management protocol
> Effective and responsive postoperative nausea and vomiting protocol
> Effective and responsive patient information programme
> Effective and responsive psychoeducational planned programme of care

Conclusion

Elective surgery has changed dramatically over the past 10–15 years. The emphasis on brief hospital stay, minimal trauma of surgical access and rapid anaesthetic recovery will continue and develop further. This is an irreversible global healthcare trend (Toftgaard 2007; Ojo et al. 2008). Consequently, many physical nursing interventions, once central to postoperative surgical care, are disappearing as they are no longer necessary in this new surgical era. Many devolved medical tasks have been taken up by the nursing profession to help fill the void created by the demise of numerous physical tasks and aid the rapid development and expansion of modern elective surgery. However, other vitally important aspects of care relating to patients' experience of brief hospital stay are now required. The nursing profession must therefore consider patients' experience of such brief episodes and provide care accordingly. This will require continued research into patients' experience of day and short-stay surgery and a change of emphasis in surgical nurse education. Surgical care must in future always embrace contemporary physical aspects of care and patient psychoeducational experiences in addition to being mindful of the continually shrinking opportunity for nurse–patient interaction.

Further reading and resources

Burden, N, DeFazio-Quinn, DM, O'Brien, D and Gregory-Dawes, BS (2000) *Ambulatory Surgical Nursing*, London: WB Saunders

Coll, AM (2006) *How Can I Make it Better: A Guide to Pain Management for Day Surgery Nurses*, Salisbury: Fivepin

Hodge, D (1999) *Day Surgery: A Nursing Approach*, London: Churchill Livingstone

Markanday, L (1997) *Day Surgery for Nurses*, London: Whurr

Mitchell, MJ (2005) *Anxiety Management in Adult Day Surgery: A Nursing Perspective*, London: Whurr

Mitchell, MJ (2006) Nursing knowledge and the expansion of day surgery in the United Kingdom, *Ambulatory Surgery*, **12**(3): 131–8

Mitchell, MJ (2010) General anaesthesia and day-case patient anxiety, *Journal of Advanced Nursing*, 66(5): 1059–71

Mottram, A (2009) Therapeutic relationships in day surgery: a grounded theory study, *Journal of Clinical Nursing*, **18**(20): 2830–37

NHS Modernisation Agency (2004) *10 High Impact Changes for Service Improvement and Delivery*, London: HMSO

Oldman, M, Moore, D and Collins, S (2004) Drug patient information leaflets in anaesthesia: effect on anxiety and patient satisfaction, *British Journal of Anaesthesia*, **92**(6): 854–58

Smith, I (2000) *Day Care Anaesthesia*, London: BMJ Books

Ambulatory Surgery Journal www.ambulatorysurgery.org

American Society of Anesthesiologists www.asahq.org

Association of Anaesthetists of Great Britain and Ireland www.aagbi.org

British Association of Day Surgery www.daysurgeryuk.org

International Association of Ambulatory Surgery www.iaas-med.org

NHS Modernisation Agency www.modernnhs.nhs.uk/threatre

National Association of Theatre Nurses (online courses) www.natn.org.uk

Pre-operative Association www.pre-op.org

Royal College of Anaesthetists www.rcoa.ac.uk

Royal College of Surgeons www.rcseng.ac.uk

Toolkit for Producing Patient Information www.doh.gov.uk/nhsidentity

2

References

Apfel, CC, Laara, E, Koivuranta, M et al. (1999) A simplified risk score for predicting postoperative nausea and vomiting: Conclusions from cross-validations between two centers, *Anesthesiology*, **91**(3): 693–700

Audit Commission for Local Authorities and the National Health Service in England and Wales, (1998) *Managing Pain after Surgery: A Booklet for Nurses*, London: HMSO

BADS (British Association of Day Surgery) (2007) *BADS Procedure Directory*, London: BADS

Bandura, A (1982) Self-efficacy mechanism in human agency, *American Psychologist*, **37**(2): 122–147

Baskerville, P (2007) Surgical Education *(medical)* in Ambulatory Surgery, 7th International Congress on Ambulatory Surgery, Amsterdam, Holland

Boore, JR (1978) *Prescription for Recovery*, London: Royal College of Nursing

Bradshaw, C, Pritchett, C, Bryce, C et al. (1999) Information needs of general day surgery patients, *Journal of Ambulatory Surgery*, **7**(1): 39–44

Broadbent, E, Petrie, KJ, Alley, PG and Booth, RJ (2003) Psychological stress impairs early wound repair following surgery, *Psychosomatic Medicine*, **65**(5): 865–69

Cahill, J (1999) Basket cases and trollies: day surgery proposals for the millennium, *Journal of One Day Surgery*, **9**(1): 11–12

Coll, AM (2006) *How Can I Make it Better: A Guide to Pain Management for Day Surgery Nurses*, Salisbury: Fivepin

Coll, AM and Ameen, J (2006) Profiles of pain after day surgery: patients' experiences of three different operation types, *Journal of Advanced Nursing*, **53**(2): 178–87

Coll, AM, Ameen, JR and Moseley, LG (2004) Reported pain after day surgery: a critical literature review, *Journal of Advanced Nursing*, **46**(1): 53–65

Cook, T, Fitzpatrick, R and Smith, I (2004) *Achieving Day Surgery Targets: A Practical Approach Towards Improving Efficiency in Day Case Units in the United Kingdom*, London: Advanced Medical Publications

Costa, MJ (2001) The lived perioperative experience of ambulatory surgery patients, *American Operating Room Nurses' Journal*, **74**(6): 874–81

Crockett, JK, Gumley, A and Longmate, A (2007) The development and validation of the Pre-operative Intrusive Thoughts Inventory (PITI), *Anaesthesia*, **62**(7): 683–9

Cuschieri, A (1991) Minimal access surgery and the future of interventional laparoscopy, *American Journal of Surgery*, **161**(3): 404–7

Darzi, A (2007) *Saws and Scalpels to Lazers and Robots: Advances in Surgery*, London: TSO

Darzi, A and Mackay, S (2002) Recent advances in minimal access surgery, *British Medical Journal*, **324**(7328): 31–4

De Andres, J, Valia, JC, Gil, A and Bolinches, R (1995) Predictors of patient satisfaction with regional anesthesia, *Regional Anesthesia*, **20**(6): 498–505

De Jesus, G, Abbotts, S, Collins, B and Burvill, A (1996) Same day surgery: results of a patient satisfaction survey, *Journal of Quality in Clinical Practice*, **16**(3): 165–73

Demir, F, Donmez, YC, Ozsaker, E and Diramali, A (2008) Patients' lived experiences of excisional breast biopsy: a phenomenological study, *Journal of Clinical Nursing*, **17**(6): 744–51

DH (Department of Health) (2005) *Treatment Centres: Delivering Fast, Quality Care and Choice for NHS Patients*, London: DH

DH (2008) *High Quality Care for All: NHS Next Stage Review Final Report*, Darzi Review, London: DH

Dewar, A, Craig, K, Muir, J and Cole, C (2003) Testing the effectiveness of a nursing intervention in relieving pain following day surgery, *Ambulatory Surgery*, **10**(2): 81–8

Douglas, CH and Douglas, MR (2004) Patient-friendly hospital environments: exploring the patients' perspective, *Health Expectations*, **7**(1): 61–73

Fetzer, SJ, Hand, MC, Bouchard, PA et al. (2004) Evaluation of the rhodes index of nausea and vomiting for ambulatory surgery patients, *Journal of Advanced Nursing*, **47**(1): 74–80

Fetzer, SJ, Hand, MA, Bouchard, PA et al. (2005) Self-care activities for post-discharge nausea and vomiting, *Journal of PeriAnesthesia Nursing*, **20**(4): 249–54

Flood, A, Lorence, DP, Ding, J et al.(1993) The role of expectations in patient's reports of post-operative outcomes and improvement following therapy, *Medical Care*, **31**(3): 1043–56

Fox, NJ (1999) Power, control and resistance in the timing of health and care, *Social Science and Medicine*, **48**(10): 1307–19

Freeman, K and Denham, SA (2008) Improving patient satisfaction by addressing same day surgery wait times, *Journal of PeriAnesthesia Nursing*, **23**(6): 387–93

Gajraj, N and Sidawi, E (1993) How painful is insertion of a spinal needle?, *Anesthesia and Analgesia*, **76**(6): 1370

Gajraj, NM, Sharma, SK, Souter, AJ et al. (1995) A survey of obstetric patients who refuse regional anaesthesia, *Anaesthesia*, **50**(8): 740–1

Gan, TJ (2006) Risk factors for postoperative nausea and vomiting, *Anesthesia and Analgesia*, **102**(6): 1884–98

Georgalas, C, Paun, S, Zainal, A et al. (2002) Assessing day-case septorhinoplasty: prospective audit study using patient-based indices, *Journal of Laryngology and Otology*, **116**(9): 707–10

Gilbert, J (1989) Nursing in a day care unit, in EG Bradshaw and HT Davenport (eds), *Day Care: Surgery, Anaesthesia and Management*, London: Edward Arnold

Gilmartin, J and Wright, K (2007) The nurse's role in day surgery: a literature review, *International Nursing Review*, **54**(2): 183–90

Gilmartin, J and Wright, K (2008) Day surgery: patients felt abandoned during the preoperative wait, *Journal of Clinical Nursing*, **17**(18): 2418–25

Hammond, C and Smith, I (2004) Day surgery design: has anyone asked the patients? *Journal of One Day Surgery*, **14**(4): 91–4

Hayward, J (1975) *Information: A Prescription Against Pain*, Series 2, No. 5, London: Royal College of Nursing

Hazelgrove, JF and Robins, DW (2002) Caring for the carer: an audit of the day surgery services for carers within the Wessex Region of England, *Ambulatory Surgery*, **8**(1): 13–18

Healthcare Commission (2005) *Day Surgery*, London: Healthcare Commission

Hein, A, Norlander, C, Blom, L and Jakobsson, J (2001) Is pain prophylaxis in minor gynaecological surgery of clinical value? A double-blind placebo controlled study of paracetamol 1 g versus Lornoxicam 8 mg given orally, *Ambulatory Surgery*, **9**(2): 91–4

Jakobsen, DH, Callesen, T, Schouenborg, L et al. (2003) Convalescence after laparoscopic sterilisation, *Ambulatory Surgery*, **10**(2): 95–9

Kleinbeck, SV and Hoffart, N (1994) Outpatient recovery after laparoscopic cholecystectomy, *Association of Operating Room Nurses' Journal*, **60**(3): 394–402

Koscielniak-Nielsen, ZJ, Rotboll-Nielsen, P and Rassmussen, H (2002) Patients' experiences with multiple stimulation axillary block for fast-track ambulatory hand surgery, *Acta Anaesthesiologica Scandinavica*, **46**(7): 789–93

Krohne, HW (1978) Individual differences in coping with stress and anxiety, in CD Spielberger and IG Sarason (eds), *Stress and Anxiety*, vol. 5, London: Wiley

Krohne, HW and Slangen, KE (2005) Influence of social support on adaptation to surgery, *Health Psychology*, **24**(1): 101–5

Lack, JA, Rollin, A-M, Thoms, G et al. (2003) *Raising the Standard: Information for Patients*, London: RCoA and AAGBI

Leino-Kilpi, H and Vuorenheimo, J (1993) Peri-operative nursing care quality, *Association of Operating Room Nurses' Journal*, **57**(5): 1061–71

Leinonen, T, Leino-Kilpi, H and Jouko, K (1996) The quality of intra-operative nursing care: the patient's perspective, *Journal of Advanced Nursing*, **24**(4): 843–52

Litt, MD, Nye, C and Shafer, D (1995) Preparation for oral surgery: Evaluating elements of coping, *Journal of Behavioural Medicine*, **18**(5): 435–59

Litt, MD, Kalinowski, L and Shafer, D (1999) A dental fears typology of oral surgery patients: Matching patients to anxiety interventions, *Health Psychology*, **18**(6): 614–24

Lorenz, SG (2007) The potential of the patient room to promote healing and well-being in patients and nurses: an integrative review of the research, *Holistic Nursing Practice*, **21**(5): 263–77

McCarthy, SC, Lyons, AC, Weinman, J et al. (2003) Do expectations influence recovery from oral surgery? An illness representation approach, *Psychology and Health*, **18**(1): 109–26

McGrath, B, Elgendy, H, Chung, F et al. (2004) Thirty percent of patients have moderate to severe pain 24 hr after ambulatory surgery: a survey of 5,703 patients, *Canadian Journal of Anaesthesia*, **51**(9): 886–91

McHugh, GA and Thoms, GM (2002) The management of pain following day-case surgery, *Anaesthesia*, **57**(3): 270–5

Mahler, HI and Kulik, JA (2000) Optimism, pessimism and recovery from coronary bypass surgery: Prediction of affect, pain and functional status, *Psychology, Health and Medicine*, **5**(4): 347–58

Mauleon, AL, Palo-Bengtsson, L and Ekman, S-L (2007) Patients experiencing local anaesthesia and hip surgery, *Journal of Clinical Nursing*, **16**(5): 892–9

Mills, RT and Krantz, DS (1979) Information, choice and reactions to stress: A field experiment in a blood bank with laboratory analogue, *Journal of Personality and Social Psychology*, **37**(4): 608–20

Mitchell, MJ (1997) Patients' perceptions of pre-operative preparation for day surgery, *Journal of Advanced Nursing*, **26**(2): 356–63

Mitchell, MJ (2000a) Psychological preparation for patients undergoing day surgery, *Ambulatory Surgery*, **8**(1): 19–29

Mitchell, MJ (2000b) Anxiety management: a distinct nursing role in day surgery, *Ambulatory Surgery*, **8**(3): 119–28

Mitchell, MJ (2004) Pain management in day-case surgery, *Nursing Standard*, **18**(25): 33–8

Mitchell, MJ (2005) *Anxiety Management in Adult Day Surgery: A Nursing Perspective*, London: Whurr

Mitchell, MJ (2007) Nursing research into modern day surgery: a literature review, *Ambulatory Surgery*, **13**(4): 1–29

2

Mitchell, MJ (2008) Conscious surgery: influence of the environment on patient anxiety, *Journal of Advanced Nursing*, **64**(3): 261–71

Moon, JS and Cho, KS (2001) The effects of handholding on anxiety in cataract surgery patients under local anaesthesia, *Journal of Advanced Nursing*, **35**(3): 407–15

Moran, S, Jarvis, S and Ewings, P (1998) It's good to talk but is it effective? A comparative study of telephone support following day surgery, *Clinical Effectiveness in Nursing*, **2**(4): 175–84

NHS Scotland (2005) *Building a Health Service Fit for the Future: A National Framework for Service Change in the NHS in Scotland* (Kerr Report), Edinburgh: Scotland

Ojo, EO, Ihezue, CH, Sule, AZ et al. (2008) The safety of day case surgery in a developing country, *Journal of One Day Surgery*, **18**(1): 13–18

Older, CG, Carr, EC and Layzell, M (2010) Making sense of patients' use of analgesics following day case surgery, *Journal of Advanced Nursing*, **66**(3): 511–21

Pai, I and Nicholl, J E (2005) Are your day-case patients adequately informed? A survey comparing day-case and inpatients, *Journal of Evaluation in Clinical Practice*, **11**(5): 509–12

Parlow, JL, Meikle, AT, van Vlymen, J and Avery, N (1999) Post-operative nausea and vomiting after ambulatory laparoscopy is not reduced by promethazine prophylaxis, *Canadian Journal of Anesthesia*, **46**(8): 719–24

Parsons, EC, Kee, CC and Gray, P (1993) Peri-operative nursing caring behaviours, *Association of Operating Room Nurses' Journal*, **57**(5): 1106–14

Perez, F, Monton, E, Nodal, MJ et al. (2006) Evaluation of a mobile health system for supporting postoperative patients following day surgery, *Journal of Telemedicine and Telecare*, **12**(1): 41–3

Pfisterer, M, Ernst, EM, Hirlekar, G et al. (2001) Post-operative nausea and vomiting in patients undergoing day-case surgery: An international, observational study, *Ambulatory Surgery*, **9**(1): 13–18

Prewett, AT, Thakkar, H and Found, P (2008) An audit of patient satisfaction with anaesthetic services in a large day surgery unit, *Journal of One Day Surgery*, **18**(1): 22–5

Rosenbaum, M and Piamenta, R (1998) Preference for local or general anesthesia, coping dispositions, learned resourcefulness and coping with surgery, *Psychology and Health*, **13**(5): 823–45

Rosenberger, PH, Jokl, P and Ickovics, J (2006) Psychosocial factors and surgical outcomes: an evidence-based literature review, *Journal of the American Academy of Orthopaedic Surgeons*, **14**(7): 397–405

Royal College of Anaesthetists (2006) *Risk Associated with your Anaesthetic*: Section 1, *Feeling Sick*, London: RCoA

Royal College of Surgeons of England (2007) *Improving your Elective Patient's Journey*, London: Royal College of Surgeons of England Patient Liaison Group

Royal College of Surgeons of England/East Anglia Regional Health Authority (1995) *New Angles on Day Surgery*, NHS Executive: East Anglia Regional Clinical Audit Office

Ruuth-Setala, A, Leino-Kilpi, H and Suominen, T (2000) How do I manage at home? Where do Finnish short-stay patients turn for help, support and company after discharge, and why? *Journal of One Day Surgery*, **10**(1): 15–18

Schroder, KE and Schwarzer, R (1998) Coping as a mediator from recovery from cardiac surgery, *Psychology and Health*, **13**(1): 83–97

Shiloh, S, Zukerman, G, Butin, B. et al. (2003) Post-operative patient-controlled analgesia

(PCA): How much control and how much analgesia? *Psychology and Health*, **18**(6): 753–70

Sinclair, DR, Chung, F and Mezei, G (1999) Can postoperative nausea and vomiting be predicted?, *Anesthesiology*, **91**(1): 109–18

Skilton, M (2003) Post-operative pain management in day surgery, *Nursing Standard*, **17**(38): 39–44

Smith, I (2006) Dissecting the myths of day surgery: the anaesthetist's view, *Journal of Perioperative Practice*, **16**(5): 244–8

Stevens, J, van de Mortel, T and Leighton, D (2001) Generating theory from the client's experience of same day laparoscopic sterilisation, *Australian Journal of Holistic Nursing*, **8**(1): 23–30

Suhonen, RA, Iivonen, MK and Välimäki, MA (2007) Day-case surgery patients' health-related quality of life, *International Journal of Nursing Practice,* **13**(2): 121–9

Teasdale, K (1995) The nurse's role in anxiety management, *Professional Nurse*, **10**(8): 509–12

Toftgaard, C (2007) World wide day surgery activity 2003, *Ambulatory Surgery*, **13**(1): 6–25

Van den Bosch, JE, Bonsel, GJ and Kalkman, CJ (2005) Does measurement of preoperative anxiety have added value for predicting postoperative nausea and vomiting?, *Anesthesia and Analgesia*, **100**(5): 1525–32

Volicer, BJ (1973) Perceived stress levels of events associated with the experience of hospitalisation: development and testing of a measurement tool, *Nursing Research*, **22**(6): 491–7

Ward, C, Varvinski, A and Montgomery, J (2007) Patients' choice of induction method: do patients prefer being given a choice of their induction method?, *Journal of One Day Surgery*, **17**(2): 33–6

Weinberg, DB (2003) *Code Green: Money Driven Hospitals and the Dismantling of Nursing*, Ithaca, NY: Cornell Press

Weltz, CR, Klein, SM, Arbo, JE and Greengrass, RA (2003) Paravertebral block anesthesia for inguinal hernia repair, *World Journal of Surgery*, **27**(4): 425–9

Williams, A, Ching, M and Loader, J (2003) Assessing patient satisfaction with day surgery at a metropolitan public hospital, *Australian Journal of Advanced Nursing*, **21**(1): 35–41

Wilson-Barnett, J (1976) Patient's emotional reactions to hospitalisation: an exploratory study, *Journal of Advanced Nursing*, **1**(5): 351–8

Wu, CL, Berenholtz, SM, Pronovost, PJ and Fleisher, LA (2002) Systematic review and analysis of postdischarge symptoms after outpatient surgery, *Anesthesiology*, **96**(4): 994–1003

Yellen, EA and Ricard, R (2005) The effect of a preadmission videotape on patient satisfaction, *American Operating Room Nurses' Journal*, **81**(4): 831–40

Lovemore Nyatanga and Brian Nyatanga

In this chapter we will explore:

> What death is
> Death and existentialism
> Caring for dying patients
> Beliefs and practices regarding death and dying
> Grief and bereavement
> Caring within the hospice setting
> Assisted dying

Introduction

This chapter presents the most elusive aspect of human existence; it is also the most challenging aspect of our ability to understand the essence of life and death. Philosophers and psychologists have, over many years, debated the issue of life and death without reaching any unanimous conclusion. Most people would agree that life is the beginning of death, while death signals the end of life. However, although we all know death is a certainty, we tend to go about our daily lives fearful of it, as if we know how it will affect us at the time. Plato (427–347 BC) captured the debate so well in *Apology,* when Socrates asserted that:

> To fear death, gentlemen, is no other than to think oneself wise when one is not, to think one knows what one does not know. No one knows whether death may not be the greatest of all blessings for man, yet men fear it as if they knew that it is the greatest of evils. And surely it is the most blameworthy ignorance to believe that one knows what one does not know. (Cooper 1997)

Given his assertion that there may be global ignorance about death, it is important to explore some of conceptions of death and dying.

What is death?

The term 'death' is itself ambiguous as it has life as a precursor (Lukacs 1978; Brown 2008). What compounds this ambiguity is that life is also a concept that is not entirely clear. In other words, each time people ask what is death, they also implicitly ask what is life because these two are linked. Although it may seem quite logical to suggest here that when life ends, death begins, the reality is that it is not as clear-cut as that. Admittedly, this is simplistic because some people view the end of life or death as the beginning of a new life, even if Sartre claims this to be 'bad faith'. Death is therefore seen as a transition to that new life. Other people view death as only referring to the body as the soul or spirit carries on living. The ending of life is one thing, and Honderich (1995) claims that this process too is ambiguous. If the ending of life is not clear, then it follows that death is equally ambiguous. In living we are dying, and our lives are progressively extinguished, until finally we are gone (dead), in a process that stretches out over a period of time. This is true and we can view death as a threshold concept, which means that a sufficiently substantial extinction of life must occur before death takes place. 'The ending of life', hence 'death', can refer either to this entire process, or solely to its last part – the loss of the very last trace of life. Thus death can be a *state*, the *process of extinction*, or the *denouement* (final completion) of that process. Because of this, it follows that other people, including patients we care for, will have different ideas and definitions of death. For some, this may either be too complex to contemplate or too frightening to think about, therefore they may choose not to engage in any talk or discussion about death in general, let alone their own. Table 11.1 provides a list of different definitions of death, and goes a long way to show the difficulty of defining death in the same way.

Table 11.1 *Different definitions of death*

Type of death	Definition
Necrobiosis	Death of individual cells (except nerve cells) of an organism over a life span. New cells replace the dead cells in a continual process throughout the life span
Necrosis	The death of many cells at once, which can result in the death of an organ or part of it. In medicine, it is referred to as an 'infarction'
Clinical death	Denoted by lack of breathing, lack of blood circulation and lack of brain activity. Clinical death begins with the onset of symptoms of death or cardiac arrest
Brain death	Death caused by depriving the brain of oxygen continuously for three to seven minutes. After that, the brain is incapable of being brought back to life
Somatic death	A complete seizure, permanent and irreversible death of an organism. Such death in humans usually follows brain death as other organs rely on the brain to function, with the exception of artificial support

Source: Nyatanga 2008. Reproduced with permission from Quay Books

Death as a part of life

In the context of death as a part of life perpective, death is seen as something that is inevitable, and therefore every person has to come to terms with it in order to live well. Heidegger ([1927]1962) considers the human condition as 'being' moving towards death and bases it on his existential argument. He views death as one of the structural features of human existence that everyone has to acknowledge or assume. He further claims that no one becomes truly adult unless they assume and accept their birth and death. It is important that the human condition (including death) is accepted if we are to be truly human (Heidegger [1927]1962). The question we need to ask is: What makes it hard for people to openly accept their impending deaths? If death is part of life, maybe we need to embrace it so that it may become easier to discuss our fears and anxieties about death.

Death as an interruption

Unlike sleep, death is a permanent interruption to life. The fact that death can interrupt a young, middle-aged or older life, including men and women, black or white, rich or poor, makes it indiscriminate and unpredictable. This may explain why people fear it to the degree of not being able to talk about it. Death signals the end of our input into our own aspirations, projects and other worthy activities. However, despite this, people tend to react in different ways by adopting attitudes, such as ignore it and live life in spite of it. Some choose to confront it and find ways of 'beating' it, as in medical advances, but with little success. If success is not possible, there are now attempts to try and slow down the process of ageing and dying, thus delaying death. These actions tend to stress the life-preserving attitude of our societies, particularly those in the Western world.

Death as a transition

The perspective of death as a transition can be thought of as attempting to quell any fear connected with death by suggesting that what really matters is the life after this earthly one. Therefore death is only a transition to that better (eternal) life. This view encourages people to embrace death and not fear it, at least for those who largely believe in a God or higher power. The other consideration in this perspective is that only the soul would be capable of surviving the body and making the transition. This raises three fundamental questions:

1 Does the identity of that person change or does it become incomplete without the body?
2 Does the body/mind dualism, as argued by Descartes, exist? According to Descartes (1591–1650), the body and mind are separate entities and the mind is the more fundamental of the two. However, Descartes could not prove completely how these two entities (body and mind) existed and indeed interacted within a person. Other philosophers, particularly the existentialists (see below), have tried to explain conceptions of death and some of the ambiguities surrounding death and dying.
3 Does the idea of a life after death act as a convenient buffer against fear of death?

Death and existentialism

There can be no better place to start the exploration of the different conceptions of human existence than existential philosophy (also popularly known as existentialism). Some of the key exponents of existentialism include Søren Kierkegaard, Martin Heidegger, Jean-Paul Sartre, Simone de Beauvoir, Friedrich Nietzsche, Gabriel Marcel, Albert Camus and Edmund Husserl. Existentialism as a philosophy has been championed by Kierkegaard (Honderich 2005) as an alternative to the rationalist philosophy of Hegel and Descartes, for example. For Kierkegaard and other existentialists, the central premise is that 'existence precedes essence' (Sartre 2003). This premise implies that an individual has no predetermined path or purpose in life beyond what the individual chooses. Through such choices, individuals create their own nature and indeed their own essence – hence the premise, existence precedes essence (Figure 11.1).

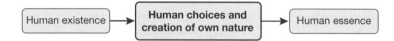

Figure 11.1 *Existence precedes essence*

Figure 11.1 signifies the existentialists' debate on the ontology of human existence. Ontology may be defined as the 'science of being' (Wyschogrod 1954) – the study of the form of things and their associations. According to Weston (1994), Heidegger uses the concept of '*Dasein*' (literally meaning 'to be there' in the world) to explore the ontology of human existence. Heidegger sees *Dasein* as existential possibilities open to people. Weston (1994) remarks on *Dasein* as the unique aspect of human existence, which interprets everyday experiences, turning them into our own unique ways of being in the world (see Figure 11.2).

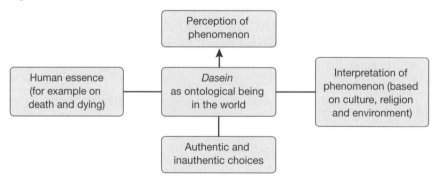

Figure 11.2 *The ontology of human existence*

Dasein has a primordial structure (also known as existential possibilities). *Dasein*'s primordial structure can be chosen and followed with great emotional investment, for example life and death. The choices people make from *Dasein*'s existential possibilities can be said to be 'authentic' if they best represent reality (albeit subjective reality) and fulfilment. Needless to say, 'inauthentic' choices are those that encapsulate self-deception and bad faith. Within this chapter, 'bad faith' has a philosophical meaning, as outlined by Jean-Paul Sartre ([1943]2003). Bad faith (*mauvaise foi*) is about individuals engaging in self-deception such as wishing to believe the falsely obvious, as when individuals wish to believe falsely that a loved one will not die when they already are in a coma. Bad faith, in this case, is inauthentic because it conspires to deceive the self and others by presenting a 'lie' as a pleasant untruth. Thus the issue of authentic and inauthentic choices becomes ontologically more pressing when death and dying are the focus of debate. The possibility that death subconsciously conjures up the greatest anxiety in human beings is stated by Pattison (1997), who cites Kierkegaard, Heidegger and Sartre. The anxiety or fear is anchored on the awareness of the possibility of not being (nonexistence) in the world. The anxiety is worsened by the possibility of nothingness, as well as the possibility of total disintegration of the self. As if this was not enough, there is the possibility of grave uncertainties regarding events that may or may not occur beyond death. For Kierkegaard and Heidegger (Weston 1994), death anxiety (or ontological anxiety) might ultimately be the fear of the possibility of not having any further existential possibilities. For some people, a futile attempt to keep death anxiety under check is to engage in ritualistic reassurances that are in themselves obviously false but mask the impulse to panic or run away from it all. Generally, some people will often use euphemisms to hide or minimise death anxiety. This psychological indulgence is important for them as a way of 'buffering' the impact of death anxiety. Table 11.2 provides some common euphemisms used in relation to someone who has died.

Table 11.2 Common euphemisms

Journey euphemisms	Rest euphemisms	Loss euphemisms
The departed Cross the great divide Go to meet one's maker Go to the happy hunting ground Joining the angels Joining one's ancestors A big send-off	Gone to eternal rest Resting in peace Gone to one's rest Now in Heaven Everlasting sleep Everlasting peace	No longer with us Will be sadly missed Society has lost … The greatest With fond memories Reported missing Unaccounted for Off the record
Reward euphemisms	**Joy euphemisms**	**End euphemisms**
No more suffering No more pain Freedom of the soul Relieved of suffering Called to rest	Peaceful In the arms of the Father United with God In Heaven In Paradise Singing with the angels	The late … No more Deceased Time or number was up Presumed dead Debt we all must pay Pull the plug

The role of euphemisms

People's tendency to use euphemisms as a defence against death anxiety is most likely to begin with their cultural and religious socialisation. For most people, their dependence on parents and society as role models may have a lot to do with the eventual inauthenticity and self-deception inherent in euphemisms. The language and the kindness of words used to describe the dead person have always been fascinating. Just like the fear of the possibility of having no further existential possibilities, euphemisms express a pervasive fear of the unknown, hence the six categories of euphemisms. The fear of the loss of a loved one and fear of *Dasein*'s own possibility of death brings about the pseudo-humbleness expressed through euphemisms. The media and in particular newspaper obituaries are a rich platform for death euphemisms. Obituaries are more than cultural rituals. They have a strong social and cultural function for most people. Nyatanga (2008), for example, argues that death is often compared to the sun that influences the natural order of things. This is yet another euphemism that prefers to see the bright side of death as opposed to the dark and feared reality that it is for most people. Euphemisms therefore help to replace fear with hope, which in turn creates a sense of order, security and meaning. Without these mental processes, death might be the most scary phenomenon, for no one knows its real consequences. To recap, euphemisms serve to soften the impact of death on a family, a people, a community and society. Also euphemisms encourage the portrayal of positive aspects within a death, while focusing on the 'good' positive aspects of the person who has died. We return later to elaborate on this last point to show the need and beliefs that perpetuate such practices.

Perceptions of death across the life span

The general view, according to existentialism, is that individuals deny their susceptibility to death even though they may privately acknowledge the inevitability of death. Because of this, it may explain how death is generally viewed as a taboo topic and people use flowery language to sweeten death talk. No one seems willing to talk directly about death, hence we have an abundance of euphemisms, as shown above. So how do children, for example, come to know about death and dying? The answer is as difficult as the question itself because:

> Children have their own existence with an emerging essence
> There are numerous sources of knowledge about death (authentic as well as inauthentic)
> Parents, according to Freud, often project their death anxiety onto their children. This projected anxiety is seen as protecting the child from the unnecessary distress of death and dying. Indeed, some parents do not think it is proper to take young children to any funeral other than, perhaps in a few instances, the child's own parent. It is, however, acknowledged that this Freudian assertion may not apply to other cultures, where all family members are expected to be present at funerals.

Nagy (1948) carried out one of the pioneering studies into children's under-standing of death. She concluded that there were at least three stages of understanding: age 3–5 – death as a faded continuation of life; age 5–9 – death as final; age 9 plus – death not only final but also inevitable. The implication of Nagy's outline is twofold:

1 There is the assumption that children younger than three do not really have a traceable conception of death. Thus, infants and some toddlers do not understand death at all, even though they can sense when there is sadness, fear, anxiety and excitement around them. These nonspecific early sensa-tions may become important when children begin to develop their understanding of death between the ages of three to five.

2 Children over the age of nine tend to have a similar understanding of death to adults. They appreciate that death is permanent and that bodily functions cease.

Nagy's model has had support from developmental psychologists (for example Vygotsky and Piaget), who believe that the understanding of death is a factor of cognitive development. Elsewhere, it has been confirmed that the 'develop-ment of the death concept' questionnaire shows significant differences in the conception of death between age groups. These differences support the cogni-tive developmental approach but are sometimes compromised by the socialised articulation of death and dying. This socialised articulation is the environmental imperative implied by Goodwin and Davidson (1991).

Caring for dying patients: a student nurse's perspective

There is a dearth of research on how student nurses feel about caring for dying patients. One recent study by Cooper and Barnet (2005) is worthy of discus-sion here, as it reported a number of aspects of caring for the dying that caused anxiety to first year student nurses. Cooper and Barnet concluded that it was more the aspects of the caring role, as opposed to student nurses' personal fear of death, that contributed to much of the anxiety experienced. Some of the aspects identified included students not being able to cope with the physical suffering of the patient they were caring for. It seems that the main aspects of difficulty were seeing physical deterioration and pain that could not be controlled.

Some student nurses reported feelings of inadequacy, when they felt unable to do more to help patients. They felt inadequate in their knowledge of inter-ventions to use and skills to communicate and offer support. Students felt, as Buckman (1990) has acknowledged, that they did not know what to say to dying patients. Another area that caused anxiety was the ending of the rela-tionship with dying patients when students finished their placements. This suggests students had already developed strong relationships with patients to a level of provoking emotional responses at the time of leaving their placements.

Students who witnessed sudden death experienced more distress than witnessing an expected death. This reaction may not be restricted to student nurses but include most people, even experienced professionals. It is possible that with sudden death, students may not have felt able to provide sensitive care that would arguably enhance the quality of life for the dying patient. Witnessing a death of younger patients was more stressful than that of older ones, as students might have identified more with the young deceased person. It is logical to suggest that students may have found rationalisation of an older person's death more comfortable than that of a younger person.

One final point from Cooper and Barnet's (2005) study was the impact of performing last offices. Last offices are an important part of completing the dying process (Nyatanga and de Vocht 2009), but for students, this was their first time of seeing, touching and washing a dead body. Students in Cooper and Barnet's study identified procedural aspects, such as the packaging of orifices, dealing with dentures and covering the dead body's head with a white sheet, as sources of their anxiety. It is clear from the findings of this study that student nurses invest emotionally when engaged in caring for dying patients. What needs emphasising is the need for mentor support, early training in communication skills, but most importantly, palliative care education before students go out on such placements.

Beliefs and practices regarding death and dying

Earlier, we discussed the existential premise that 'existence precedes essence'. It is this essence that creates our beliefs about death. It is also this essence that governs the practices associated with death and related bereavement behaviour. This section links, where possible, cultural or religious beliefs, care of the dying and possibilities beyond death. Human beliefs about death and what happens next are often expressed through chosen euphemisms. According to Murray Parkes et al. (2003), cultural and sometimes religious beliefs heavily influence beliefs and customs relating to death. Religion has certainly had an impact on the possibility of life beyond death as well as the issues of body, soul and spirit. The following sections present some of the common beliefs and practices regarding death in four major belief systems.

Christianity

Christians are religious people who follow the teaching of the Holy Bible. They see the life and work of Jesus Christ as an example of how they should live their lives (hence Christianity). Jesus himself is said to have been born in Nazareth (Israel). During his life on Earth, Jesus had 12 disciples specially chosen to form the essence of his work and teachings. It is therefore not surprising that the earliest followers of Christianity were Jews. The Jews believed Jesus to be the Messiah (saviour of mankind) as exemplified by his death on Good Friday and resurrection on Easter Sunday. Before Jesus himself went to heaven, it is thought he had the Last Supper with his disciples. At the Last Supper, Jesus is said to have given them bread and wine as symbols of his body and blood respectively. In John 6:54, Jesus is said to have told his disciples that: 'Whoever eats my flesh and drinks my blood has eternal life, and I will raise him up at the last day.' This, for many Christians, is reassurance that death in this world may not be the absolute end.

However, not all Christians view death in the same way (Nyatanga 2008). For example, Christians such as Roman Catholics and Protestants in Ireland tend to celebrate the death of a loved one. The celebration is also another way of thanking God for the life of the deceased. The World Council of Churches (Cracknell and White 2005) came into being in 1948 as a recognition of the different interpretations of scriptures. It also believed that the diversity of interpretations may have been endorsed within the New Testament of the Holy Bible. The book of Acts 10:34–35 says: 'I truly understand that God shows no partiality, but in every nation anyone who fears him and does what is right is acceptable to him.'

Judaism

Judaism or the Jewish practice of death and dying is based on a number of biblical interpretations. For example, Genesis 3:19 states: 'For you are dust and to dust shall you return.' For Judaism, this suggests that since human beings came from the earth, it is appropriate that they return to it at death. This interpretation also explains why cremation is not a favoured Jewish option. Another aspect that distinguishes Judaism from other practices is the speed with which the dead are buried. It seems that the urgency of burial is based on another interpretation of the Bible. Deuteronomy 21:23 states: 'His body shall not remain all night … you shall bury him on that day.' The belief here is that the soul returns to God immediately after death. There is therefore no reason to hang on to the body any longer than it is humanly possible to bury it. If the soul goes to God immediately, the body must be returned to earth immediately.

Attending to the body and soul of the dead is another important aspect of Judaism. Normally the body of a dead person is never left unattended, and whoever is with the dead person at the point of their death does not leave until burial. It is considered respectful to watch over the dead person's body during the transition from this life into the next. In terms of last offices (final preparation of the body after death), the mouth and eyes of the dead person should be closed and a sheet should cover the face. The dead person's feet should be positioned such that they are facing the doorway. The last offices may include the religious process of cleansing and purifying the body (taharah), normally carried out by culturally qualified and knowledgeable burial society personnel.

Hinduism

Much of what is believed in Hinduism comes from the doctrine of karma. Karma means action or the effects of action. The actions are rather moralistic in the sense that good actions have good effect while bad actions have bad effect. Since good actions and good effect are the ultimate goal of existence, Hinduism believes that people with bad actions die but reincarnate until they finally gain respite (moksha). To gain moksha, the person must live a life without sin. In cases of death through illness, the dying person should be lifted out of bed and gently put onto the floor. Their head is normally turned towards the north. To die in this way signifies respect for the earth (where life began) and facilitates the departure of the soul from the body after death. Part of the dying process involves relatives specially called to perform death rites such as dipping leaves of sweet basil in holy water from the River Ganges. Water drops from the leaves are then placed on the lips of the dying person. During this process, relatives also sing holy songs and read from the Vedas (the sacred scriptures of Hinduism). From a medical viewpoint, it is important to appreciate that Hindus may refuse medication when they believe they are about to die. This refusal is based on the belief that it is of great importance to die with all our senses clear. As medication may alter one's state of consciousness, some Hindus may decline medication.

Following death, the body is washed and anointed with special fragrances before being dressed in pure white. The body is then placed in a coffin. When other protocols have been fulfilled, the coffin is then taken to the crematorium. At the crematorium, the main mourner (usually the oldest son or such designated person), will light a candle placed on top of the coffin. This lit candle signifies the lighting of the crematorium pyre. Cremation releases the soul while the ashes of the dead person are usually scattered over the River Ganges or equivalent. Hindu funerals mark the transition from this life to another and death is the beginning of that great journey.

Islam

Muslims believe in Allah and his messenger Muhammad. The teachings of Allah are contained in the Koran (Qur'an) and those who abide by the Koran will have eternal life. For those who are dead, Islam asserts they will wake up on Judgement Day. Until Judgement Day, the dead remain in their graves. Allah will judge each person according to how well they lived their earthily lives.

In terms of the dying process, it is normal for relatives and friends to gather around the dying person. The gathering is about giving comfort to the dying person. Relatives and friends also cite verses from the Koran, and ask for final forgiveness. Ideally, a Muslim's last words are: 'I bear witness that there is no god but Allah.' This is the final declaration of faith in this life and life after death (that starts on Judgment Day).

Following death, the eyes should be closed and the body covered with a clean white sheet. As part of the last offices, the family will normally wash the dead body with clean and sometimes scented water. The washed body is then shrouded and wrapped in a kafan (clean white burial sheet). Use of the kafan does not apply to martyrs as they are normally buried in the clothes in which they died.

Grief and bereavement research

Grief and **bereavement** tend to be considered as ways of resolving one's loss and adapting to life without the 'thing' or person. Loss is a common experience in human existence. Throughout life, it is possible that one might have experienced a number of losses, resulting in what we now call 'cumulative loss'. Major loss tends to stimulate personal growth and social readjustment; however, the opposite is true where there is poor management of these processes.

Over many years, studies on loss, grief and bereavement have been carried out, which have resulted in the formulation of theories and models used to support bereaved people. Table 11.3 sketches some of these studies from the 1930s onwards.

Table 11.3 Research studies on loss, grief and bereavement

Author(s)	Date	Innovation	Area studied
Eliot	1930	Family grief	Identified need for studies on family grief
Eliot	1933	Social psychology of bereavement	Identified the need for research into social psychology of bereavement
Lindemann	1944	Psychiatric	Study of acute grief responses of survivors of night club fire deaths
Irion	1954	Mourning as adaptation	Studied perspectives on mourning as a process of adaptation to loss
Freud	1957	Psychoanalysis	Proposed that grief is a process to resolve loss
Marris	1958	Structuralist	Studied women's responses to death of their spouses
Murray Parkes	1964	Assumptive worlds	Effects of bereavement on widows' mental and physical health
Peretz	1970	Psychoanalysis	Reactions to loss and separation as tied to psychic conflicts in children
Kübler-Ross	1970	Adaptation	Identified five-stage reaction people go through following knowledge of impending death
Bowlby	1973, 1980	Attachment	Grief as adaptive response taking account of present and past meanings of loss
Schoenberg et al.	1974	Anticipatory grief	Study of anticipatory grief and impact on spouses

Author(s)	Date	Innovation	Area studied
Rosenblatt et al.	1976	Cultural	Studied cultural variations in bereavement
Worden	1982	Grief work	Developed a staged model to work through grief
Murray Parkes and Weiss	1983	Bereavement outcomes	Study on predictor variables for estimating bereavement outcomes
Prunkl and Berry	1988	Four-room model of the dying and grieving process	Reported that each room in the model characterises a particular reaction to dying and the grieving process
Doka	1989	Grief	Explored the concept of disenfranchised grief
Balk	1990, 1996	Adolescents	Studied sibling bereavement in adolescents
Davies	1991	Adolescents	Studied sibling bereavement in adolescents
Rando	1992/93	Mourning	Examined impact of complicated mourning
Stroebe et al.	1995	Alternative outcomes of bereavement	Reported different viewpoint about the outcome of bereavement. Introduced the dual process model of bereavement
Tonkin	1996	Growth around grief model	Concluded that the size of grief does not reduce with time, but remains the same. The bereaved person grows and develops around the grief and deals with it effectively (see Figure 11.3)
Worden and Silverman	1996	Child adjustment	Studied the effects of parental death on child adjustment

As can be seen from Table 11.3, research studies were carried out in relation to loss, grief and bereavement of different age groups and circumstances. Some studies focused on children, while others focused on adults. Interest in the study of death led to systematic research in many disciplines, which also led to the development of death education for both lay and professional people (Pine 1977). Research on loss and bereavement was closely associated with the emergence of the 'death movement' in the 1950s (for example Irion 1954; Jackson 1957; Marris 1958; Murray Parkes 1964; Doka 1989, 2007). Murray Parkes (1972) was instrumental in developing knowledge of bereavement in adult life, which included the identification of variables that predicted bereavement outcomes following the death of a spouse (for example Murray Parkes and Weiss 1983; Laungani and Morgan 2005).

Kübler-Ross (1970) identified five reaction stages people may go through when faced with impending death: denial, anger, bargaining, depression and acceptance. Because these reactions depend on different people's feelings and perceptions of death and what it means, it is possible that the sequence of reactions is not always linear. The suggestion is that some people may deny death one minute and then accept it and later on be angry about it. On another day, they may be bargaining for more time, before getting angry again and so on.

In the 1980s, bereavement models were multidimensional and process oriented (Diamond 1981; Murphy 1983; Demi 1984). Studies focused on all types of loss and bereavement, including parental bereavement guilt, loss of pregnancy (Swanson-Kauffman 1986), adolescent sibling bereavement, to just name a few.

Up until the 1990s, there was consensus on the process and outcomes of bereavement, that is, that it is mainly to help the bereaved to work through the chaos created by the loss. However, differences began to emerge with stimulating debate from Stroebe et al. (1995) on the myths and misconceptions associated with loss and bereavement. Stroebe et al. (1995) argued that there was a dual process at each given time of bereavement, and that the bereaved could oscillate between the loss- and restoration-oriented dimensions of bereavement. The dual process enables the bereaved to seek new ways of restoring their lives, while being able to reflect on the loss and perhaps putting it into its rightful perspective. This process is contrary to Freud's ideas that, in order for the bereaved to restore normal life, they must completely 'withdraw' their energies/thoughts from the deceased, thereby suggesting a clear separation between grief work and new life without the deceased. (See Nyatanga 2008, Ch. 11, p. 251, for a more detailed explanation of the dual process model of bereavement.)

Misconceptions of bereavement

Some models of bereavement suggest that grief is something the bereaved should 'work through' in stages or in a linear type of progression. The idea is for the bereaved person to regain some order in their life. What we want to stress here is that setting time frames for the bereaved to move through is not helpful. Suggesting and advocating that bereaved people create some 'order' in their life seems insensitive to their particular needs. One possible explanation might be that when carers feel unable to 'deal' with the chaos of the emotional, cognitive, spiritual and behavioural outburst from the bereaved, they distance themselves by applying models, as they seem safer than chaos. Bayliss (2008) has challenged carers and professionals to forget 'order' and work with chaos, because chaos is what is happening and real for the bereaved person at that time.

There is another suggestion that with time grief will subside enough to allow the bereaved to live their life again. Considering a recent study by Tonkin (1996), this suggestion is a misconception. Figure 11.3 represents Tonkin's findings. In 11.3a, soon after the loss, the grieving person feels overwhelmed by the loss, and with time, it is suggested that the grief would diminish (11.3b), and the person feels able to function again. According to Tonkin, what actually happened over time was that the size of the grief remained the same but the bereaved person grew in strength and stature to develop around the grief (11.3c) and was able to function again. At this point, 11.3c, the bereaved tend to understand themselves better and their relationship with others including the deceased. This gives them the ability to function again and at appropriate moments to think about the deceased. This is not to disregard the complexity of grief, but to label such grief as pathological, because it does not conform to the models we have come to know, may well be to deny the positive effects it can have (Bayliss 2008).

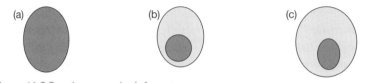

Figure 11.3 *Growing around grief*
Source: Tonkin 1996. Reproduced with permission

The changing face of bereavement

Loss and grief gained wide acceptance as a cause of serious human suffering, and therefore interventions and support programmes were developed. The cause of loss was much more predictable, like cancer and other illnesses. However, the rapid pace of social and technological change has created a new environment where human beings are more vulnerable to drug misuse, virulent microorganisms, AIDS, violence and murders (Benoliel 1997). The global picture today is characterised with death and loss brought about by human pursuits such as warfare, greed, terrorism, genocide, torture and racism. There is also increased environmental pollution, and this too is a cause of death. This picture suggests the world today is increasingly inhabited by people experiencing multiple losses, and therefore multiple bereavements. Benoleil (1997) claims that in most developed countries, bereavement services are slow to develop as they do not always fit with the organising framework of disease and treatment. Funding for bodies that can provide bereavement support such as hospices is minimal, leaving it to voluntary organisations like charities to provide bereavement care. Such care is patchy and often concentrates on extreme cases only, leaving the mild cases to develop to extreme, and the cycle goes on. There is an argument to ensure that high-quality care is given to people before they die, which would in turn 'pave the way' for healthy bereavement processes (Nyatanga 2008).

Nurses have been major players in confronting the challenges of loss and bereavement over the past 50 years (Benoliel 1997). The new global picture of loss and bereavement requires all healthcare professionals to engage in loss and bereavement support. This call also comes with challenges for the training of all healthcare professionals to a level where they can effectively help someone through loss and bereavement. We shall now briefly discuss some of the care available to dying patients and their families.

Care for the dying within hospice settings

During medieval times, the word 'hospice' was used to denote a place where travellers could find rest and shelter on their journey (Saunders 1978). These places were run and maintained by religious orders, and even today some hospices have remnants of religion influencing their care. In the nineteenth and twentieth centuries, the Irish Sisters of Charity began to use the word 'hospice' to refer to homes for dying patients (Saunders 1978). In time, hospices started to offer nursing and medical care for very ill and dying patients. The modern hospice movement was developed by Dame Cicely Saunders, based at St Christopher's Hospice, Sydenham, London. The main remit for the hospice was to improve quality of life for cancer sufferers, but it later diversified into what we now call **palliative care**, a term that suggests care for dying patients regardless of disease.

The World Health Organization (WHO 2004) strongly believes that any care given to dying patients should take into account the needs of relatives and family of the patient, and hence the term 'significant others' is commonly used. Caring for significant others is seen as helping the dying patient's peace of mind while ensuring a smoother bereavement period for families. The overall aim of the philosophy is to return to a more human, family-oriented care that improves the quality of the remaining life of the patient (Lattanzi-Licht and Connor 1995). Because hospices are, by nature, small places where only a few patients at a time can access care, efforts are under way to develop the palliative care philosophy and its principles into the fabric of every healthcare system around the world (WHO 2004). Palliative care is therefore, in essence, a philosophy, and not a facility, that should be applied to all settings caring for dying patients, whose main goal is to achieve a dignified death (Twycross 1997; WHO 2004; Nyatanga 2008).

The practice of palliative care

Palliative care takes place in hospices, hospitals, nursing homes, residential homes and even the patient's home. Palliative care is normally delivered by well-trained nurse specialists, who support dying patients with their emotional as well as physical needs, including pain and symptom control. There are strong emotional reactions encountered at the end of life (Brennan 2010) and therefore palliative care professionals are now being trained to support people with psychological as well as spiritual needs (Twycross 1999; Nyatanga 2008).

Although it is well documented that most people prefer to die at home (Higginson 2003), a large proportion continue to die in hospitals (Field and James 1993; Davies et al. 2006). A study by Davies et al. (2006) showed that a small proportion of patients die in hospices or in their own homes. Nursing homes accounted for the smallest number of all deaths (see Table 11.4). An understanding of the different settings where patients die is important in order for palliative care to be delivered to all patients and their families.

Table 11.4 *Preferred and actual place of death*

Study	Hospital	Hospice	Own home	Nursing home
Actual				
Field and James 1993	54%	4%	23%	13%
Davies et al. 2006	44%	20%	30%	8%
Preferred				
Higginson 2003	11%	24%	56%	Unknown

Hospitals have many advantages in terms of caring as they have most caring facilities under one roof, that is, staff expertise, multidisciplinary diversity, nursing equipment like oxygen and hoists, and readily available medicines and therapies. Caring for patients in the community allows for patients to be cared for in their home and, in a way, health professionals are guests in this setting.

One final thought is that there are patients who, because of a terminal illness, might have contemplated ending their own life with help, only to realise that assisted dying is illegal in the UK and indeed most Western countries. We will now briefly outline why this position seems out of step with such patients' needs.

Assisted dying

In democratic countries like Britain, people are free to do almost anything, with rights that include the freedom of speech, movement, association, marriage and even committing suicide. However, when it comes to asking for assisted dying (AD), especially for those with unbearable terminal suffering, the law of the land does not permit this practice. Lord Joffe has tried unsuccessfully on numerous times to introduce a Bill in Parliament that would legalise AD in this country. However, despite these setbacks, the debate on legalising AD seems to be gaining momentum (at least in the UK). This may be due to recent media coverage of high-profile cases of people travelling abroad to Switzerland for AD. We know of Dan James, a 23-year-old rugby player who was paralysed after a scrum collapsed on him; Craig Ewert, a 59-year-old university lecturer with end stage motor neurone disease; and Dr Anne Turner, long-term sufferer with progressive terminal supranuclear palsy. Anne Turner died with assistance four years ago in Switzerland, but her last moments of life were dramatised in *A short stay in Switzerland* on BBC 1 in January 2009. Recently, Debbie Purdy, who suffers with multiple sclerosis, sought assurance that her husband Omar would not be prosecuted when he accompanies her to Switzerland for assistance when her condition deteriorates. This assurance may have signalled a slight shift in UK legal thinking around AD, but more is needed.

Given that all these people are intelligent, articulate and knew exactly what they wanted or want with their lives, it remains incomprehensible that we continue to deny terminally ill, mentally competent adults suffering unbearably the choice of AD in this country and many other Western countries. Proponents of AD believe in giving people the ability to control their destiny. Those against AD argue that this would open the door to euthanasia and lead to a slippery slope where the vulnerable old are made to feel a burden, and eventually forced into AD. Both secular and religious arguments emphasise the value of life and therefore the need to prolong it or adopt palliative care practices. Recent arguments from palliative care have changed the temperature of the debate by insisting that AD is killing and euthanasia is murder, and therefore have no place in palliative 'care'.

While these arguments seem persuasive, they sadly exclude the voices of the very people they purport to protect, who are faced with the ultimate decision of whether and how to end their lives. Evidence from recent surveys suggests that 80% of Europeans would prefer to have the option to die with assistance (Becker 2006; Cohen et al. 2006). Therefore, continued opposition to AD is not only counterproductive in advancing the debate, but ignores the wishes of patients and surrenders our potential leadership role to shape the future of AD and create necessary safeguards for the vulnerable. The reality is that if we, the healthcare professionals, do not lead, someone else will and this would be irreconcilable with our claim to palliative 'caring'. Most of us now openly accept that even optimal palliative care cannot relieve all suffering in all dying patients. Besides, not every patient is fortunate enough to access the service. People who have travelled abroad, paying up to £3,000 for assistance, are true testimony to the argument that the law needs changing. What we do not know, or maybe admit to, is what happens to those who cannot afford to go abroad. One suggestion is that nearly 20,000 people are being helped to die in the UK alone (see Biggs 2005), either illegally or under double effect practices (when one's otherwise legitimate act, for example relieving a terminally ill patient's pain, will also cause an effect one would normally be obliged to avoid, for example the patient's death). De Vocht and Nyatanga (2007) warned that not legalising AD only creates an illusion that it will not happen.

There is no denying that more and more people will travel abroad for assistance, and we cannot afford to ignore this momentum. We need real debate and the slippery slope argument is becoming an unfortunate metaphor, while the use of alarmist language like killing and murder is not only regressive, but a clear sign of tired arguments. Indeed, legalising AD will not be comfortable but at least it supports the wishes of suffering patients. We are best placed to influence governments to close the passage to Switzerland by legalising AD. This will mean:

> All people, and not just those who can afford to pay, have the choice of AD, which is closely monitored, without the cost and stress of travelling abroad.
> Stringent guidelines are written to protect the vulnerable.
> Dying people can have more time before having to end their life here at

home. At present, they have to travel much earlier while they are still competent to sign papers and so on.

> Upholding unconditional caring, which is also a central philosophy in palliative care.

Good palliative care must therefore empower terminally ill patients to control their own destiny. In some situations, AD can be a dignified end to good palliative care (de Vocht 2008). It is possible that having the option of AD may improve patients' psychological outlook and quality of life to the extent that some may not even use this option. We believe there is good evidence to now legalise AD as a simple act of kindness to those in unbearable suffering.

Take some time to complete the activities below.

Activity 11.1

My own death wishes

If you knew just one week in advance that you were going to die and you had the power and resources to plan your own death, what are the five most important things that you would want before you die?

Share your ideas with others and discuss the possible psychological factors that made you identify your list of five things.

The activity is quite personal and indirectly teases out a person's death anxiety and general attitude to death. This reflective activity can also help nurses and other health professionals in their understanding of contemporary fears and attitudes to death and dying. The important thing about this reflective exercise is that healthcare professionals will most likely reflect or project their death anxieties to the patients and colleagues under their influence. There is nothing wrong in influencing other people, after all, that is what care delivery practice is often about. The issue is whether or not that influence is informed by contemporary research or is evidence based. If not evidence based, then one likely consequence is that patients and professionals alike may perpetuate the myths of death and dying and may themselves be unable to cope with the inevitability of death. It is critical for nurses and other healthcare professionals to reflect on their own perceptions and attitudes to death and dying. In particular, before nurses can help other people to overcome their fear of death and dying, it is imperative that they examine not only their own perceptions but also the death and dying conventions of others including cultural and personal experiences.

Activity 11.2

The good death as a euphemism

If you knew that you were going to drop dead within 24 hours, what are the five most important things that would best prepare you for such a death?

Share your ideas with others and discuss the possible psychological factors that made you identify your list of five things.

The good death may well be argued as one of the newer euphemisms popularised in the twenty-first century. What seems most fascinating about the idea of the good death is that thanatologists (those who study death and dying) and other researchers have concluded that the 'good death' is defined differently by doctors, nurses, patients, families and friends. This means it is a personal euphemism that affords psychological harmony or tranquillity for specific people in specific circumstances. Thus:

> A good death depends on cultural imperatives
> A good death depends on perceived psychological harmony
> A good death is about closure – saying goodbye and sorting out unfinished business
> A good death is about dying surrounded by loved ones
> A good death is about dignity and a pain free end
> Individualistic societies promote the personal autonomy of the dying, including palliative care and voluntary euthanasia.

If the group is mixed age and culture, then this could be a rich source of comparative experiences and ideologies.

Conclusion

The definition of death offered in this chapter acknowledges the difficulty that still exists in finding a unitary view. Despite the various definitions, nearly every culture has perceptions of death and dying. Each culture also tends to have conceptions of the different types of death and whether normal or abnormal. Kellahear (1990), for example, discusses conceptions of an 'acceptable death' and a 'good death'. He argues that an acceptable death is nondramatic, disciplined and with very little emotion. This conception relates to institutional settings such as hospitals, particularly in Western cultures. By contrast, Kellahear (1990) argues that a good death is one that allows for social adjustments and personal preparation by the dying person and their family. This is a time when the dying person attempts to complete unfinished tasks, to say farewells, and for the family to begin to prepare for life without the dying. The point to make, which also makes the understanding of ideas such as a good death elusive, is that there are different perceptions of a good death depending on whether it is the perception of the dying person, relatives, professionals like doctors or society at large. The characteristics of a good death are not universal, therefore there are going to be differences. However, we can suggest here that if we are to ensure a good death, then it has to be from the dying person's perspective in the first instance. However, if you view a good death in terms of the impact it has on the family, then van Gennep's idea may be persuasive. Van Gennep (1960) considers a good death as the funeral that the dying give to the living so as to enable the family to gradually disengage from the dying person as an active part of the family's life. The care offered to dying patients generally falls under palliative care, which aims to ensure that each death is unique and dignified. There are different settings, including hospices, where such care is delivered. However, an important point we raised is that the principles of palliative care should be seen as a philosophy, which should be possible in any setting that cares for dying patients. It was emphasised that an added bonus of providing high-quality care to dying patients is that bereaved families may have a 'healthy' bereavement process, free from complications or pathology.

References

Balk, DE (1990) The self-concept of bereaved adolescents: sibling death and its aftermath, *Journal of Adolescent Research*, 5: 112–32

Balk, DE (1996) Models for understanding adolescent coping with bereavement, *Death Studies*, 20: 367–87

Bayliss, J (2008) Rethinking loss and grief, in B Nyatanga (ed.) *Why Is It So Difficult To Die?* (2nd edn), Dinton: Quay Books

Becker, R (2006) The moral maze of assisted dying, *International Journal of Palliative Nursing*, **12**(6): 251

Benoliel, JQ (1997) Death, technology, and gender in postmodern American society, in S Strack (ed.), *Death and the Quest for Meaning*, Northvale, NJ: Jason Aronson

Biggs, HM (2005) The Assisted Dying for the Terminally Ill Bill 2004: will English law soon allow patients the choice to die?, *European Journal of Health Law*, **12**(1): 43–56

Bowlby, J (1973) *Separation*, New York: Basic Books

Bowlby, J (1980) *Loss*, New York: Basic Books

Brennan, J (2010) *Cancer in Context: A Practical Guide to Supportive Care*, Oxford: Oxford University Press

Brown, G (2008) *The Living End: The Future of Death, Aging and Immortality*, Basingstoke: Palgrave Macmillan

Buckman, R (1990) *I Don't Know What to Say: How to Help and Support Someone Who is Dying*, London: Papermac

Cohen, J, Marcoux, I, Bilsen, J et al. (2006) European acceptance of euthanasia: socio-demographic and cultural factors associated with the acceptance of euthanasia in 33 European countries, *Social Science and Medicine*, 63: 743–56

Cooper, J (ed.) (1997) *Apology*, trans. G Grube, in *Plato, Complete Works*, Indianapolis: Hackett

Cooper, J and Barnet, M (2005) Aspects of caring for dying patients which cause anxiety to first year student nurses, *International Journal of Palliative Nursing*, **11**(8): 423–30

Cracknell, K and White, SJ (2005) *An Introduction to World Methodism*, New York: Cambridge University Press

Davies, B (1991) Long-term outcomes of adolescent sibling bereavement, *Journal of Adolescent Research*, 6: 83–96.

Davies, E, Linklater, KM, Jack, RH et al. (2006) How is place of death from cancer changing and what affects it? Analysis of cancer registration and service data, *British Journal of Cancer*, 95: 593–600

Demi, AS (1984) Hospice bereavement programs: trends and issues, in SH Schraff (ed.), *Hospice: The Nursing Perspective*, New York: National League for Nursing

De Vocht, HM (2008) Dying by euthanasia: an easy thing to do?, in B Nyatanga (ed.) *Why Is It So Difficult To Die?* (2nd edn), Dinton: Quay Books

De Vocht, HM and Nyatanga, B (2007) Health professionals' opposition to euthanasia and assisted suicide: a personal view, *International Journal of Palliative Nursing*, **13**(7): 351–5

Dimond, M (1981) Bereavement and the elderly: a critical review with implications for nursing practice and research, *Journal of Advanced Nursing*, 6: 461–70.

Doka, KJ (ed.) (1989) *Disenfranchised Grief: Recognizing Hidden Sorrows*, Lexington, MA: Lexington Books

Doka, KJ (2007) *Living with Grief: Before and After the Death,* Washington DC: Hospice Foundation of America

Eliot, TD (1930) The adjustive behavior of bereaved families: a new field for social research, *Social Forces*, 8: 543–9.

Eliot, TD (1933) A step toward the social psychology of bereavement, *Journal of Abnormal and Social Psychology*, 27: 380–90.

Field, D and James, N (1993) Where and how people die, in D Clark (ed.), *The Future of Palliative Care*, Buckingham: Open University Press

Freud, S ([1917]1957) Mourning and melancholia, in J Strachey (ed. and trans.), *The Standard Edition of the Complete Works of Sigmund Freud*, vol. 14, London: Hogarth

Goodwin, C and Davidson, P (1991) A child's conception of death, *Early Childhood Education Journal*, **19**(2): 21–4

Heidegger, M ([1927]1962) *Being and Time*, trans. J Macquarrie and E Robinson, Oxford: Blackwell

Higginson, I (2003) *Priorities and Preferences for End of Life Care in England, Wales and Scotland*, London: National Council for Palliative Care

Honderich, T (ed.) (1995) *The Oxford Companion to Philosophy,* Oxford: Oxford University Press

Honderich, T (ed.) (2005) *The Oxford Companion to Philosophy* (new edn), Oxford: Oxford University Press

Irion, PE (1954) *The Funeral and the Mourners*, Nashville, TN: Abingdon Press

Jackson, E (1957) *Understanding Grief*, Nashville, TN: Abingdon Press

Kellahear, A (1990) *Dying of Cancer: The Final Year of Life*, London: Harwood

Klass, D (1988) *Parental Grief: Solace and Resolution*, New York: Springer

Kübler-Ross, E (1970) *On Death and Dying*, New York: Tavistock

Lattanzi-Licht, M and Connor, S (1995) Care of the dying: the hospice approach, in H Wass and RA Neimeyer (eds), *Dying: Facing the Facts*, Washington DC: Taylor & Francis

Laungani, P and Morgan, J (eds) (2005) *Death and Bereavement around the World*, vol 3: *Death and Bereavement in the Americas*, New York: Baywood

Lindemann, E. (1944) Symptomatology and management of acute grief, *American Journal of Psychiatry*, 101: 141–8

Lukacs, G (1978) *The Ontology of Social Being*, Merlin Press: London

Marris, P (1958) *Widows and their Families*, London: Routledge

Murphy, SA (1983) Theoretical perspectives on bereavement, in PL Chinn (ed.), *Nursing Theory Development*, Rockville, MD: Aspen

Murray Parkes, C (1964) The effects of bereavement on physical and mental health: a study of the case records of widows, *British Medical Journal*, 2: 274–9

Murray Parkes, C (1972) *Bereavement: Studies of Grief in Adult Life*, New York: International Universities Press

Murray Parkes, C and Weiss, R (1983) *Recovery from Bereavement*, New York: Basic Books

2

Murray Parkes, C, Laungani, P and Young, B (2003) *Death and Bereavement across Cultures*, New York: Brunner-Routledge

Nagy, M (1948) The child's theories concerning death, *Journal of Genetic Psychology*, 73: 3–27

Nyatanga, B (2008) *Why Is It So Difficult To Die?* (2nd edn), Dinton: Quay Books

Nyatanga, B and de Vocht, HM (2009) When last offices is more than just a white sheet, *British Journal of Nursing*, **18**(7): 1028

Pattison, G (1997) *Kierkgaard and the Crisis of Faith: An Introduction to his Life and Thought*, London: SPCK

Peretz, D (1970) Development, object-relationships, and loss, in B Schoenberg, AC Carr, D Peretz and AH Kutscher (eds), *Loss and Grief: Psychological Management in Medical Practice*, New York: Columbia University Press

Pine, VR (1977) A socio-historical portrait of death education, *Death Education*, 1: 57–84.

Prunkl, PR and Berry, RL (1988) *Death Week: Exploring the Dying Process*, Basingstoke: Hemisphere

Rando, TA (1992/93) The increasing prevalence of complicated grief: the onslaught is just beginning, *Omega*, 26: 43–59

Rosenblatt, PC, Walsh, PC and Jackson, D (1976) *Grief and Mourning in Cross-cultural Perspective*, New Haven, CT: Human Relations Area Files Press

Sartre JP ([1943]2003) *Being and Nothingness: A Phenomenological Essay on Ontology*, trans. H Barnes, London: Routledge

Saunders, C (1978) Hospice care, *American Journal of Medicine*, 65: 726–8

Schoenberg, B, Carr, AC, Kutscher, AH et al. (eds) (1974) *Anticipatory Grief*, New York: Columbia University Press

Stroebe, M, van den Bout, J and Schut, H (1995) Myths and misconceptions about bereavement: the opening of a debate, *Omega*, 29: 187–203

Swanson-Kauffman, KM (1986) Caring in the instance of unexpected early pregnancy loss, *Topics in Clinical Nursing*, **8**(2): 37–46

Tonkin, L (1996) Growing around grief: another way of looking at grief and recovery, *Bereavement Care*, **15**(1): 10

Twycross, RG (1997) The dying patient, *British Medical Journal*, 315: 1365–8

Twycross, RG (1999) Palliative care in the past decade and today, *European Journal of Pain*, **3**(suppl 1): 23–9

Van Gennep, A (1960) *The Rites of Passage*, Chicago: University of Chicago Press

Weston, M (1994) *Kierkegaard and Modern Continental Philosophy*, London: Routledge

WHO (World Health Organization) (2004) *The Solid Facts: Palliative Care*, E Davies and I Higginson (eds), Copenhagen: WHO Regional Office for Europe

Worden, JW (1982) *Grief Counseling and Grief Therapy*, New York: Springer

Worden, JW and Silverman, PR (1996) Parental death and the adjustment of school-age children, *Omega*, 33: 91–102

Wyschogrod, M (1954) *Kierkegaard and Heidegger: The Ontology of Existence*, London: Routledge & Kegan Paul

part 2 glossary

Attention Selectively concentrating on some aspect of the environment.

Attitude A mental state whereby people, concepts and events are evaluated.

Aversion therapy A behavioural therapy where a negative reaction occurs to a pleasurable stimulus, object or behaviour because it has been paired with a negative stimulus (such as nausea).

Behaviour The action or reaction of an organism.

Behaviorism A psychological approach emphasising the scientific and objective study of behaviour and learning.

Behaviour therapy A therapy in which learning is said to determine behaviour, so learning is used to increase positive behaviours or decrease negative behaviours.

Bereavement A multifaceted response to loss, particularly to the loss of someone or something to which a bond was formed.

Chlamydia An atypical bacteria that is able to cause a sexually transmitted disease.

Cholecystectomy Surgical removal of the gall bladder.

Cholesterol An essential lipid (fatty) substance. Excessively high levels of cholesterol are known to increase the chance of heart attack and stroke.

Classical conditioning Learning that uses a reflex behaviour as a neutral response and pairs it with a neutral stimulus to create a newly learned behaviour.

Code of conduct A set of professional standards and morals that a person follows.

Cognition Refers to the processes of knowing, attention, memory and reasoning.

Cognitive therapy A therapy that attempts to change feelings and behaviours by changing the way a person thinks.

Consciousness A state of being conscious or aware.

Culture The norms (socially acceptable human performance), beliefs, attitudes and moral beliefs of a society or group within a society.

Curative A healthcare approach that essentially focuses on curing disease as opposed to preventing ill health.

Defibrillator A machine that delivers an impulse of electricity to an affected heart muscle, which is usually administered by a professional person, for example a nurse, to a patient who is believed to have suffered a heart attack.

2

Discrimination Unfavourable and unequal treatment based on prejudice.

Efficacy A measure of the effectiveness of a treatment.

Emotion A combination of physiological arousal, feelings, cognitive processes and behavioural reactions to produce emotional sensation.

Empowerment The act of enabling a patient to take control of a situation and used in healthcare to describe the improved opportunity of vulnerable or disadvantaged people. This includes increased choice for patients and a stronger voice in decision making.

Episodic memories A form of long-term memories for autobiographical events.

Ethics Moral principles that you follow.

Expert patient A patient who suffers a chronic condition who has become 'expert' in the management of their condition.

Gastrointestinal surgery Surgical intervention pertaining to the upper or lower gastrointestinal tract. (The upper gastrointestinal tract consists of the mouth, pharynx, oesophagus, stomach and duodenum. The lower gastrointestinal tract consists of most of the intestines and anus.)

Genitourinary surgery Surgical intervention pertaining to the genital and urinary organs.

Global society The actual, or trend towards, linking all humanity through a common culture and systems of communication, whether face to face, or mediated through written and technological/electronic mechanisms.

Health education Any activity that promotes health through learning, that is, some relatively permanent change in an individual's capabilities or dispositions.

Health promotion Any planned and informed intervention that is designed to improve physical or mental health, or prevent disease, disability or premature death.

Herd immunity The protection of a small number of non-immunised people by the immunisation of the majority of a population. In most common infectious diseases, it is believed that if 80% or more of a population choose to have an immunisation, the remaining 20% who choose not to have the immunisation are still protected by herd immunity.

Human performance The behaviours, thoughts and emotions that individuals possess.

Humanistic perspective An approach to psychology that focuses on the human experience, the here and now, personal growth and self-actualisation.

Learning A process of acquiring skills and knowledge.

Long-term memory (LTM) A part of memory that retains information over a long period of time.

Medicalisation The increasing trend for medical and allied health disciplines to intervene in the everyday life of individuals.

Memory The mental capacity to encode, store and retrieve information.

Neurosurgery Surgical intervention per taining to the treatment of disorders of the brain, spinal cord and peripheral nerves.

Operant conditioning Learning that uses voluntary behaviours as a naturally occurring response which is then paired with a naturally occurring stimulus to create a newly learned behaviour.

Orthopaedic surgery A branch of surgery relating to conditions involving the musculoskeletal system.

Palliative care The care that focuses on reducing the severity of symptoms of serious conditions. It is often linked with terminal illnesses but is actually the care of people with life-threatening conditions to improve the quality of their lives and includes conditions that are both curable and terminal.

Postoperative After operation.

Preoperative Before operation.

Prejudice Lacking impartiality and showing bias.

Primacy effect When a person has better recall of words at the beginning of a list.

Procedural memory A form of long-term memory for how things are achieved.

Professional Belonging to a profession and being competent in that role.

Psychodynamic theory A psychological model in which abnormal behaviour is explained in terms of conflict between unconscious driver and past experiences.

Psychology The scientific study of thought, behaviour and emotion.

Recency effect When a person has better recall of the words towards the end of a word list.

Schema An internal representation of the world such as clusters of knowledge about people or situations.

Sensory memory An initial store for memory, which is similar to attention, a large amount of information is processed quickly, irrelevant information is lost, but relevant information from the sensory memory is sent to short-term memory.

Short-term memory (STM) A form of memory with a limited capacity, which stores information for a short amount of time before it is lost or sent to long-term memory.

Social learning theory A learning theory that emphasises observation and modelling the behaviour of others.

Sociological imagination The way(s) in which sociologists understand the world based on robust theories and research.

Sociology The rigorous study of society using robust theories and research.

Statins Drugs that lower blood cholesterol levels and hence are effective in reducing the incidence of heart disease and stroke.

Stereotyping Placing a person in a certain group, regardless of any substantial information.

Stress A physiological reaction, but also feelings and thoughts that occur when harmful, challenging or threatening events challenge one's perceived ability to cope with the demands of the situation.

Stressor An agent (either internal or external) that causes stress.

Thyroidectomy Surgical removal of part or all of the thyroid gland.

2

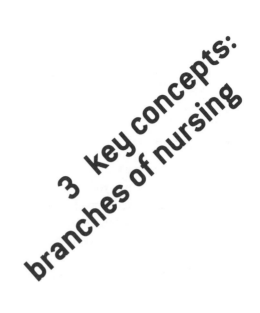

3 key concepts: branches of nursing

3

Introduction

The third part of *The Nursing Companion* introduces and describes key concepts relating to the main branches of nursing. Chapters 12–15 address the four established branches, while Chapter 16 is on caring for older people. There is a growing population of older people who live active and fulfilling lives but a significant number will require nursing and social care, in their own homes, in hospital or in longer term residential settings. Nursing plays a vital role in the care of older people no matter where it occurs, hence its inclusion in *The Nursing Companion.*

During your time spent in training, you will experience caring in each of these branches. As you progress, it will become noticeable that styles of caring differ markedly in each branch but knowledge gained from previous chapters dealing with core topics will prove useful in understanding essential basic principles that guide caring in any situation. For example, you will recognise how nursing across the branches requires an ability to communicate effectively. You will most certainly utilise knowledge of sociology and health promotion when caring for people with mental health problems, those with a learning disability or older people. When caring for children and young adults, you will call upon skills and knowledge derived from an understanding of managing pain, health promotion and issues relating to palliative care.

As you move through each of these branches, the specialist knowledge and skills will become apparent. Adult nursing takes you into a host of situations where you may be caring for a person living with cancer, or someone who has experienced a stroke or a heart attack. You may nurse people who are affected by the onset of dementia or those recovering from surgery. The nature of adult nursing is such that it identifies dimensions of care that cross over into other branches, yet each area is a specialism in its own right requiring detailed study.

While the importance of acquiring generic skills and knowledge cannot be overemphasised, nursing children and young people or those with a learning disability or mental health problems will require you to develop highly professional approaches specific to each branch. Part 3 offers a broad approach and is designed to help you gain confidence in understanding the essence of care that underpins these specialist areas. It will contribute towards making sense of what is experienced in the practice areas and be available as an enhancement of theoretical perspectives as and when they are required.

12 adult nursing

Nancy-Jane Lee and Jean Parnell

In this chapter we will explore:

> The nature of adult nursing
> Origins of, and key influences on, contemporary adult nursing
> Several nursing specialisms and the role of the adult nurse within them

Introduction

This chapter introduces adult nursing and considers some of the common health issues that adult nurses may encounter. Inevitably, there is overlap with other chapters in the book, so the chapter is designed as a taster. It is written for the student nurse, or prospective student nurse, to dip into and use as a basis for personal development planning and further learning. It is the starting point and not the end point for the study of adult nursing.

The nature of adult nursing

Nursing is regulated in the UK by the Nursing and Midwifery Council (NMC, www.nmc.org.uk/). The NMC is responsible for maintaining a professional register of nurses and for maintaining quality and standards of nursing while protecting the public from harm. In order to practise, a registered nurse must have:

> met the standards of proficiency for pre-registration nurse education
> been declared of good health and good character
> paid the registration fee
> their name on the NMC register as a person who is capable of safe and effective practice as a nurse (NMC 2008a).

All nurses work within *The Code: The Standards of Conduct, Performance and Ethics for Nurses and Midwives* (NMC 2008b).

For professional registration purposes, there are four 'branches' of nursing in the UK – child health, mental health, learning disabilities and adult nursing. It is fair to assume that child health nurses work with children, young people and their families, mental health nurses work with people who have mental health issues, and learning disabilities nurses work with individuals with learning disabilities. Do adult nurses therefore work with adults who have purely physical as opposed to mental health or psychosocial needs? Does the notion of adulthood range from the age of 18 to the end of life and exclude any contact with children and young people? The reality of nursing practice does not have the boundaries of the nursing branches. Adults also have mental health issues that may predispose to physical health breakdown. Alternatively, the consequences of long-term physical illness can contribute to poor mental and psychosocial wellbeing for the adult concerned and their family or significant others. Prolonged illness, sudden death and/or trauma have an impact on families and social groups as a whole and not just the adults who succumb to illness. In summary, adult nursing is concerned with the physical and psychosocial aspects of health and illness that impact upon people and their significant others throughout their life course.

The origins of, and key influences on, adult nursing

The history of nursing is associated with Florence Nightingale (1820–1910), particularly her work at Scutari hospital, Turkey, during the Crimean War and the introduction of training for nurses. Rafferty (1996) provides a thorough analysis of nursing history. There are, however, other significant influences on the development of nursing, for example the work of Mary Seacole (1805–81), who campaigned and raised awareness regarding conditions in the Crimean War, in the face of racial adversity and discrimination. Her contribution has been overlooked or ignored until comparatively recently. Anionwu (2006) provides a comprehensive history of the life and work of Mary Seacole.

In contemporary times, some of the values and beliefs that underpin nursing have been informed by Virginia Henderson. One of her major contributions was her philosophy of nursing, which was adopted by the International Council of Nurses in 1966:

> The unique function of the nurse is to assist the individual, sick or well, in the performance of those activities contributing to health, or its recovery (or to a peaceful death) that they would perform unaided if they had the necessary strength, will or knowledge. (Henderson 1966)

The work of Virginia Henderson in relation to nursing is iconic, and although written some years ago, is still pertinent to nursing practice today (Henderson [1978]2006).

The rest of the chapter gives an overview of many nursing specialisms and highlights the role of the adult nurse in each area.

Cancer nursing

An overview

Cancer will affect the lives of one in three people. Four types of cancer account for 50% of all cases – lung, breast, bowel and prostate. The mortality and incidence of cancers are linked to social deprivation and inequalities (DH 2004).

Successive governments have worked to address the so-called 'postcode lottery' of care where service access, provision, treatment and care have varied according to geographical region. These inconsistencies have been highlighted and policies are now in place to address them. Examples of some key policies that influence cancer nursing include:

> *The NHS Cancer Plan: A Plan for Investment, A Plan for Reform* (DH 2000a) – details the government's strategic plan for cancer care in relation to prevention, screening and treatment
> *The Nursing Contribution to Cancer Care* (DH 2000b) – considers requirements in relation to education and training, nurse leadership and service delivery for cancer services
> *The NHS Cancer Plan and the New NHS: Providing a Patient-centred Service* (DH 2004) – outlines progress to date with service provision.

The role of the adult nurse

Within cancer care policies, there is a distinction between the different levels of cancer care and the nurse has a role at all stages (DH 2004):

> Level 1, *self-management:* the nurse has a role with health prevention and health education in relation to smoking, diet and nutrition, maintenance of a healthy lifestyle, weight management, exposure to sunlight, all identified in government policies as key factors influencing health.
> Level 2, *disease management:* there is increased emphasis on the consistency of care geographically, the implementation of evidence-based practice, and the development and application of care guidelines as produced by the National Institute for Clinical Excellence.
> Level 3, *case management:* there is guidance relating to the development of specialised cancer services and individual patient/client assessment according to need, and the role of the nurse is to work as part of an interprofessional team to deliver a range of services. Specialist oncology nurses and Macmillan nurses will work with the adult nurse in hospital and community settings.

While excellent communication and support is vital within all levels of nursing care, it is especially so if individualised care is to be realised. Nurses will also address patient/client needs in relation to the management of side effects from chemotherapy and radiotherapy treatments, surgery and the prevention and management of side effects such as nausea and vomiting, profound fatigue, the prevention and management of oral hygiene problems and mouth ulcers, the prevention and management of pain, psychosocial support for the patient/client and others, service user involvement in care planning and decision making, along with communication and support for the family and social groups.

3

Cerebrovascular accident

An overview

Commonly known as a stroke, a cerebrovascular accident is caused by a clot or bleeding within the brain. It is estimated that stroke is the third highest cause of death in the UK, and 110,000 people in England will have a stroke every year (DH 2007a). The government's *National Stroke Strategy* aims to improve service and reduce deaths from stroke; however, it is suggested that one of the key targets to reduce strokes in people under the age of 75 years by 40% by 2010 has already been achieved (DH 2007a). Stroke is often associated with older people but it can also occur in younger people.

Stroke is characterized by the following:

> Weakness or numbness of the face, arm or leg on one side of the body
> Blurred vision or loss of vision in one or both eyes
> Difficulty communicating or difficulty understanding
> Confusion
> Sudden severe headache with no immediately apparent cause
> Dizziness, unsteadiness or a sudden fall for no reason
> Nausea (DH 2009a).

As stated earlier, the incidence of stroke and associated complications has been reduced. 'Clot-busting' or thrombolytic drugs can be administered in accordance with treatment protocols if the stroke is caused by a blood clot, minimizing complications and improving patient recovery. Furthermore, in order to improve rapid access to treatment, the government has launched a media campaign to educate the public and raise awareness of stroke and the importance of early diagnosis and treatment.

The role of the adult nurse

The nurse can play an important role educating people about the risk factors associated with stroke, and in providing ongoing support. For example, nurses can educate people about smoking and run smoking cessation clinics. They can advise about the need for a sensible and reduced alcohol intake, along with a low salt, high fibre diet, with a good intake of fruit and vegetables. Regular exercise and stable weight management, along with maintenance of blood pressure and low cholesterol, are all key factors in stroke prevention.

Improving Stroke Services: A Guide for Commissioners (DH 2006a) outlines the areas where nurses have a key role to play as part of a multidisciplinary team (MDT) involved with early diagnosis and treatment, followed by rehabilitation and support in the community setting tailored to individual need. The following elements are identified as good practice:

> Opportunities for health education and prevention among the population
> Treatment of early warning signs of stroke

> Rapid admission to a specialised stroke unit and a head scan within 24 hours to aid diagnosis and decisions regarding treatment. Thrombolytic or clot-busting drugs may be given in accordance with treatment guidelines and protocols. There should be monitoring of the patient to assess and manage their condition, according to the protocols

> There should be specialist multidisciplinary rehabilitation in hospital, transferred into community settings

> There should be information and empowerment for service users, with involvement at all stages (DH 2006a).

Community nursing

An overview

'Primary healthcare' is an umbrella term used to describe those services organised and delivered in the community, as opposed to the secondary or hospital setting. Primary care includes community nursing, GPs, pharmacists, opticians and health professionals such as physiotherapists and **podiatrists** working in the community.

The importance of community care has been emphasized in reports, for example *Our Health, Our Care, Our Say* (DH 2006b). In 2007, a major review of the NHS was commissioned by the government and undertaken by Lord Darzi – *Our NHS, Our Future* (DH 2007b) – which identified the need for comprehensive community services. The development of polyclinics was proposed in *Healthcare for London* (DH 2007c). Polyclinics are described as large clinics in the community, which would provide a comprehensive range of services not traditionally associated with primary healthcare, for example minor surgery, clinical investigations, consultation with medical specialists, treatment options. The development of polyclinics is thought to provide greater choice for health service users, with more flexible opening times and access.

The role of the adult nurse

In order to work in the community, adult nurses need to have excellent communication skills and great sensitivity to the fact they are entering and working in people's own homes and meeting and working with family members and others who make a significant contribution to care. In addition to good knowledge of individual patients, their families and others, community nurses need to understand the profile of their local area, have a working knowledge of the other agencies, voluntary and statutory, that work in the area and the health profile of the community.

There are a number of roles in the community:

> **Community nurses**: perhaps better known originally as 'district nurses', they deliver care in people's homes. The community nursing sister is

responsible for the initial assessment of care need and care planning, while a team comprising staff nurses and support workers may be involved in care delivery.

> *Practice nurses:* they work in GP services and have a range of roles in the clinics there. They are involved in health promotion and the development of smoking cessation clinics for example, they will be involved in vaccination programmes and the development of screening services, for example cervical screening. Practice nurses also run clinics for wound care and other treatments.

> *School nurses:* they work in schools and have a major role to play with issues such as health screening, health education and promotion, health checks and immunisation.

> *Specialist nurses:* a range of specialist nursing services are offered in the community. Macmillan nurses, for example, provide invaluable support for families experiencing cancer, providing specialist services for them and for the nursing teams based in the community. Admiral nurses provide support for families and others caring for those with **dementia**.

> *Community matrons:* they are highly specialised nurses who, after additional training, take on responsibility for the care of those with complex health needs. Community matrons make an initial comprehensive assessment of need; they can undertake physical examinations and order specialised investigations and treatment. Community matrons provide a comprehensive service to enable those with chronic health problems to remain in the community and avoid continual hospital admissions due to complications, for example.

> *Health visitors:* they have originally been nurses or midwives and after further specialist training they work predominantly with health promotion and prevention issues. Traditionally associated with child health, care of the newborn and under fives, health visitors also come into contact with a range of people in the community, given their contribution to health promotion and public health issues.

Activity 12.1

Make a list of the number of services offered within your local health centre. For example, how many different nursing roles are there, who else works there, is there a pharmacist, what kinds of services do they offer? Make notes on the range of roles and services you can identify.

Coronary heart disease

An overview

Coronary heart disease was the biggest killer in the country in 2000, with 110,000 deaths in England and 300,000 people having a heart attack. Social deprivation had a key link, with the disease being three times higher in unskilled than professional men, for example. There was also a higher incidence of coronary heart disease in men born on the Indian subcontinent, 38% higher and 43% higher for women (DH 2000c).

In response to the high mortality rate and inequalities in service provision and treatment on a geographical basis, the *National Service Framework for Coronary Heart Disease* was introduced (DH 2000c). This highlighted 12 standards to improve services and healthcare outcomes, focusing on:

> Reducing heart disease in the population
> Preventing coronary heart disease in high-risk patients in primary care
> Treating heart attacks
> Investigating and treating stable angina
> Revascularisation
> Managing heart failure and providing palliative care
> Cardiac rehabilitation (DH 2000c).

As part of the above developments, prompt response from the emergency services was enhanced with the introduction of 'first responders'. These are community volunteers trained to respond in emergency situations and to provide support and treatment at the earliest opportunity. This kind of response helps coronary heart disease patients have access to thrombolytic drugs within an hour of calling help, thus saving lives and preventing long-term complications. In addition, the use of drugs such as aspirin and statins has done much to improve the health and wellbeing of the population. Similarly, improved risk calculators and equations have helped to better identify those people at risk from coronary heart disease and to take early measures to improve health.

The role of the adult nurse

As with stroke, there is a key role for nurses as regards health education and prevention of disease and measures to address long-term complications.

Dementia

An overview

Dementia is described as 'a syndrome due to disease of the brain, usually chronic or progressive in nature' (WHO 2001). There are over 100 types of dementia, the most common form is Alzheimer's disease followed by vascular dementia (Alzheimer's Society 2007). Alzheimer's disease is characterized by changes in the structure and function of proteins in the brain, which destroy brain tissue. This results in memory loss, and as the disease progresses, the ability to carry out basic skills becomes increasingly impaired (Burns et al. 1997). Vascular dementia is where either multiple small infarcts or larger infarcts affect small vessels in the brain, resulting in a decline in communication and concentration. By 2025, there will be over a million people with the disease. The financial cost of dementia to the UK is over £17bn a year. This does not include support from family and friends who save the government over £6bn a year (Alzheimer's Society 2007).

Role of the adult nurse

Most people with dementia live in the community and, to varying degrees, have problems with thinking clearly, remembering things, communicating and doing day-to-day things like cooking or getting dressed. These and other problems associated with dementia, such as **depression**, mood swings, aggression, wandering and getting lost, involve input from **community psychiatric nurses**. Physical health problems can also occur and patients' nursing needs will be met by adult nurses both in primary and secondary care settings. Nurses in the acute setting will have to consider the impact of so-called normal routines on the patient with dementia. Nutrition, hydration, continence, hygiene and sleep patterns are often disrupted when the person with dementia is admitted to hospital. Involving the patient and their carers in planning care can reduce stress and confusion by keeping to familiar routines as far as possible (Fortinash and Holoday-Worret 2007).

Organisational impositions such as the number of bed moves, for example, should be kept to a minimum and if possible avoided to reduce the impact of hospital admission. Frequent moves can increase confusion and cause a great deal of stress to the person with dementia, disrupting routines and frameworks that they use to help them function (Cunningham and Archibald 2006). In the community, consideration should be given to patients' and carers' normal routines in order to cause less distress and disturbance.

Key policies that influence nursing practice

The Department of Health has published plans for improving the provision of health and social care services for people with dementia and their carers in *Living Well with Dementia: A National Strategic Policy* (DH 2009b). The document sets out how the government wants to improve care in the acute, intermediate, care home and community settings by identifying three key steps to improve the quality of life for people with dementia and their carers:

> Better knowledge about dementia and removal of the stigma
> Early diagnosis, support and treatment for people with dementia, their family and carers
> Development of services to meet changing needs better.

This document will influence nursing practice in the care of people with dementia.

Emergency nursing

An overview

Emergency nursing has evolved from 'casualty', where 'casual' attendees would present at an outpatient department, often being seen by whichever physician was around, to the complex specialty of emergency medicine, as it is known today.

The emergency nurse accepts, without prior warning, people of any age requiring healthcare. Patients may present with problems that originate from one or more sources – medical, social, spiritual, cultural or psychological – and the emergency nurse is a clinical decision maker, identifying and prioritising those who attend.

Role of the adult nurse

The emergency department (ED) is often separated geographically into distinct areas:

> *Triage*, meaning to sieve or sort, is often the first place, when a patient presents to the ED, where they will be assessed. An emergency nurse uses advanced assessment and decision-making skills, often with the aid of a triage tool, such as an electronic version of the Manchester triage system (Manchester Triage Group 2006) to assign a priority to the patient. The system uses the standard five-point triage scale (developed by the RCN A&E Association and the British Association for Emergency Medicine), which consists of colours and categories to represent priority: red – immediate, orange – very urgent, yellow – urgent, green – standard, blue – non-urgent. An important note to remember is that triage is a dynamic process. If a patient begins to deteriorate while in the waiting area, after being initially categorized as an 'urgent', they should be reassessed, and retriaged accordingly. As a result of the government's A&E targets, many departments changed this assessment process, to include a doctor as well as a nurse, so that early investigations could be initiated, and those patients who needed minimal care could be seen and treated and discharged at this point.

> The *majors* area is for patients who are unwell and need further investigations.

> The *resuscitation* room is for those who may deteriorate, such as patients with acute cardiac chest pain, or those who have sustained major trauma, or require resuscitation. Trauma care is managed using the advanced trauma

life support guidelines, which use an A–E assessment of the patient in order to identify life-threatening injuries, and to manage these before moving on.

> The *minor injuries* area is often managed by nurse practitioners, who have undergone further training to assess, investigate, diagnose and treat this group of patients autonomously.

The ED can be a busy scene of organized activity, which can be alarming, as equipment is often unfamiliar, and the variety of professionals who work within the department or who come to see patients vary – from the ED staff to the various specialties that patients may be referred to and other members of the MDT.

The important things to remember as a student nurse are to:

> Ask – ask if you can help, ask if you don't understand
> Observe – observe and listen to what is happening, learn from observation and ask if you don't understand
> Do not be afraid to learn, and practise your clinical skills under supervision
> Utilise the MDT expertise within the department to enhance your knowledge.

There may be times when decisions are made that you may not understand or agree with. Ethical dilemmas are challenging in any clinical situation, and can be more frequent in the emergency setting. Remember to keep a notebook in your pocket, document your questions, if inappropriate to ask at the time, as your mentor can then explain when you both have the time to discuss such matters.

Endocrinology

The endocrine system comprises glands situated throughout the body that secrete hormones. Hormones circulate around the body and target key organs bringing about physiological changes. This section focuses on the pancreas and the prevention and management of diabetes, which has an increasing impact upon many people's lives.

The pancreas: an overview

The pancreas produces the hormone insulin, which has a vital role in controlling blood glucose levels. Interference with the production of insulin will lead to the development of diabetes mellitus. Diabetes affects 2.35 million people in England and this is expected to increase by a further 2.5 million in the future. Diabetes is associated with heart attacks, stroke, blindness, kidney problems and amputation due to circulatory problems (DH 2006c). As such, diabetes is a major risk to health and wellbeing, if not diagnosed and managed correctly to prevent complications. It is described as a global pandemic, given the increase in childhood and adult obesity, and poses a greater risk for black and minority ethnic groups (DH 2006c). There are two types of diabetes:

> *Type 1 diabetes* is not preventable and arises when the body cannot produce insulin at all. It manifests itself quickly, with rapid onset of signs and symptoms.

> *Type 2 diabetes* may not be so obvious, and arises when the body cannot produce enough insulin. It is preventable and is associated with weight gain and obesity.

The signs and symptoms of diabetes include increased thirst and a tendency to pass urine more frequently, tiredness, weight loss and blurred vision. A family incidence of diabetes and a history of high blood pressure or stroke are indicators of diabetes development, according to Diabetes UK (www.diabetes.org. uk).

As with other key health issues, a National Service Framework has been developed to raise the standards and consistency of care for those people with diabetes and serves to raise prevention issues (DH 2001). A series of reports since then have identified progress in relation to diabetes care, for example *Supporting People with Long Term Conditions to Self Care* (DH 2006d) identified four elements for development by health and social services:

1 Skills and training
2 Information
3 Tools and devices
4 Support networks.

The role of the adult nurse

Adult nurses have a key role to play with health education and prevention measures in relation to diabetes. Wherever nurses encounter patients and others, there are opportunities for assessment and education regarding issues such as diet and exercise. These opportunities extend to those with either type 1 or type 2 diabetes. With the former, people will need education and support in relation to the administration of insulin and monitoring of blood sugar levels, along with advice about diet, exercise and lifestyle. With type 2 diabetes, people will need support relating to weight management and the administration of medication to control diabetes, if this is used.

In both situations, there are possible long-term complications for people with diabetes, and health promotion to prevent complications is essential. Two areas are vitally important:

> *Eye care:* people with diabetes need regular eye check-ups and should maintain healthy blood sugar levels to minimize complications, as poor eyesight or blindness are associated with diabetes that is poorly managed in the long term.

> *Foot care:* people with diabetes should wear well-fitting shoes, and maintain good foot health. Toe nails should be cut carefully, with the involvement of the podiatrist to prevent long-term complications. Poor circulation caused

by ill-fitting shoes, and poorly managed blood sugar levels, along with long-term infection, can result in serious problems, with amputation in the severest cases.

People with diabetes are cared for in the community or they may access specialist clinics and support networks. Consultant nurses may run clinics for those with diabetes to complement medical care and to provide specialist health promotion advice, diabetes management and support. There is increasing emphasis on self-care for those with long-term conditions such as diabetes and initiatives such as expert patients provide advice and support from people with diabetes as well as helping to establish networks for those with diabetes.

Infection control

Activity 12.3

Reflect for five minutes and make a list of the infections you, your family or friends have experienced within the last 12 months and how they impacted on physical and psychosocial wellbeing. You will be returning to this activity at the end of this section.

An overview

All nurses, regardless of the branch of study, have a professional responsibility and duty in relation to the protection of patients/clients, their families and other health workers through preventive and management measures for infection. The impact of infection is such that it is a responsibility of all health workers, from hospital consultants to the porters and facilities management staff, to apply infection control measures. The standard of hospital cleanliness and the diligence of staff are the subject of intense media and political interest. Infection prevention and control is once again a key preoccupation, as it was before the development of antibiotics.

The Health and Social Care Act 2008: Code of Practice for the Prevention and Control of Healthcare Associated Infection and Related Guidance (DH 2009c) states clearly that NHS organisations have a legal requirement to protect patients and staff from the risks of healthcare associated infection.

Role of the adult nurse

Nursing knowledge and expertise for infection control is summarised in Table 12.1.

Table 12.1 Nursing interventions and practical applications

Nursing intervention	Practical application	Additional evidence
Practice skill – hand washing	For self, for patients, especially those confined to bed, before and after meals, after toileting, after contact with body fluids, when moving between patients Visitors should be educated about the importance of hand washing	Healthcare associated infection costs the NHS at least £1bn a year and causes at least 5,000 deaths
Practice skill – asepsis	Principles of wound healing, wound management, catheter care, suction care should be known and applied. Application of infection prevention techniques in nursing practice, skills to care for the patient with an infection, suitable administration of antibiotics and antipyretics as prescribed, fluids to maintain hydration, maintaining personal hygiene and comfort for the patient, accurate recording of nursing observations, communication and explanation for the patient and their family, help with diet to promote healing, documentation of nursing care given and reporting of progress for healthcare workers	See Iggulden et al. 2009 for further information and nursing care
Nursing observation	Assessment skills to observe the signs of localised infection include redness, pain, tenderness, oozing/exudate. Other signs include increased temperature, pulse and respiration, enlarged and tender glands, tiredness, lethargy, reduced appetite, nausea, flushed skin, sweaty, hot and cold, shivering. Wound assessment skills should be used	See Iggulden et al. 2009
Nursing knowledge	Health promotion and education for all involved in nursing care, including other health workers, patients and their families Knowledge of national and local policies relating to infection prevention and management How to deal with body fluids safely, universal precautions for infection control Understanding the role of the hospital infection control team, safe disposal of sharps, wound dressings, soiled and infected linen, infection control policies	

Nursing intervention	Practical application	Additional evidence
Professional behaviour	Adherence to the local uniform policy, clean hair tied back as appropriate, no rings or wristwatches, cuts and abrasions covered up, wearing of correct apron according to procedure, all the above issues	Apart from the serious issues of infection and cross-infection, patients and their families want and expect trust and due professional behaviour from nursing staff

Activity 12.4

Return now to your initial list of illnesses and categorise them according to those caused by bacteria, viruses, fungi and parasites.

Older people

An overview

A person is said to be elderly between the ages of 60–74, old between the ages of 75–89 and very old when they are over 90. Life expectancy in good or fairly good health, free from a limiting illness and disability, has increased for both men and women over the past 23 years. Although the population has been living longer, the added years are not necessarily spent in good health. In 2004, men could expect to live 14.3 years with a limiting illness or disability and women 17 years (National Statistics Online 2008). Due to age-related changes in the way older people's bodies function and the associated health problems as people age, nursing care for older should be adapted to older people's particular needs and circumstances. The Nursing and Midwifery Council produces guidance on the care of the older person and describes three main elements to providing the fundamentals of care (NMC 2009, p. 11):

> *People:* the skills and qualities of nurses who provide compassionate care and who challenge poor practice
> *Process:* how staff care for people, including assessment of need, respect for privacy and dignity, and equal partnerships with the older person
> *Place:* the diverse environments where care is delivered should be appropriate, adequately resources and effectively managed.

Not following such guidance can be considered as abuse of the older person.

Role of the adult nurse

Nursing care is often organised using nursing models and the nursing process. There are many physiological changes that occur as a person ages that will affect how the nurse organises care to fulfill the older patient's needs. Using the activities of living (Holland 2008), the following points illustrate the differences in needs that the older person may have:

> The thirst stimulus is reduced as we age, so it is important that the nurse ensures the patient is adequately hydrated.
> The gait of older people may become unsteady, and together with a reduction in visual acuity, they may become susceptible to falls. Nurses would then need to consider the level of lighting and ensure that the environment was free of clutter.
> The immune system also becomes less efficient with age, making people more prone to infection, which, coupled with a reduced ability of the body to respond to infections, can cause an unusual presentation to a chest infection, for example. This might result in the older patient presenting with confusion, rather than complaining of feeling unwell or a high temperature.

Activity 12.5

Access and read the Royal College of Nursing publication *Nursing Assessment and Older People* by following the link http://www.rcn.org.uk/_data/assets/pdf_file/0010/78616/002310.pdf.

Operating theatres

An overview

Surgery is performed in many areas, from minor procedures in health centres to more complicated procedures on short-stay surgical units and operating theatres in hospital settings. Surgical procedures can be carried out as an emergency or they can be **elective**. The involvement of nurses in surgery can be divided into three areas; preoperative, **intraoperative** and postoperative. In order to care effectively for patients who may not be fully alert, it is important that nurses who work in theatre have a good understanding of the physiology and pathophysiology associated with surgical procedures and anaesthetics. All operating theatre nurses are responsible for updating patients' nursing notes.

Role of the adult nurse

The adult nurse's primary responsibility to a patient undergoing surgery is to ensure the wellbeing of the patient and should act as the patient's advocate from the time they enter the operating suite to the time they leave. Care commences when the receiving nurse in the operating theatres greets the patient and takes the handover from the nurse who has accompanied the patient:

> The *anaesthetic nurse* is involved in the care of the patient undergoing an anaesthetic. The anaesthetic nurse prepares equipment and drugs for the induction, maintenance and reversal of anaesthesia.
> The *scrub nurse* is responsible for the maintenance of a safe environment throughout surgery for both staff and patients. This includes monitoring

temperature, the positioning of the patient in such a way as to avoid tissue and nerve damage while allowing access for surgery, as well as maintaining a sterile field. The scrub nurse is responsible for instruments and equipment during surgery and is the person who maintains a count of the numbers of swabs and instruments used during surgery; confirming that the numbers preoperatively and postoperatively agree, which will indicate that none have been left in the patient.

> The *recovery nurse* monitors patients' recovery. The ABCDE method of assessment is a methodical way to do this; it is used to identify any aspects of a patient's condition that may indicate areas of concern following anaesthesia and surgery (American College of Surgeons 2004). Following many procedures, **patient-controlled analgesia** is routine; the recovery nurse may need to remind patients how to use this. The recovery nurse, together with other nurses in theatre, is responsible for updating patients' nursing notes.

Postoperative nursing care

Postoperative care begins when the nurse receives the patient's handover from the theatre nurses and establishes that it is safe for the patient to return to their bed area. Here the nurse is responsible for caring for the patient's wound, monitoring pulse, blood pressure and temperature to establish that the patient is recovering. Pain management is an important aspect of nursing care during the recovery period and involves pain assessment and administration of medication. This period ends when the patient is discharged home, discharged with follow-up or into the care of nurses in the community.

Following surgery and recovery from sedation or anaesthetic, the nurse is responsible for ensuring that the patient's records are updated, and for giving a comprehensive handover, including information regarding the patient's condition, the surgery that has been performed and the care needed over the next few hours, to the receiving nurse, who will escort the patient back to their bed area. The nurses on the ward will then continue with the ABCDE assessment until the patient is recovered.

Activity 12.6

Find out more about the ABCDE method of assessment in a book or journal article on caring for the acutely ill patient.

Orthopaedic nursing

An overview

The term 'orthopaedic' is derived from the Greek *orthos* meaning straight and *paedos* meaning child. The specialty developed from helping children who had musculoskeletal problems. These problems were congenital, developmental or traumatic. As healthcare has improved and congenital, developmental and childhood infections have been recognised and treated earlier, fewer children have ongoing problems into adulthood. With changing demographic trends, such as increased life expectancy, people are presenting with degenerative conditions such as osteoporosis and osteoarthritis. As people live longer, the associated traumatic fractures associated with falls and osteoporosis may occur. Osteoarthritic changes in joints are found in 15% of people over the age of 55 (Hakim and Clunie 2002). Osteoarthritis in joints may lead to the need for joint replacement. Changes in working patterns have meant that there is an increase in leisure time, with an increased possibility of musculoskeletal trauma related to sporting activities.

Role of the adult nurse

This specialty in nursing has moved from a medical to a nursing model of care, (Kneale and Davis 2005). Care settings for orthopaedic nursing are also changing. In the past 20 years, the length of stay for inpatients has reduced and is predicted to reduce even more in future (DH 2008). Adult nurses caring for patients in the community will need to develop knowledge and skills in caring for people with orthopaedic conditions in varied locations, from patients' own homes to intermediate care, nursing and care homes. Minor surgery, formerly undertaken in secondary care, such as the removal of ganglions, increasingly occurs in general practice. The adult nurses' role in all settings is to promote evidence-based practice and ensure that their practice reflects this (NMC 2008a).

Nurses in A&E, outpatient departments, elective and trauma wards in secondary care will also encounter people with orthopaedic problems. In A&E departments, specialist nurses acting as trauma coordinators and fractured femur coordinators oversee the care and progress of patients through the department from admission through to discharge or transfer to an orthopaedic ward. Orthopaedic wards are generally separated into elective and trauma areas. Trauma orthopaedic nursing includes the care of patients with musculo-skeletal injuries caused by a variety of incidents, which can include injury to bone, joints and soft tissue such as tendons, ligaments and muscles. Patients who have been admitted to hospital for planned treatment such as surgery to replace a joint are admitted to an elective ward area. With the increase in short-stay surgery, adult nurses specialising in orthopaedic nursing will have a duty to influence, educate and inform nurses who work on short-stay surgical units in order to ensure that patients receive evidence-based care that is safe and tailored to their condition. Patients with orthopaedic conditions may need therapeutic restriction of their mobility. Common forms of restriction include traction, external or **internal fixation**, **casts**, **splints**, bandages and **strapping**. These forms of therapeutic restriction can be used to prevent further injury or damage and to promote healing, but may also predispose the patient to other risks, for example the development of pressure ulcers and the psychological aspects of restricting a person's mobility. The role of the nurse in these situations is in information giving, health promotion and teaching self-care.

Rheumatology

An overview

Rheumatoid diseases primarily affect the body's connective tissues and are classed as autoimmune diseases of unknown cause. The most widely known disease is rheumatoid **arthritis**. This is characterised by recurrent inflammation involving the **synovium**, or lining of the joint, leading to destruction of the joint tissue and consequent pain, deformity and loss of function. Less common forms of arthritis are associated with skin conditions such as psoriasis and joint problems such as gout. Others can follow infections, particularly viral infections, and gut infections that cause diarrhoea and food poisoning. Some arthritic diseases can affect other organs as well as joints, for example the eyes, skin, heart, lungs, kidneys and nerves (Isaacs 1998). Rheumatoid arthritis mainly affects smaller joints such as those in the hands and feet, but other joints such as the elbow can be affected too. Joints become swollen, red and painful and feel warm to touch. Rheumatoid arthritis is often accompanied by general ill health including fatigue, anaemia, **nerve entrapment** neuropathies, dry mucous membranes and involvement of the lymph and vascular systems. There are approximately 20,000 new cases of rheumatoid arthritis each year and 400,000 adults with ongoing problems (Wiles et al. 1999; Symmons et al. 2002). Juvenile idiopathic arthritis affects approximately 2,500 children each year, with approximately 15,000 children having ongoing problems (Sacks et al. 2007; Riise et al. 2008).

Role of the adult nurse

Patients with rheumatoid disease often have complex needs, and for this reason nurses often work as part of a MDT, which might include a consultant rheumatologist, GP, rheumatology nurse specialist, pain nurse specialist, nurses in acute and community settings, occupational health nurses, physiotherapists and podiatrists.

The main aims of nursing a patient with a rheumatoid disease is to inform and educate the patient; this can be a two-way process, with the patient teaching the nurse their own coping strategies. The nurse assesses plans, implements and evaluates care, offering care for the physical, emotional and social needs of the patient. Advice on the control of pain and the promotion of comfort using non-pharmacological strategies is an integral part of nursing care. Together with the patient, occupational health nurses and physiotherapists, the nurse initiates strategies that maintain nutrition, skin integrity, mobility, muscle power, function and independence. The nurse provides information regarding drugs that might be used to control symptoms and how these can limit the progress of the disease. Medication might include non-steroidal anti-inflammatory drugs, analgesia, corticosteroids and disease-modifying antirheumatic drugs. The nurse monitors and records the effect of treatment, liaises with and orchestrates care with other members of the MDT.

Activity 12.6

Access the Arthritis Research Campaign's website following the link http://www. arthritisresearchuk.org/arthritis_information/information_for_medical_profes.aspx.Click on each of the four areas under 'Information for' and read one item from each section.

Conclusion

This chapter has introduced some key areas for adult nursing. Increasingly, within the work of the adult nurse, there is an emphasis on health promotion and education. This is important to help prevent a range of health problems that will impact upon the quality of people's lives. These are often linked to lifestyle issues such as diet, alcohol consumption and smoking, exercise and weight management, along with stress management. The contribution of social deprivation to people's health breakdown is now well documented, and government policies increasingly exist to promote equality of health access and opportunity.

It may be a surprise to some readers that health promotion is an important aspect of adult nursing. This is because popular media stereotypes emphasise the care of patients in hospital, within acute and critical settings. However, government policies, the Darzi Review, changing demographics and population health profiles are increasing the need for primary care services, community-based services, readily accessible and local to people's homes. This chapter has also explored a range of adult nursing roles. Following pre-registration education, adult nurses can specialise in a wide range of settings. Roles exist from staff nurse to consultant nurse, and can be found in education and research settings. At all levels of delivery, knowledge of research evidence is important to develop and apply evidence-based practice and develop the quality of care expected in the twenty-first century.

Further reading and resources

DH (Department of Health) (2001) *National Service Framework for Older People*, available online at http://www.dh.gov.uk/en/Publicationsandstatistics/Publications/PublicationsPolicyAndGuidance/DH_4003066, accessed 26/05/09

DH (2001) *Reforming Emergency Care*, http://www.dh.gov.uk/

DH (2004) *Transforming Emergency Care in England*, http://www.dh.gov.uk/

DH (2006) *The Direction of Travel for Urgent Care*, http://www.dh.gov.uk/

DH (2006) *The Eighteen Week Patient Pathway: An Implementation Framework and Delivery Resource Pack*, available online at http://www.dh.gov.uk/en/Publicationsandstatistics/Publications/PublicationsPolicyAndGuidance/DH_4134668, accessed 26/05/09

DH (2007) *National Service Framework for Older People: Annual Report, Standard 6*, available online at http://www.dh.gov.uk/en/Publicationsandstatistics/Publications/PublicationsPolicyAndGuidance/Browsable/DH_4901891, accessed 21/05/09

DH (2009) *Prevention Package for Older People*, available online at http://www.dh.gov.uk/en/SocialCare/Deliveringadultsocialcare/Olderpeople/Preventionpackage/DH_106149, accessed 21/05/09

Resuscitation Council (2008) *Medical Emergencies and Resuscitation*, available online at http://www.resus.org.uk/pages/MEdental.pdf, accessed 21/05/09

Arthritis Research Campaign www.arc.org.uk

Cancer Research UK www.cancerresearchuk.org

Macmillan Cancer Support www.macmillan.org.uk/

Marie Curie Cancer Care www.mariecurie.org.uk/

The Stroke Association www.stroke.org.uk/

The Stroke Research Network www.uksrn.ac.uk/

National Dementia Strategy www.dh.gov.uk/dementia

Alzheimer's Society www.alzheimers.org.uk/site/

Faculty of Emergency Nursing http://www.fen.uk.com/

St Emlyns http://www.stemlyns.org.uk/

Emergency Nurses Association http://www.ena.org/

Diabetes UK www.diabetes.org.uk/

National Diabetes Support Team www.diabetes.nhs.uk/

Health Protection Agency www.hpa.org.uk

Hospital Infection Society www.his.org.uk

National Resource for Infection Control www.nric.org.uk

NHS Evidence – Surgery, Anaesthesia and Critical Care http://www.library.nhs.uk/theatres/

Nursing Information Research Exchange (Wound Management Resources) http://www.nire.ie/index.asp?locID=247&docID=-1

NHS North West Critical Care Institute http://www.gmskillsinstitute.nhs.uk/#/aim-course/4515409031

Acknowledgement

The authors and publishers wish to acknowledge the contributions from Annabella Gloster and Ian Jones.

References

Alzheimer's Society (2007) *Dementia UK*, London: Alzheimer's Society

American College of Surgeons (2004) *Advanced Trauma Life Support Program for Doctors* (7th edn), Chicago, IL: ACS

Anionwu, E (2006) *About Mary Seacole*, available online at http://www.maryseacole.com/maryseacole/pages/aboutmary.html, accessed 21/05/09

Burns, A, Howard, R and Pettit, W (1997) *Alzheimer's Disease: A Medical Companion*, Oxford: Blackwell Science

Cunningham, C and Archibald, C (2006) Supporting people with dementia in acute hospital settings, *Nursing Standard*, **20**(43): 51–5

DH (Department of Health) (2000a) *The NHS Cancer Plan: A Plan for Investment, A Plan for Reform*, London: DH

DH (2000b) *The Nursing Contribution to Cancer Care*, London: DH

DH (2000c) *National Service Framework for Coronary Heart Disease*, London: DH

DH (2001) *National Service Framework for Diabetes*, London: DH

DH (2004) *The NHS Cancer Plan and the New NHS: Providing a Patient-centred Service*, London: DH

DH (2006a) *Improving Stroke Services: A Guide For Commissioners*, London: DH

DH (2006b) *Our Health, Our Care, Our Say*, London: DH

DH (2006c) *Turning the Corner: Improving Diabetes Care*, London: DH

DH (2006d) *Supporting People with Long Term Conditions to Self Care: A Guide to Developing Local Strategies and Good Practice*, London: DH

DH (2007a) *National Stroke Strategy*, London: DH

DH (2007b) *Our NHS, Our Future*, London: DH

DH (2007c) *Health Care for London*, London: DH

DH (2008) *High Quality Care for All: NHS Next Stage Review Final Report*, Darzi Review, available online at http://www.dh.gov.uk/en/Publicationsandstatistics/Publications/PublicationsPolicyAndGuidance/DH_085825, accessed 21/05/09

DH (2009a) *What you Need to Know about Strokes*, London: DH

DH (2009b) *Living Well with Dementia: A National Strategic Policy*, available online at http://www.dh.gov.uk/en/Publicationsandstatistics/Publications/PublicationsPolicyAndGuidance/DH_094058, accessed 21/05/09

DH (2009c) *The Health and Social Care Act 2008: Code of Practice for the Prevention and Control of Healthcare Associated Infection and Related Guidance*, London: DH

Fortinash, KM and Holoday-Worret, PA (2007) *Psychiatric Nursing Care Plans* (5th edn), London: Mosby

Hakim, A and Clunie, GP (eds) (2002) *Oxford Handbook of Rheumatology*, Oxford: Oxford University Press

Henderson, V (1966) *The Nature of Nursing: A Definition and its Implications for Practice and Education*, New York: Macmillan

Henderson, V ([1978]2006) The concept of nursing, *Journal of Advanced Nursing*, **53**(1): 21–34

Holland, K (ed.) (2008) *Applying the Roper Logan Tierney Model of Nursing in Practice* (2nd edn), Edinburgh, Churchill Livingstone/Elsevier

Iggulden, H, Macdonald, C and Staniland, K (2009) *Clinical Skills: The Essence of Caring*, Buckingham: McGraw-Hill/OUP

Isaacs, JD (1998) *Clinical Drawings for your Patients: Rheumatology* (2nd edn), Abingdon: Health Press

Kneale, J and Davis, P (eds) (2005) *Orthopaedic and Trauma Nursing*, London: Churchill Livingstone

Manchester Triage Group (2006) *Emergency Triage*, K Mackway-Jones, J Marsden and J Windle (eds), Cambridge, MA: Blackwell

National Statistics Online (2008) *Older People: Health and Wellbeing, Living Longer, More*

3

Years in Poor Health, available online at http://www.statistics.gov.uk/cci/nugget. asp?id=2159, accessed 30/05/09

NMC (Nursing and Midwifery Council) (2008a) *What is a Registered Nurse?*, London: NMC

NMC (2008b) *The Code: Standards for Conduct, Performance and Ethics for Nurses and Midwives,* London: NMC

NMC (2009) *Guidance for the Care of Older People*, available online at http://www.nmc-uk. org/aDisplayDocument.aspx?DocumentID=5593, accessed 30/05/09

Rafferty, AM (1996) *The Politics of Nursing Knowledge*, London: Routledge

Riise, OR, Handeland, KS, Cvancarova, M et al. (2008) Incidence and characteristics of arthritis in Norwegian children: a population based study, *Paediatrics,* **121**(2): e299–306

Sacks, JJ, Helmick, CG, Luo, YH et al. (2007) Prevalence of and ambulatory health care visits for pediatric arthritis and other rheumatologic conditions in the United States in 2001-2004, *Arthritis and Rheumatism*, **57**(8): 1439–45

Symmons, D, Turner, G, Webb, R et al. (2002) The prevalence of rheumatoid arthritis in the United Kingdom: new estimates for a new century, *Rheumatology*, **39**(12): 1403–9

WHO (World Health Organization) (2001) *Alzheimer's Disease: The Brain Killer,* WHO: Geneva

Wiles, N, Symmons, DP, Harrison, B et al. (1999) Estimating the incidence of rheumatoid arthritis: trying to hit a moving target? *Arthritis and Rheumatology*, **41**(7): 1339–46

13 nursing children and young people

**Barbara Elliott, Eileen Wake, Jeremy Jolley,
Susan Jolley, Linda Shields and Rhona Williams**

In this chapter we will explore:

> The background to children's nursing
> Models and contexts of children's nursing
> Promoting health for children and young people
> Issues at specific stages of childhood
> Safeguarding children
> Healthcare needs of children and young people in various settings
> The future of children's nursing

Introduction

This chapter is an overview of the many and varied aspects of nursing sick children and their families. Children's nurses care for sick children from birth through childhood and adolescence to young adulthood. Thus they are required to have extensive knowledge of child development and health issues at particular ages as well as an understanding of the needs of children when they are ill and those of their families and how these needs can be met. In addition to caring for children when they are sick, children's nurses have a role in the prevention and early detection of ill health and in the care of children who are not sick but who may be particularly vulnerable due to specific disabilities or social circumstances.

Children's nurses work in a wide range of settings including hospital wards, outpatient departments, community clinics, schools and family homes. Most of the core skills of children's nursing are learned in hospitals, although community children's nursing is developing rapidly (Myers 2005). An increasing number of children are treated in their own home, including children requiring highly specialised care, and community children's nurses are required to provide parents with skilled support. Children's nurses work in close collaboration with other healthcare professionals such as health visitors, doctors, physiotherapists, pharmacists, dieticians as well as social services, education and voluntary organisations. However, children's nurses must also work independently, as they have a unique role to perform for which they alone are responsible.

A chapter such as this cannot give the full range and detail of the knowledge required by children's nurses and there are many excellent textbooks available that do fulfil this role. Rather, this chapter gives a flavour of children's nursing and introduces the reader to the key issues of this extremely rewarding and challenging field of nursing.

Background to children's nursing

From the beginning of history, people have chosen to live in social groups. Inevitably, these social groups included children, some of whom would have been sick and injured. For the most part, the task of caring for sick and injured children has rested with parents and, even today, it is the child's family and immediate carers who provide much of the day-to-day care required by children and young people when they are ill. However, through most of history, there have been people who offered more specialist care to children. Much of this work has not been recorded and much of what has been recorded is difficult to relate to in terms of today's modern context of technical care. We know, for example, that Thomas Phaire (1510–60) practised as a kind of child physician, although much of his practice would have to be regarded as art rather than science and much of his work was about 'care' rather than 'treatment' (Phaire 1545).

There is little evidence of an organised discipline of children's nursing until the last quarter of the nineteenth century. Paediatric nursing, as it became known, is a relatively new phenomenon, born out of the development and increasing number of children's hospitals during the latter half of the nineteenth century. Physicians were appointed as 'consultants' to this new generation of hospitals. These consultants usually had their own private practices and could not be present in the hospital throughout the day, so a body of people needed to be invented who would be present throughout the patients' day and who would provide care to those patients unable to care for themselves. It is in this way that nursing as we know it today was born. The first children's hospital, Great Ormond Street Hospital for Children, London, opened in 1852 and became a template for the development of many more children's hospitals during the following half-century. It soon became clear that sick children needed a special kind of care, a special kind of nurse. In 1888, Catherine Wood, then Lady Superintendent of Great Ormond Street Hospital for Children, wrote:

> I commence by stating two propositions first, that sick children require special Nursing ; and, second, that sick children's Nurses require special training ... Let us put into the arms of a young Nurse some poor little neglected babe. It is to be her charge by day, and she is to do her best with it; her pride will be aroused, especially if some other young Nurse also has a case, and a generous rivalry between the two will be to the manifest advantage of the babes. Suppose that this babe improves in the marvellous

way that babes do, with love and intelligent care, then that Nurse will have learnt a lesson in the care of young infants that will abide by her always. (Wood 1888, p. 510)

Professional nursing of sick children has always been a unique mix of skill, learning and care. The first two qualities can be learned by anyone, but the ability to 'care' for sick children requires a special kind of person. Wood (1888) made it clear that not everyone could nurse sick children, and this is just as true today. To nurse a sick child is to get inside their head, to allow oneself to be a child again, to feel what the child is feeling and to possess an urge to make things better.

Some might try to measure human achievement by the progress of science and medicine. However, it is the *care* of the weak and vulnerable that defines civilisation. Where such care is lacking, civilisation is diminished commensurably. Consider the tragedy of modern warfare; war is technical, skilled and scientific but it so often reflects the debasement of humanity. In the horror of war, it is the few examples of care, of a stronger person helping a weaker other, that illustrate the continuing presence of humanity and civilisation. So it is that providing 'care' to sick children is a defining measure of society. Care is not a simple skill but a deep, complex and ancient human quality, the practice of which helps to define us as human beings.

Among the nursing disciplines, children's nursing is unique in its relationship with the family. Every child is part of some sort of family, whether it is a nuclear family of mother, father and children, a family with just one parent, or a family where parental responsibility is shared between many adults. With the increasing rate of divorce, many children live in reconstituted or blended families, spending time in different homes with biological and step-parents and step- and half-siblings. Whatever their family, the most important principle in the care of sick children is that when a child is sick, it is never just the child who is affected, but the whole family (Shields et al. 2003).

Wherever children's nurses work, they take with them this core philosophical approach, that care must be focused on an understanding of the needs of the child as a child and as a member of a family. The nurse acts as the child's advocate in situations where healthcare is busy and highly complex. It is easy for those focused, for example, on the treatment of a fractured bone or the management of a hospital department to forget that the sick child is a special kind of person, a vulnerable and easily damaged person, a person who is an integral part of a family. Children's nurses ensure that the child's needs as a human being are not forgotten and that in the busy, technical and scientific environment, the child and family's need for human care is given due priority.

Models and contexts of children's nursing

The models of care, or the ways of organising nursing care, in use today are based on the principle that the family is an essential part of a child's life and so must be included in care. Three popular models of children's nursing are described below:

> **Care-by-parent** is when children and their family members stay in a special area, with rooms with a bed for the parents and en-suite facilities, furnished in a comfortable, home-like style (Goodband and Jennings 1992). There are tea and coffee-making and laundry facilities, dining and play areas, and a treatment room. Parents live with the children and provide care in conjunction with the nurses. What the family can do is decided according to the wishes of the parents and children. Care-by-parent units are particularly beneficial for babies who are being breast-fed, for children with chronic serious diseases such as cystic fibrosis or cancer, when the treatment can be particularly frightening, and when privacy is important, for example when a child is dying.

> **Partnership in care** is another popular nursing model (Casey 1995). It is based on the idea that nursing care for a sick child can be given by the child or parents with support and education from the nurse, and that family or parental care can be given by the nurse if the family is absent. The role of the family, or parent, is to take on the everyday care of the child, while the role of the children's nurse is to deliver clinical care, teach and support the child and family and, if necessary, refer the family to other professionals such as physiotherapists or social workers. In high-dependency care, nurses may be providing most of the care the child receives, while in community nursing, it is the parents who provide the bulk of the hour-by-hour care required by the child.

> **Family-centred care** is the most common model of care in children's nursing today. This is a way of caring for children and their families within health services, which ensures that care is planned around the whole family, not just the individual child, and all the family members are recognised as care recipients (Shields et al. 2006). In other words, care cannot be given just to sick children, rather the whole family is the 'body' to which care must be given. Members of the family all have different ways of coping with what is happening to their child. They may be anxious, frightened and upset, or they may be calm and well able to cope. Whatever their coping style, it is important for nurses to recognise this and support them.

Parents must always be considered when planning care, and be included in any decision making about their child. They should be asked if they want to participate in giving care or if they would rather all care be carried out by nurses. Parents' wishes about this must be respected, as being included in caring while their child is sick will help some parents but others may find it frightening.

Play

Play is not something that children do because they have nothing better to do, it is the prime activity of children and it is through play that they discover and make sense of the world. It would be easy to consider that playing with children is solely the role of the play specialist and that nurses have more important issues to attend to such as medicines or dressings. However, the skilled children's nurse is able to utilise highly developed communication skills, which include an ability to play at the child's level, to facilitate assessment, diagnosis and treatment and so have an influential role in the child's recovery. Play in hospital was first formally recognised in the Platt Report (Ministry of Health 1959) and the right of children to play and have access to play facilities has been cited in many government reports since as essential for children's care (DH 1991, 2002; DfES 2003; DH/DCSF 2009).

Play is vital to any child, but for those who find themselves in the unfamiliar world of illness and/or hospital, play is a key source of comfort and familiarity and a way through which they can make sense of and understand their situation. Play is the prime method by which health professionals can communicate with children and which can hasten their recovery and adaptation to new situations (Elliott 2009). The organisation Action for Sick Children (2004) supports the importance of play and identifies the significance of the role of families and the maintenance of normality as far as possible when a child is sick.

Play takes many forms, depending on the age of the child, from the solitary play of the toddler to the interactive activities of the school-aged child, but children of all ages are able to relax and find comfort in familiar toys and activities. It is important that children's nurses consider the most appropriate type of play for individual children to prevent regression and loss of skills and also so that it can be incorporated into preparation for procedures, distraction and also post-procedural activities to aid understanding of the processes undergone.

Play must always focus on the whole family, for it is through working with the parents, siblings and other family members that true understanding and acceptance may occur. Parents will generally welcome the chance to play with their child and nurses can assist them to integrate this into their child's care needs. Play presents a sense of normality for all the family in an often unfamiliar and chaotic world and is essential in providing reassurance, distraction and comfort. The Children's Play Information Service (2009) provides a useful factsheet on the importance and types of play undertaken with children in hospital.

Cultural diversity

We live in an increasingly multicultural society with people from many countries and cultures coming to live together. This makes life rich and interesting for all and enables people to develop their understanding of others and become more tolerant. Children's nursing is just as affected by these changes in society as every other profession and terms such as 'multicultural nursing', 'transcultural nursing' and 'cross-cultural nursing' are used.

In a multicultural environment, the health service culture is usually based on the norms of the dominant cultural group. However, people from different ethnic and cultural backgrounds who use the health services need to be able to express their own way of living, their own beliefs and values. How much health services allow people to do that causes much debate. Most hospitals and health services ensure that ward routines and the way people work take into account the cultural values of the people who use the service. However, some people argue that it is not done well enough, and there are many problems that arise from allowing all cultural groups to do things their own way (Shields 1999). It may not be possible to take into account all the cultural needs of every family, but staff, including children's nurses, must develop a quality known as **cultural competence**, that is, behaviours and attitudes that enable them to work effectively in cross-cultural situations (Arnold 2007).

Sensitivity to cultural constructs is important in nursing but encountering different religions and cultures can make people (both staff and patients and families) feel uncomfortable and threatened. Lack of understanding can lead to uncertainty and fear, which may be manifested as difficult, withdrawn or confrontational behaviour. It is important that nurses caring for children are aware of these issues and take them into account so that communication with and understanding of children and parents from all cultural and ethnic groups are enhanced. This leads to better interaction between children, parents and nurses, and in turn leads to good healthcare delivery and a happy health service experience for the child and the whole family.

Promoting health for children and young people

All professionals involved with children work towards enabling children to be healthy through a variety of measures, including health promotion, **disease prevention**, **health protection** and health education. Further exploration of these issues can be found in Hall and Elliman (2007).

Children's nurses have an important role in promoting and maintaining the health of children and young people in their care. Good health in childhood is not only important during childhood per se but there is increasing evidence that healthy lifestyles during childhood and adolescence have an impact on health and wellbeing well into adulthood. A number of recent initiatives have highlighted the importance of health and health promotion for children. 'Being healthy' is the first of the five outcomes for all children set out in *Every Child Matters* (DfES 2003):

> Being healthy
> Staying safe
> Enjoying and achieving
> Making a positive contribution
> Economic wellbeing.

Children's nurses have a role in all five outcomes, but their focus is obviously on the first. The first standard in the *National Service Framework for Children,*

Young People and Maternity Services (DH/DfES 2004) is also concerned with promoting health and wellbeing, identifying needs and intervening early. In February 2009, the government published the strategy for children and young people's health *Healthy Lives, Brighter Futures* (DH/DCSF 2009), which sets out how world-class health outcomes, services of the highest quality and excellent experiences in using services will be achieved for children and their families and how health inequalities will be minimised.

Targeted health promotion and improved access to services are important strategies in reducing health inequalities. Children's nurses are often in contact with the most vulnerable children and young people, such as those who are homeless or living on low family incomes, those involved in risk-taking behaviour or looked after by local authorities. Such children and young people, who may also suffer from acute or chronic illnesses, have an equal if not greater need for health promotion strategies as well children. However, their ability to access such services may be limited due to their illness and/or circumstances.

Promoting health and wellbeing in children and young people is an integral part of children's nursing. The *Healthy Child Programme* (DH 2009a, 2009b, 2009c) includes screening tests, developmental reviews and immunisations and is delivered by a range of healthcare practitioners working together. Children's nurses may be directly involved in this and in other aspects of multiagency health promotion and encouraging healthy lifestyles. Children's nurses must ensure that families, children and young people take responsibility for and make informed choices about their lifestyle. Listening to and respecting children's views as well as providing timely and appropriate information are important skills for children's nurses. There is a huge range of health issues across the life span from birth to adolescence, of which children's nurses must be aware in order to promote good health. For example, children's nurses need to be aware of the issues involved in promoting breast-feeding, immunisation programmes, early detection of developmental delay and growth problems, injury prevention, healthy diets, physical activity, oral health and sexual health, including teenage pregnancy and sexually transmitted diseases.

Activity 13.1

Laura is eight years old and was admitted to hospital for observation having fallen off her bike. She appears to be overweight and when the nurse records her height, weight and body mass index, it is clear that she is well above expected levels for her age. Her mother says that Laura is teased at school because of her size and that she complains of having no friends. When the nurse asks about her diet, Laura's mum says she is a fussy eater and tends to fill up on crisps and biscuits because she does not like the meals prepared for the family.

Think about the physical, emotional and social issues for Laura and her mother. Consider how the children's nurse might help this family during Laura's stay in hospital and by making referral to appropriate professionals after discharge.

Weight is a sensitive and complex issue and the children's nurse must respond to the concerns of Laura and her mother in a supportive and caring way. For the majority of growing children, strict diets and weight loss are not recommended, rather a change in dietary habits and increase in physical activity levels are sufficient. There are many materials available to help families make healthy changes to their lifestyle and the nurse could introduce Laura and her mother to some of these materials such as the initiative *Change 4Life* (NHS 2010). The nurse might discuss healthy alternatives for snacks and the use of fun activities such as sticker charts for recording healthy food choices. The importance of family mealtimes should be discussed and reasons why Laura does not want to eat with the family will need to be explored and possibly followed up by the school nurse. Increasing physical activity should be discussed and again there are suggestions for fun activities and videos showing ideas for games to encourage children to be active (NHS 2010). Having fallen off her bicycle, Laura will need to build her confidence in cycling again and the children's nurse should offer advice regarding use of cycle helmets and undertaking cycling proficiency training at school. The children's nurse would discuss her concerns with medical colleagues, as referral to a dietician and/or specialist follow-up may be required. Support from the school nurse and health visitor should be considered on discharge, as achieving and maintaining healthy weight is a long-term issue with which Laura and her mother may need ongoing support.

Issues at specific stages of childhood

Children go through different developmental stages and this affects how their care is planned. Giving nursing care to an adolescent with a broken leg from falling off his bike is different to caring for a 9-year-old girl who is having her tonsils removed, or a toddler who is vomiting, or a baby who has pneumonia. All these children and their families have different physical, emotional and social needs and children's nurses ensure that all these needs are taken into account when planning care.

This section considers some of the specific nursing issues in relation to different age groups of children. Detailed consideration of child development can be found in books such as *The Developing Child* (Bee and Boyd 2010) and discussion of the nursing care required by children with specific medical and surgical conditions can be found in edited textbooks such as Glasper and Richardson (2006).

Neonates

A **neonate** is a baby in the first 28 days of life. At the time of birth, many organs and systems of the body are immature and neonates are dependent on others for the provision of food, warmth, comfort and safety. The neonate has a high metabolic rate and undergoes rapid growth and development. A neonate can readily lose temperature due to factors such as a large surface area to body weight ratio, limited ability to shiver and deficiency of subcutaneous fat tissue. If the temperature is not maintained, the colder the neonate becomes, the more oxygen and glucose is used in the process of generating heat. Eventually, this can cause breathing difficulties and low blood glucose as energy reserves are used up. Such energy must be supplied in the form of milk, or if the baby is ill and unable to feed, via intravenous fluids. Nutrition is essential to supply energy and nutrients for growth and development. Therefore much of the care of neonates is directed towards ensuring adequate warmth and nutrition.

Neonates are vulnerable to infections due to their immature immune system, and when infected they can deteriorate rapidly, necessitating prompt recognition and treatment (Boxwell 2010). Approximately 10% of neonates require observation and care above that normally needed and are admitted to specialised neonatal units (NAO 2007). Reasons for admission include prematurity, low birth weight, respiratory illnesses and infection. Maternal use of illicit drugs is relatively common in some countries, resulting in a number of neonates being at risk of withdrawal symptoms once they have been born as they are no longer exposed to the drugs via the mother's bloodstream (Johnson et al. 2003). This condition, known as 'neonatal abstinence syndrome', requires careful observation and medical treatment, sometimes for months, and the babies may suffer additional problems after discharge (Johnson et al. 2003).

Most of the neonates nursed in neonatal units are born prematurely, the smallest and sickest of these can only breathe effectively with the aid of machinery and require intensive care. Many are not yet able to suck and are fed via a tube into the stomach, or, if unable to tolerate this, via an intravenous infusion. Such neonates are susceptible to brain damage, and must be nursed with great care and sensitivity. Any disturbance such as handling, loud noises or bright lights can cause stress and discomfort and cause deterioration in the neonate's condition (Boxwell 2010). Those involved with these extremely vulnerable neonates must have highly developed observational skills. Since premature neonates have limited ability to communicate, nurses must be alert to cues in their behaviour that may indicate pain, discomfort or a change in condition and be proactive in pre-empting problems as they arise and in seeking support from the multidisciplinary team. Parents are extremely concerned about their infants and may feel helpless within the highly technological environment. Therefore nurses must have good communication skills in order to listen to and acknowledge their anxieties and encourage parents to participate in care at their own pace.

Infants

An **infant** is a child from birth to one year of age. Infants tend to lose weight in the first week of life but by the end of the second week have regained their birth weight. After this, infants gain approximately 140–200 g per week, doubling their birth weight by four to seven months of age. The rate at which infants gain weight then progressively declines, so that the birth weight is trebled by the first birthday (Kelsey and McEwing 2006).

Breast milk is the ideal source of nutrition for young infants and continues to provide valuable nutrients as part of a mixed diet even after weaning has taken place. There are many advantages to breast-feeding for the baby, including protection from infection, and the mother. There are also huge benefits to society from the reduction of health problems such as gastroenteritis in breast-fed babies. Diarrhoea and pneumonia are more common and more severe in children who are bottle-fed, and are responsible for many deaths in developing countries (WHO 2009). Other acute infections such as otitis media and urinary tract infections are less common and less severe in breast-fed infants, and global studies suggest that breast-fed infants are far less likely to be admitted to hospital than bottle-fed babies (WHO 2009). Children's nurses should therefore always encourage and facilitate breast-feeding in infants even when they are sick and hospitalised. The Baby Friendly Initiative (UNICEF 2009) outlines standards to promote successful breast-feeding and it is recommended that, whether working in hospitals or the community, professionals follow guidelines to support and encourage breast-feeding mothers (NICE 2006). However, care should be taken not to make those who choose to bottle-feed their infants feel inadequate or guilty. Milk does not satisfy all the nutritional requirements from the age of six months onwards. Weaning takes place when foods other than milk are gradually introduced.

Most hospitalisations during infancy are due to infections. It is important to take into account the infant's stage of development, and to be aware that the infant may regress to an earlier stage while sick and in an unfamiliar environment. To try to reduce these stresses, parents are encouraged to stay with their infants, but it should be appreciated that this can be challenging when there are siblings at home. Children's nurses need to promote the continued normal development of infants as well as recovery from their illness (Scanlon and Sorrentino 2006). Many infants requiring additional healthcare, particularly of a long-term nature, remain with their families in the community with support from a team of healthcare professionals including children's nurses, being admitted to hospital only when essential.

In the UK, infants undergo health surveillance at birth, and at set ages such as six weeks and eight months in the community. However, any contact with a health professional such as a visit to the doctor is an opportunity to assess the infant's progress. The purpose of routine examinations at the above stages is to detect problems at an early age and to enable appropriate support and interventions to be provided (DH 2009a). Particular attention is paid to general health, feeding, growth and development. Immunisations are also offered to prevent infectious diseases.

Preschool children (one to four years)

From approximately one year onwards, babies become 'toddlers' and, as their muscles and coordination develops, their gross and fine motor skills increase. During this period, children learn to walk, climb, run, hop, hold a pencil, build bricks and so on. At the same time, their cognitive and language skills are developing as well as their social skills. During these few years, children develop from helpless babies dependent on others to meet all their needs to relatively independent human beings who can dress themselves, help themselves to food when hungry, make friends and learn simple social rules such as taking turns and sharing. These great achievements in terms of development are not without risk and children in this age group are particularly vulnerable to accidents as they explore their world, often unaware of the dangers.

Children's nurses working in A&E units will encounter children who have suffered a range of accidents or unintentional injury. Most accidents are preventable and, while nurses should not accuse or blame parents or carers or indeed the child in the immediate aftermath of an incident, when they may already feel desperately guilty, nurses need to be aware of the importance of accident prevention strategies and give appropriate and timely advice. Children from lower socioeconomic backgrounds are more at risk of sustaining unintentional injuries (Towner 2002) and nurses need to be sensitive to the stresses and issues facing such families in order to provide appropriate care and support.

Falls are the most common reason for children attending A&E and may be relatively minor, resulting from children falling over on the pavement or playground, or more serious if they fall or are dropped from a height such as falling downstairs or out of a window. Falls and other unintentional injuries such as burns and scalds, poisoning and drowning are frequently the result of children exploring a dangerous world with ever increasing ability. Children's nurses need to be familiar with normal child development in order to ensure that parents, carers and their own workplace provide a stimulating but safe environment for young children to develop.

School children (5–11 years)

As children's independence grows and their world expands beyond the immediate home and family environment, risks to their health change. For example, pedestrian road traffic accidents replace accidents in the home as a major cause of morbidity, particularly for boys under 10 years. The relationship between social deprivation and rates of childhood illness, in particular infections and accidents, continues (Towner 2002).

Children of all ages and social backgrounds may suffer from chronic illness and there is evidence that some illnesses such as asthma and diabetes mellitus are increasing. Diagnosis of a chronic illness can result in the child and family suffering many losses dependent on the age and stage of development of the child (Lowes 2007). One of the challenges for children's nurses is to enable children and their families to find ways to manage the illness in such a way that any impact on education and social interactions is minimised. A term often used when discussing the impact of chronic illness on children is 'quality of life' and a number of instruments have been developed to measure the quality of life of children with specific diseases (Eiser 1997). Such instruments are used to assess the effectiveness of both medical and nursing interventions. Children's nurses are involved in teaching children self-management of their chronic illness in order for them to gain greater control of their disease, increase their independence and so improve their quality of life. It is important that nurses understand children's perspectives of their illness and that of their parents, as this will influence their response to advice and education.

Children's nurses not only work with children with chronic illnesses and their families but they may be involved, with the child and family's permission, in educating teachers, friends and others such as Brownie and Cub leaders about the child's illness and treatment. In this way nurses enable children with chronic illness to enjoy the same social support and interactions as their healthy peers.

Adolescents (11–16 years)

A child becomes an adult through a process or transition known as 'adolescence'. There are a number of definitions of adolescence and a variety of ages at which it is considered to start and finish. There are clearly physiological changes from the appearance of secondary sexual characteristics, known as 'puberty', to full sexual and reproductive maturity. However, key social, emotional and intellectual changes also take place. In many cultures, the physical changes occur before the social and legal markers of adulthood such as the ability to vote, marry and engage in sexual relationships. The confusion about status and roles can create tensions for young people and their families and for those caring for them.

A useful definition of adolescence is given by the World Health Organization:

> Adolescence is a dynamic period of growth and development that bridges childhood to adulthood, while being distinctly different from both groups. Adolescence is characterised by many rapid, interrelated changes of body, mind and social relationships. (Brumbaugh Keeney et al. 2004, p. 15)

Adolescence may be divided into three stages of early (11–14 years), mid (15–17 years) and late (18–21 years) adolescence. Children's nurses are generally only involved in the early and mid stages, although occasionally young people with particular illnesses or disabilities may remain with paediatric services into late adolescence. The needs of young people vary depending on their stage of adolescence and level of maturity. A common mistake is to fail to recognise the needs of young people in early adolescence because their changes in physical appearance and social status are minimal. For example, an 11-year-old girl may be placed in a mixed sex bay on a children's ward and yet she may be more embarrassed about her developing body and more in need of privacy than a 15-year-old who has become accustomed to her new shape and sexuality.

Adolescents have to achieve a number of tasks or goals in order to become independent adults (Christie and Viner 2005). Developing a clear identity of self, as a separate and independent person, in relation to others is perhaps the key task of adolescence. For many, the achievement of this task is relatively painless and problem free, but for others it can be a major source of turmoil and they encounter the 'storm and stress' frequently associated with the teenage years. Adolescents who are or become sick have additional challenges as their ability to master these normal tasks of adolescence, such as becoming independent of parents, may be limited.

Adolescents make up approximately a quarter of paediatricians' workload and yet interest in this age group has been sadly lacking in the UK compared to other countries such as Australia and North America, where the speciality of adolescent health is well established (Payne et al. 2005). Young people have specific health needs, many of which remain unmet. Current healthcare for adolescents is discussed in detail in the policy initiative *Bridging the Gaps: Health Care for Adolescents* (RCPCH 2003). This document describes young people's frustrations with health provision including:

> lack of information
> difficulties accessing help for confidential issues
> lack of expertise and continuity of care by professionals
> failure to respect the validity of young people's views
> young people in hospital having to be accommodated either in a children's ward or with a population they regard as elderly.

The ideal of specific adolescent units, as discussed by Viner and Keane (1998), has not been achieved, with very few hospitals having designated adolescent units. However, many children's wards have specific adolescent bays or areas and employ staff who have specific experience and education with this age group.

Young people with specific issues such as disability, poverty, ethnicity, being looked after and sexual orientation have particular difficulties with access to services (RCPCH 2003). Strategies to improve and monitor health services for young people in the UK have been set out and children's nurses are well placed to ensure that young people's views are listened to and improvements made.

Preparation for hospital and procedures

When a child comes into contact with health services, the experience can be strange, uncomfortable and sometimes painful and frightening. Because of this, part of a nurse's role is to make the child as comfortable as possible, so that the encounter causes the child minimal pain, distress and worry. Children's nurses achieve this through delivering sensitive care structured around an appropriate model, as described earlier, and which includes adequate preparation of the child and family.

Activity 13.2

Think about your earliest memory of seeing a doctor or visiting a hospital or surgery. Were you frightened or excited? Were the people you met kind and welcoming or did they seem stern and distant? Were your parents with you? What do you remember of the experience – the smell, the food, being upset, fantastic new toys?

Our first encounters with healthcare settings can influence our reaction to them for the rest of our lives. Children who are prepared for the encounter/ visit, are welcomed by happy, friendly staff, given interesting and exciting toys and activities and whose parents or carers are involved in their care are far less likely to be frightened by the experience and tend to be more willing to cooperate and return happily if required.

Effective preparation requires an understanding of the child's stage of development and sound communication skills and may involve specific play materials such as books, dolls, games and dressing-up clothes. It is important that those preparing children have the knowledge and confidence to answer their questions honestly and the communication skills to ensure that the information is understood (Elliott 2009). Many children are admitted to hospital as emergencies following accidents or sudden onset of acute illness. For these children, there is no time to offer planned preparation and detailed explanations so it is important that all children are encouraged to have some understanding of what hospitals are like and a positive view of them as places where most people are made well again. It is crucial that nurses, doctors, hospitals and specific treatments, such as injections, are never used to threaten children. Television programmes, particularly 'fly on the wall' documentary series, have done much to demystify hospitals and educate the public including children about what happens there. However, such programmes may give false impressions or cause a new set of fears for children and it is essential that children's nurses discover what each individual child understands about their admission to hospital and correct any misconceptions.

Many hospitals have organised programmes to prepare children for admission to hospital. Some hospitals have a play hospital (National Association of Hospital Play Staff 2000), where children can come and play with the equipment that they will see when they are admitted. Certain hospitals have pre-admission visits, so children and their families can visit the ward and meet the nurses and other staff who are going to care for them. Visits to the operating theatre if the child is going to have an operation or to the X-ray department if they are having a radiological procedure may be included.

Teenagers also require consideration when thinking about preparation for hospitalisation and procedures. As well as the tumultuous emotions to be dealt with during normal adolescence, sick and hospitalised teenagers have their own specific concerns. They need preparation, and this can be done in a variety of ways, either by parents, the local doctor or the school nurse. Open and honest communication is vital to prepare a teenager for hospital or a health service visit. Many children's hospitals have interactive websites for children of all ages but these may be especially useful for adolescents who are particularly at ease with this form of communication (see for example www.childrenfirst. nhs.uk). Consideration also must be given to the preparation of young people with chronic illnesses for transfer from paediatric to adult services. Children's nurses have a key role in ensuring that not only the young person and their family are adequately prepared for the transfer but that the adult services receiving the young person into their care are fully informed and prepared (RCN 2004a).

Effective preparation of children and their families for hospitalisation and medical procedures is essential not only to reduce their anxiety and gain their cooperation but also to ensure that they have sufficient information, appropriate to their age and stage of development, to make informed decisions and consent to treatment.

Informed consent

Informed consent from children and their families is required to ensure that children receive the best care possible to meet their needs. It is required in a healthcare context for any treatments, investigations, nursing care and in relation to record keeping and sharing information (DH 2001a, 2001b, 2001c; GMC 2007). However, where there are concerns regarding the safety of the child, where significant harm is suspected or has happened, then the need for informed consent to share information is superseded by the duty of care to protect the child (RCPCH 2004; DCSF 2008a; Wake 2009a). The law in relation to capacity to consent and parental responsibility differs in each country and children's nurses should ensure they are familiar with the relevant legislation for the country in which they work.

In English law, young people are considered to be adults at the age of 18 years (Children Act 1989, 2004). Young people from the age of 16 years are presumed to be competent to make their own healthcare decisions, although there are some limitations when there is evidence that the young person does not fully comprehend the nature of the treatment/nontreatment (Mental Capacity Act 2005).

Informed consent is inherently complex, particularly for young people under the age of 16 years where the chronological age alone is insufficient to identify whether a young person fully understands the nature of the proposed treatment or nontreatment. The term 'Gillick competence' is used to identify children and young people who have 'reasonable understanding' of the decision-making process regarding their health and enables them to give informed consent to varying degrees. Alongside this, the term 'Fraser guidelines' focuses on contraceptive advice and young people under 16 years old (DH 2004; Wheeler 2006; GMC 2007). However, ascertaining what is 'reasonable' in terms of a child's understanding is not always clear. Children should always be involved in the decision-making process in accordance with their developmental abilities. Every effort should be made to communicate with and for the child in a developmentally appropriate manner to ensure that this happens and to work in partnership with the family to enable this to occur (Children Act 1989, 2004).

An important element of decision making in relation to informed consent is that of 'best interests' (Children Act 1989, 2004; BMA 2001). Any treatment and/or care prescribed has to be in the child/young person's best interests. However, this can lead to some difficulties in relation to agreements as to what is in the child's best interests and has led to a number of high-profile court cases in the UK.

In addition, neonates, infants, young children and some older children who have a profound learning disability, for example, are unable to give informed consent. As it is impossible to ascertain their wishes, surrogate decision making takes place. Every opportunity must be taken to involve children with profound learning disabilities in decision making through the use of familiar augmentative and alternative communication strategies. The surrogate decision making is usually undertaken by someone who has parental responsibility; however, this in itself is complex in terms of the need to ensure that the best interests of the infant/child are always paramount. Parental responsibility in terms of who can give informed consent for such children can be complicated and readers are advised to consider the excellent guidance available via the Children's Legal Centre (2010). When there is lack of agreement regarding what is in the child's best interests, it is important that the courts are involved as advocates. The courts appoint an advocate who seeks to strengthen the child's voice in terms of what is in their best interests.

Children have a right to be safe, to be heard and for their care and treatment to always be in their best interests. Informed decision making in relation to the healthcare of children and young people must have their best interests at the forefront. Children and young people should always be part of the decision-making process in accordance with their developmental abilities. Children's nurses have a duty of care to ensure this happens and need to work in real partnership with children, young people and their families, listening actively to their wishes and concerns and supporting them in the complex decision-making process in relation to healthcare (DfES 2004; NMC 2008).

Children and young people undergoing surgery

Children, who are smaller and less physically and emotionally developed than adults, have different visual and psychological perspectives. The environment of the operating theatre looks different to a child than to an adult. Also, children lack rationalisation skills to help them to recognise their environment in specific contexts, and so may become frightened (Shields and Waterman 2002). Figure 13.1 shows what a child sees from the operating table, while Figure 13.2 shows what an anaesthetic mask looks like when it is about to be placed over a child's face. If you are very small, these things can look especially frightening.

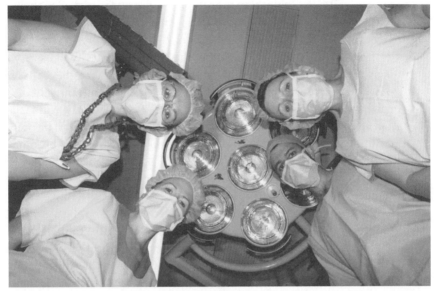

Figure 13.1 Child's eye view from the operating table
Source: Glasper and Richardson 2006. Reproduced with permission from Elsevier Limited

3

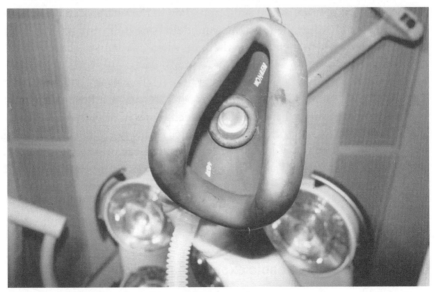

Figure 13.2 Child's eye view of an anaesthetic mask
Source: Glasper and Richardson 2006. Reproduced with permission from Elsevier Limited

Operating theatres where children and young people have surgery should be as 'child friendly' as possible, with pictures and cartoons on the walls and ceilings, bright curtains and colourful mobiles (Shields and Waterman 2002). Toy cars are fun for children to ride from the ward to the operating theatre, or trolleys dressed up as boats or other fun vehicles. It is best for children if they are admitted to the operating theatre wearing their own clothes, usually pyjamas, rather than special operating theatre gowns. Before coming to the operating theatre, children usually have a local anaesthetic cream applied to their hand so that a needle can be inserted into a vein without any pain, and drugs and fluids given intravenously (Shields and Tanner 2010).

If a child is having an operation, the child's parent(s) will usually accompany them to the anaesthetic room and stay until the anaesthetist has inserted the intravenous cannula and administered the general anaesthetic. Unless parents are well prepared for this, the rapidity with which the child falls asleep can be frightening (Shields and Waterman 2002). Parents must be prepared by ensuring that they know what their child will look like as they become unconscious, that they are told everything that will happen, and that they are escorted out of the theatre before the operation commences and given appropriate reassurance (McAlister 2010).

Following surgery, children are transferred into the recovery unit while they are still fully anaesthetised and sound asleep. Here they wake up, as the anaesthetic wears off, under the care of specialist nurses who ensure that the children are breathing effectively and are not in pain or bleeding. Because children's metabolism is fast, they wake from anaesthetic much more rapidly than adults, and can become quite active. For this reason, there is always one nurse for every patient in a paediatric recovery unit. Children remain in the recovery unit until they are awake and responding to their name, can breathe properly, pain is fully controlled and the wound dressing is dry and intact. Children are only returned to their bed on the ward when their nurse is happy that they are awake and safe.

Day surgery is used increasingly for operations on children as it avoids overnight admission and reduces the distress of hospitalisation. Major advances in surgical and anaesthetic techniques in recent years have led to less invasive surgery, shorter operation times and better pain control, so enabling more children to be discharged home on the day of surgery. The benefits for the child and family as well as reduction in waiting lists and costs for healthcare providers cannot be denied but if day-case surgery is to be a positive experience for the child and family, considerable assessment to ensure appropriate patient selection, planning and education, to ensure families feel able to cope, is required (Morse 2007).

Children and young people experiencing pain

Children suffer pain for a number of reasons; sometimes pain is caused by injury, for example a fracture, by disease processes such as inflammation and sometimes by treatment itself, for example surgery. It is sometimes necessary for children's nurses to cause pain in order for a particular therapeutic intervention to be carried out. This alone presses a particular responsibility on nurses to ensure that pain is treated as effectively as possible. Children's nurses are often the practitioners most closely involved with child patients and in the best position to observe, assess and treat children's pain.

Children's nurses need to be ever vigilant for signs of pain because it may be poorly communicated by children. Young children and babies may be unable to vocalise their pain and are often unable to provide a verbal account of the pain's characteristics, such as intensity, duration and location. Even older children may fail to communicate their pain in a manner that is easily understood by adults. Pain may be an important indicator of disease but it is also important to appreciate that pain itself can have a serious and deleterious effect on children, including their physiological stability. Pain will increase respiratory and cardiac rate and oxygen consumption. In this way, pain makes an important demand on children's physiological resources. Very ill babies and children may simply not be able to meet the additional demand caused by pain. In this situation, their condition can deteriorate rapidly; it should be understood, therefore, that pain management is an important part of children's care and treatment.

There are a number of pain assessment scales used by children's nurses to enable them to assess and record children's pain as accurately as possible. They allow nurses to assess children's pain even where the child is not able to describe the pain verbally. There are three types of pain assessment tools:

1 *self-report tools* – enable children and young people themselves to indicate on a chart or a series of pictures the level and location of their pain
2 *behavioural tools* – enable nurses and carers to assess the child's level of pain through the behaviour they exhibit, such as crying, movement and facial expression
3 *physiological tools* – assess the child's physiological responses to pain such as heart and respiratory rates. This is particularly useful for children with cognitive impairment who cannot always express their pain.

Clinical practice guidelines are available for children's nurses that review the evidence base for the different pain assessment tools and make recommendations for the management of pain in babies and children (RCN 2009).

Pain can be treated in a number of different ways. Analgesic drugs are useful and it is important to remember that drugs such as morphine and other powerful narcotics can be used on children who are very ill and even on very small babies. Powerful narcotics are safe as long as they are used under controlled situations and where children are monitored for central nervous system depression.

Drugs are not the only way to manage childhood pain. It has long been known that anxiety can exacerbate pain. Children's nurses can do much to ensure that children are not exposed to unnecessary anxiety. Children can be frightened of things that are real and things that are imagined. The 'atmosphere' in which children are nursed can be as important as any drug. An atmosphere that is quiet, calm and reassuring can do much to help. Such an atmosphere is almost certain to contain parents' anxiety and they too need their fears addressed if they are to be able to help their child. The management of pain is never simple, and it is necessary to understand the relevant pharmacology and physiology of pain. Just as important, however, is a knowledge of the child's developmental stage and of the psychology of pain as it applies to children.

Critical care

Children are successfully receiving high-dependency/intensive care on an ever increasing basis. More and more children are surviving neonatal illness and prematurity and have long-lasting effects that often require intensive care or high-dependency management. High-dependency and **critical care** services for children were outlined and recommendations made for future developments within the document *Paediatric Intensive Care: A Framework for the Future* (DH 1997). Within this document, levels of care are identified so that children have access to some immediate care within their local hospital but where their needs are greater, for example for respiratory support, then the regional centre will provide assistance and may possibly transfer the child to that regional unit.

Children's critical care services are not only located in hospital environments but also within the community setting. Many children's community nursing teams support families to care for children with highly technical equipment such as ventilators and continuous intravenous infusions for nutrition. Courses exist that are specifically arranged to prepare children's nurses to work in the community with critically ill children and their families – thus providing care within the familiar, safe environment of the home, which is generally less disruptive than the hospital environment.

Children's nurses must possess many qualities such as compassion, **empathy**, technical awareness, advanced anatomical knowledge and skills of independent care delivery and management. Qualified nurses must be able to make independent decisions and utilise competent assessment skills to work within the professional competence framework to meet the needs of critically ill children and their families (NMC 2008). Current developments related to the assessment of potentially deteriorating children have reinforced the importance of competent skills in early assessment, to determine those children most at need of critical care (Egdell et al. 2008). However, highly skilled paediatric critical care nurses are in short supply, because of the specialised nature of the work and the small number of critical care facilities within the country.

Common conditions associated with high-dependency and critical care management include unintentional injuries, infections, congenital disorders and surgical and medical conditions that require high levels of technical support. All these conditions have many similarities with regard to the role of the nurse and the management of the condition. Competent assessment skills and awareness of the importance of oxygen and fluid therapy are essential.

Children's response to illness varies with each child and their age. Very young children, under one year of age, have a high surface area of skin in relation to their size and weight and this makes them prone to dehydration and hypothermia. As a consequence, children under one have difficulty tolerating illness because of their fragility and many who have suffered severe illness have growth impairment and the consequences of lack of oxygen such as learning difficulties.

Critical care management of infants and children centres on:

> stabilisation of the respiratory system to enable adequate oxygen to be delivered to the cells of the body
> administration of fluids to ensure that circulation is maintained, which will allow oxygen to be delivered to all of the body
> supporting all the systems of the body such as cardiac and renal to enable them to function effectively to undertake all the normal functions as well as cope with the abnormality caused by the illness/disorder.

Many drugs are required in the critical care environment to support the body in its functions and critical care paediatric nurses must have a good knowledge of these drugs and an ability to undertake calculations to ensure the correct dose is administered.

Safeguarding children

Nearly 31,000 children were registered on child protection registers in England alone in 2005 (DfES 2006) and this increased to 34,000 in 2008 (DCSF 2009a). While statistics only offer one aspect of a complex picture, they should make everyone consider how children and childhood are viewed and that protecting all children is everyone's responsibility.

The death of Victoria Climbié in 2000 and Baby P in 2007 highlighted once again that children and young people are vulnerable and that the risk of significant harm or even death has not reduced. From the resultant inquiries (Laming 2003, 2009; Haringey Local Safeguarding Children Board 2008) and earlier reports, the government formulated *Every Child Matters* (DfES 2003) and the *Children's Plan* (DCSF 2007, 2008b, 2009b) and made provisions for the recommendations within the Children Act 2004 to ensure that safeguarding children became a priority. *Every Child Matters* (DfES, 2003, 2004) identified five key areas, which need to be addressed in order that every child is able to reach their potential. In terms of safeguarding children, it focuses on staying safe – ensuring children are protected from harm and neglect as well as being healthy and enjoying childhood. Thus practitioners in all agencies have a duty to cooperate together to promote the wellbeing of children and to ensure that services to safeguard and promote their welfare are in place (HM Government 2006; DCSF 2008b).

Children may experience harm physically, emotionally and/or sexually, with neglect often also an issue. There are complex factors that may make a child more vulnerable to harm, such as poor parenting capacity, domestic violence, poverty and social exclusion (Corby 2006). This requires practitioners, including children's nurses, to have a sound understanding of child development and parenting in order to ensure identification of children at risk and early detection and prevention of harm. Nurses are seen to be in a prime position to achieve this (RCN 2004b) but do not always do so for a variety of reasons, such as not thinking the unthinkable (May-Chahal et al. 2004). Other problems such as not referring families early enough to ensure adequate support and ongoing subjective debates regarding what is good enough parenting and indeed what is harm prevent children receiving the care and protection they require.

One of the key ongoing issues is that of poor communication between agencies. A large number of reports (including Luce 2003; Laming 2003, 2009; NSPCC 2008) have criticised communication as a key reason why children are not adequately protected and appear to fall through gaps in provision. There is an increasing emphasis on integrated working to improve communication between the different professional groups involved in the care of children and to improve outcomes for all children. **Integrated working** is where everyone supporting children and young people work together effectively to put the child at the centre, meeting needs and improving lives (CWDC 2009a). Integrated working is achieved through collaboration and coordination at all levels, across all services, in both single and multiagency settings. A key aspect of integrated working is the Common Assessment Framework, which was introduced to help early identification of need, promote coordinated service provision and reduce the number of assessments that some children and young people go through (CWDC 2009b).

The consequences of harm for children and young people cannot be stressed enough – the ultimate consequence may be their death. Children and young people may experience short-, medium- and long-term physical and emotional difficulties as a result of harm they have suffered, including difficulties relating to peers and significant others, school performance and running away from home. Children who have experienced harm have low self-esteem and self-worth, as well as fear and anxiety in relation to potential subsequent harm. They are more at risk of developing mental health needs such as depression and more serious and enduring mental illness later in life (Corby 2006; Parry-Langdon 2008). The impact on children or young people is too complex to discuss in this short section; however, what is clear is the duty owed to children, that every child does matter and everyone is responsible for ensuring this.

The mental health needs of children and young people

Emotional wellbeing for children and young people is an important part of overall health. The term 'emotional resilience' is used when reflecting on the capacity of children and young people to cope better with change and problems and 'bounce back' from difficult situations that cause them distress. Factors that affect children's ability to develop resilience include temperament, social skills and locus of control, as well as factors within the family such as warm and supportive parenting and good friendships (Carr 2006).

Children and young people who have developed positive emotional resilience skills are more able to learn, play, make friendships and cope with many of the problems that children may experience. However, one in five children and young people have promotional health needs (Mental Health Foundation 2005), and surveys (Parry-Langdon 2008, for example) highlight that 1 in 10 children (9% of the UK child population) under the age of 15 years have a mental health disorder, and it is likely that there are more children and young people who are vulnerable in terms of their emotional wellbeing (Maughan et al. 2004; Office for National Statistics 2008). It is therefore important that children's nurses give consideration to the emotional needs of children and young people accessing services.

Health professionals working together to meet the emotional needs of children and young people must ensure that they are actively listened to and their needs are considered in the context of their families, family functioning and the physical and social environment (Carr 2006). Some children and young people are considered to be more at risk of mental health problems; however, all children and young people are vulnerable and even children who are considered to have sound emotional resilience skills can experience significant distress and difficulties (Wake 2009b).

Factors that cause children and young people to be more at risk of mental health problems may be related to the family, for example rigid parenting styles and bonding and attachment difficulties. In such families, children may not be loved or love is conditional and/or inconsistent. Children for whom there is family breakdown and/or domestic violence or where there are parental mental health problems are also considered to be more at risk of anxiety and depression (Kurtz and Thornes 2000; Office for National Statistics 2008). In addition, children and young people who have experienced harm, emotionally, physically or sexually, are also extremely vulnerable.

Additional risk factors include being cared for within the looked after system (Meltzer et al. 2003), including those children and young people in residential and foster care and also those who are being detained within the criminal justice system. There is evidence of a high incidence of mental health problems for these young people in relation to self-harm and depression (Flood-Page et al. 2000; Mental Health Foundation 2006). Children and young people who have been bullied are vulnerable because of the impact on their self-esteem and the incidence of depression is higher among such children (Bond et al. 2001). There is also an increased incidence of mental health problems among those young people who substance misuse (Meltzer et al. 2003; National Treatment Agency for Substance Misuse 2009).

Sound knowledge of child development is vital as children and young people may demonstrate their difficulties through their behaviour, for example becoming withdrawn, loss of interest in playing or refusing to go to school (DfES 2001). Young people may demonstrate additional signs in terms being self-critical and having mood swings (Young Minds 2003). Mental health problems can appear as **anxiety disorders**, depression, eating disorders, self-harm, para-suicide and suicide (NICE 2004a, 2005). The early signs may be detected in a number of social settings, such as nursery and school as well as at home, and children's nurses need to work in partnership with families and professionals working in these areas (DfES 2001). An awareness of these early signs and the impact of the additional stress of long-term health problems and struggling to attain academic requirements is essential for those working with children.

Services for children and young people tend to be offered at primary, secondary and tertiary level in tiers of provision, which can include residential support within tier four. Most child and adolescent mental health service provision is offered in partnership with other services at primary level, with specialist input from therapists and healthcare professionals being available in a range of settings in tier two and three provision.

Healthcare needs of children with profound and multiple disabilities

Children with learning disabilities are not ill and many children never need to access child health services beyond the usual child health surveillance and childhood ailments appropriate to their chronological age. However, some children do have additional health needs, in particular children with profound and multiple disabilities (PMD) and these children are more likely to access child health services. The incidence of children with PMD has increased (Nessa 2004; Emerson 2009) due to a variety of complex factors including technological advances leading to survival of extremely premature infants.

Children are children first and foremost and this is of paramount consideration when working with children and their families. Children's needs and wishes must be acknowledged at all times, particularly children with complex disabilities as they are more reliant on carers to meet their everyday needs. Children with PMD often have significant communication difficulties, which may mean that they are reliant on augmentative communication strategies. Healthcare practitioners, including children's nurses, need an understanding of such strategies in order to ensure that children's needs are met. In addition, they need to be aware that a number of children with PMD have dual sensory impairments (DH/DfES 2003). It is important therefore that all children with PMD receive regular child health surveillance, which may be overlooked if professionals focus on the child's disability rather than the child as a whole. Indeed, children with PMD are likely to need more specialist screening than that used for children in general to ensure that their needs are effectively met (Every Disabled Child Matters 2007; NHS Confederation 2009). If sensory impairments are not detected, children may demonstrate self-stimulatory behaviour as a result of others being unable to meet their communication needs (RNIB 2000; Wake 2009b).

In working with children with sensory impairment, it is important that play incorporates multisensory approaches; however, this needs to be given careful consideration in terms of planning which equipment will enhance the child's experiences and avoid sensory overload.

In addition to communication needs, most children with PMD have mobility problems that affect their lives on a daily basis. Children with such needs must be referred as early as possible to physiotherapy and occupational therapy services in order to maintain and improve their functional ability and comfort. This in turn enhances their ability to physically interact with their environment through play. Children with PMD have an increased risk of developing additional mobility-related problems such as contractures and even pressure sores and must have regular reassessment to meet their physical, growth and cognitive needs. Children with such complex mobility needs may access healthcare for elective treatments such as surgery. Therefore children's nurses need to be aware of the importance of risk and comfort assessment in relation to positioning and ensure that sleep systems, specialist mattresses, specialist equipment and therapies that children may require are always available.

Children with PMD often have an increased incidence of chronic health problems, including epilepsy, cardiac and respiratory conditions and nutritional problems (DH 2001d). However, many children have health needs and it is important not to ascribe all health problems in children with PMD to their disability. Epilepsy in children, particularly those under five and those with PMD, is often complex and can be difficult to treat. These children must have their epilepsy care managed through specialist tertiary services to ensure they receive the best care possible (NICE 2004b).

Feeding and nutritional problems are often associated with PMD and may be linked to health problems such as respiratory distress and infections. As a consequence, children with PMD may require feeding through a tube into the stomach either via the nasogastric route or through a small incision in the abdomen. Children's nurses are involved in administering such feeds and teaching parents and other carers how to deliver them safely and need to be aware of the current National Patient Safety Agency (NPSA) guidance in relation to enteral feeding (NPSA 2004, 2005a, 2005b).

Family-centred care and support is a vital aspect of caring for children with PMD, particularly given the increased incidence of stress-related problems that families experience in caring for their child at home. However, services are still poor and tend to be fragmented (Warner 2006). Support for the family has to be for all family members including siblings and the extended family where appropriate and should include family-based short-term breaks where wished in order to support the family to function as a family. This is essential if families are to have quality time with all their children rather than daily life focusing on the physical elements of caring for their child with PMD. Play and leisure is important for everyone, and this must include children with PMD, as children are children first and foremost, as stated above.

Palliative care

The death of a child is relatively rare in Western society and it may have taken place suddenly as a result of an emergency but most typically it will occur following a period of prolonged care and management. Ensuring that children and their families receive the highest quality care throughout this period is the prime purpose of palliative care. Paediatric palliative care services have developed alongside other paediatric services with the notion that children and their families deserve holistic care and management by qualified children's nurses who put children and their families at the centre of care.

The UN Convention on the Rights of the Child (UNICEF 1989) insists that nurses who work with children should be trained in such a speciality and this is particularly important in symptom management and care when the child has a life-limiting condition. The palliative care environment is one within which children and their families are facilitated to live each moment to the full, with respite care being provided for the duration of the disease process as well as at the end of life, including bereavement support.

In the UK, it is estimated that there are currently 16 in every 10,000 children between 0–19 years old who are affected by a life-limiting condition (DH 2007). Around half of these children will require palliative care at some time (ACT/RCPCH 2003). Improved techniques of care within the acute nursing and medical sector mean that there are increasing numbers of children who survive but who do so with the threat of early death and the need for symptom management and daily care. The numbers of young people currently requiring this care between 0–24 years of age is estimated at 23,500, with this number expected to rise further (DH 2007). The majority of palliative care for children within the UK is centred on one of 44 children's hospices, which are specifically designated for children from birth to adulthood (usually identified as 19 years of age; however, some young people's hospices provide care up to 25 years of age). The first children's hospice in the world opened in 1982 in Oxford.

According to the Association of Children's Hospices (ACH 2005), children's palliative care services are provided for a range of conditions, such as:

> cancer when the treatment has failed

- cystic fibrosis when the child may have long periods of normal activity but where there will be episodes of deterioration resulting in the need for specialist assistance prior to early death
- muscular dystrophy, which is progressively degenerative, where the treatment is exclusively palliative because no curative treatments are available
- severe cerebral palsy where the condition is irreversible but nonprogressive, although the condition causes susceptibility to other health complications and many result in early death.

Specialist care for children and their families for respite, emergency and end of life treatment can occur within the hospice environment or the home, and the staff working within these environments form a team comprising many disciplines, including nursing, play and social work. The essence of the team approach is to ensure that all staff working with children receiving palliative care and their families have the opportunity to engage with them to provide support as needed and to complement each other. This may, for example, centre on the hospice cook with whom the family may have a special bond and to whom the other team members may turn in order to elicit crucial information.

The role of children's nurses within this environment is focused on ensuring that holistic care, both physically and spiritually, is provided, with the specific, individual needs of each child and family being met (Price and McNeilly 2009). Spirituality has an ever growing emphasis with paediatric palliative care services (McSherry and Jolley 2009). The management of complex drug regimens to aid pain management, as well as facilitate mobility, ensures that nurses work closely with children and their families and become integrated within the family support structure. The challenge for children's nurses within the palliative care arena is to meet the needs of children and their families in the way that they wish, while ensuring high-quality care and management. The essence is to guarantee that the final days or years of a child's life are of the highest quality and families are assisted to cope with the challenges they face both immediately and in the future.

The future of children's nursing

Children's nursing offers a wide range of possibilities for work with sick children and their families in hospitals and in the community. Work within healthcare management and in academic nursing is also possible for those who wish to gain further experience and to progress their studies. The development of children's trusts, which bring together all services for children and young people in an area, and extended schools, which offer children and families a range of services within school buildings, are providing increased opportunities for children's nurses to work in the ever expanding area of integrated children's services.

Nurse education is based in universities and from 2013, all nurses, including children's nurses, will be educated to degree level (DH 2009e). University education provides opportunities for academic study at undergraduate and postgraduate level, as well as funded research in children's nursing. This research is an important way in which children's nurses can ensure that the care to which sick children are exposed is the care they need and based on sound evidence.

The introduction of nurse consultants (Woodward et al. 2006) and advanced nurse practitioners is an indication of the demand for children's nurses to become both more specialised and more skilled. This development is in response to the reduction in junior doctors' working hours, government policies, increased A&E attendance and the need to reduce waiting times (Heward 2009), but may well be at the expense of 'basic' nursing care. The boundaries between medicine and nursing are becoming increasingly blurred, leading to more nurses working as clinical specialists in relation to the delivery of highly specific healthcare interventions. Initially, specialist children's nurses were responsible for the management of particular diseases, diabetes and epilepsy for example. However, the future will see children's nurse specialists in pain and symptom management – a development that is more consistent with nursing's traditional focus on care. The ability of children's nurses to prescribe drugs has enabled a new level of independence in practice as well as offering benefits to children and families (Lilley et al. 2005).

It is important that children's nursing continues to deliver a service that is 'therapeutic' in its orientation and focused on the delivery of human care. These characteristics will be ever more valuable in a health service that seeks to be cost-effective, focused on treatment outcomes and increasingly medically oriented (Brook and Crouch 2004). Healthcare is becoming large, complex and confusing for those who seek treatment and care. It is important that the needs of children should not be forgotten. Sick children and their families need 'care' as well as treatment. It may be that children's nursing possesses new opportunities to develop and grow, but the discipline needs to retain its historical orientation to the needs of the sick child and the family. Children's nursing in the future should be directed out of a concern to provide human care, to ameliorate suffering and not just to cure disease and mend traumatised tissue. In pursuance of this, children's nursing needs to retain its unique focus on the child and family's feelings, their discomfort, their pain and their grief. This is old magic in a world sparkling with 'science' but nursing is the most important of all the healthcare disciplines and it will continue to be both valued and rewarding.

Conclusion

This chapter is not an exhaustive account of children's nursing but rather a comprehensive review of the many and varied aspects of caring for children and young people when they are sick or have health needs. It provides insight into the various roles available to nurses working with children and young people and the key issues involved in delivering sensitive, therapeutic and family-centred care. Further reading into this fascinating field of nursing is provided in the References below.

References

ACH (Association of Children's Hospices) (2005) *Children's Hospice Services: A Guide for Professionals*, London: ACH

Action for Sick Children (2004) *Action for Sick Children: Millennium Charter*, available online at http://actionforsickchildren.org/index.asp?ID=156, accessed 19/01/10

ACT/RCPCH (Association for Children with Life-threatening or Terminal Conditions and their Families/the Royal College of Paediatrics and Child Health) (2003) *The Guide to the Development of Children's Palliative Care Services* (2nd edn), Bristol: ACT

Arnold, E (2007) Intercultural communication, in EC Arnold and K Underman-Boggs (eds), *Interprofessional Relationships: Professional Communication Skills for Nurses,* (5th edn), St Louis, MO: Saunders Elsevier

Bee, H and Boyd, D (2010) *The Developing Child* (12th edn), Boston: Pearson/Allyn & Bacon

BMA (British Medical Association) (2001) *Consent, Rights and Choices in Health Care for Children and Young People*, London: BMA

Bond, L, Carlin, JB, Thomas, L et al. (2001) Does bullying cause emotional problems? A prospective study of young teenagers, *British Medical Journal*, 323: 480–4.

Boxwell, GB (ed.) (2010) *Neonatal Intensive Care Nursing*, London: Routledge

Brook, S and Crouch, R (2004) Doctors and nurses in emergency care: where are the boundaries now?, *Trauma*, **6**(3): 211–16.

Brumbaugh Keeney, G, Cassata, L and McElmurry, BJ (2004) *Adolescent Health and Development in Nursing and Midwifery Education*, Geneva: WHO

Carr, A (2006) *The Handbook of Child and Adolescent Clinical Psychology: A Contextual Approach* (2nd edn), London: Routledge

Casey, A (1995) Partnership nursing: influences on involvement of informal carers, *Journal of Advanced Nursing*, 22: 1058–62

Children Act (1989) available online at www.opsi.gov.uk/acts/acts1989/Ukpga_19890041_en_1.htm, accessed 20/1/2010

Children Act (2004) available online at www.opsi.gov.uk/acts/acts2004/20040031.htm, accessed 20/1/2010

Children's Legal Centre (2010) *The Competence and Capacity to Consent to Medical Treatment*, available online at http://www.childrenslegalcentre.com/Legal+Advice/Child+law/Youngpeopleandmedicaltreatment/thecompetenceandcapacitytoconsenttomedicaltreatment, accessed 20/1/2010

Children's Play Information Service (2009) *Factsheet 6: Play in Hospital*, National Children's Bureau, available online at http://www.ncb.org.uk/cpis/cpis_factsheet6_hospitalplay_20090824.pdf, accessed 20/1/2010

Christie, D and Viner, R (2005) Adolescent development, *British Medical Journal,* 330: 301–4

Corby, B (2006) *Child Abuse: Towards a Knowledge Base* (3rd edn), Maidenhead: Open University Press

CWDC (Children's Workforce Development Council) (2009a) *Integrated Working Explained,*

3

available online at http://www.cwdcouncil.org.uk/assets/0000/2970/Integrated_Working_Explained.pdf, accessed 28/01/2010

CWDC (2009b) *The Common Assessment Framework for Children and Young People,* Leeds: CWDC

DCSF (Department for Children, Schools and Families) (2007) *The Children's Plan: Building Brighter Futures,* London: DCSF

DCSF (2008a) *Staying Safe: Action Plan*, London: DCSF

DCSF (2008b) *The Children's Plan: One Year On – Progress Report*, London: DCSF

DCSF (2009a) *Referrals, Assessment and Children Subject to a Child Protection Plan, England, year ending 31st Mar 2008*, available online at www.dcsf.gov.uk/rsgateway/DB/SFR/s000811/index.shtml, accessed 20/1/2010

DCSF (2009b) *The Children's Plan: Two Years On – Progress Report*, London: DCSF

DfES (Department for Education and Skills) (2001) *Promoting Children's Mental Health within Early Years and School Settings,* Nottingham: DfES

DfES (2003) *Every Child Matters,* London: DfES

DfES (2004) *Every Child Matters: Next Steps. Working In Partnership,* London: DfES

DfES (2006) *Statistics of Education: Referrals, Assessments and Children and Young People on Child Protection Registers: year ending 31 March 2005,* London: TSO

DH (Department of Health) (1991) *Welfare of Children and Young People in Hospital,* London: HMSO

DH (1997) *Paediatric Intensive Care: A Framework for the Future*, London: DH

DH (2001a) *Reference Guide to Consent for Examination and Treatment*, London: DH

DH (2001b) *Seeking Consent: Working with Children*, London: DH

DH (2001c) HSC 2001/023: *Good Practice in Consent: Achieving the NHS Plan Commitment to Patient-centred Consent Practice*, London: DH

DH (2001d) *Valuing People: A New Strategy for Learning Disability for the 21st Century*, London: DH

DH (2002) *Getting the Right Start: National Service Framework for Children, Young People and Maternity Services – Standard for Hospital Services*, London: DH

DH (2004) *Best Practice Guidance for Doctors and Other Health Professionals on the Provision of Advice and Treatment to Young People under 16 on Contraception, Sexual and Reproductive Health*, London: DH

DH (2007) *Palliative Care Statistics for Children and Young Adults*, London: DH

DH (2009a) *Healthy Child Programme: Pregnancy and the First Five Years of Life*, London: DH

DH (2009b) *Healthy Child Programme: the two year review*, London: DH

DH (2009c) *Healthy Child Programme: from 5-19 years old*, London: DH

DH (2009d) *Improving the Health and Wellbeing of People with a Learning Disability*, London: DH

DH (2009e) *Nursing Set to be All Graduate Entry by 2013*, available online at http://www.dh.gov.uk/en/News/Recentstories/DH_108359, accessed 31/01/2010

DH/DCSF (Department of Health/Department for Children, Schools and Families) (2009) *Healthy Lives, Brighter Futures: The Strategy for Children and Young People's Health*, London: DH

DH/DfES (Department of Health/Department of Education and Skills) (2003) *Together from* the Start: Practical Guidance for Professionals Working with Disabled Children (Birth to Third Birthday) and their Families, London: DH/DfES

DH/DfES (2004) National Service Framework for Children, Young People and Maternity Services, London: DH

Egdell, P, Finlay, L and Pedley, D (2008) The PAWS score: validation of an early warning scoring system for the initial assessment of children in the emergency department, Emergency Medicine Journal, 25: 745–9

Eiser, C (1997) Children's quality of life measures, Archives of Disease in Childhood, 77: 347–54

Elliott, B (2009) Communicating with children, young people and families in health care contexts, in A Dunhill, B Elliott and A Shaw (eds), Effective Communication and Engagement with Children, Young People, their Families and Carers, Exeter: Learning Matters

Emerson, E (2009) Estimating Future Numbers of Adults with Profound and Multiple Learning Disabilities in England, Lancaster: Centre for Disability Research

Every Disabled Child Matters (2007) If I Could Change One Thing, London: National Children's Bureau

Flood-Page, C, Campbell, S, Harrington, V and Miller, J (2000) Youth Crime: Findings from the 1998/9 Youth Lifestyles Survey, Home Office Research Study 20, London: Home Office

Glasper, A and Richardson, J (2006) A Textbook of Children's and Young People's Nursing, Edinburgh: Churchill Livingstone

GMC (General Medical Council) (2007) 0-18 Years: Guidance for all Doctors, London: GMC

Goodband, S and Jennings, K (1992) Parent care: a US experience in Indianapolis, in J Cleary (ed.) Caring for Children in Hospital: Parents and Nurses in Partnership, London: Scutari Press

Hall, D and Elliman, D (eds) (2007) Health for All Children (rev. 4th edn), Oxford: Oxford University Press

Haringey Local Safeguarding Children Board (2008) Haringey Serious Case Review: Child A, Executive Summary, available online at http://www.haringey.gov.uk/scr_executive_summary_a_-_final.pdf, accessed 12/1/ 2010

Heward, Y (2009) Advanced practice in paediatric intensive care: a review, Paediatric Nursing, 21(1): 18–21

HM Government (2006) Working Together to Safeguard Children: A Guide to Interagency Working to Safeguard and Promote the Welfare of Children, London: DfES

Johnson, K, Gerada, C and Greenough, A (2003) Treatment of neonatal abstinence syndrome, Archives of Disease of Childhood, Fetal Neonatal Edition, 88: 2–5

Kelsey, J and McEwing, G (2006) Physical growth and development in children, in A Glasper and J Richardson (eds), A Textbook of Children's and Young People's Nursing, Edinburgh: Churchill Livingstone

Kurtz, Z and Thornes, R (2000) Health Needs of School Aged Children, London: Young Minds

Laming, Lord (2003) The Victoria Climbié Inquiry: Report of an Inquiry by Lord Laming, Cm 5730, London: TSO

Laming, Lord (2009) The Protection of Children in England: A Progress Report, London: TSO

Lilley, M, Marshall, J, McIntosh, N et al. (2005) Independent nurse prescribing in an acute hospital setting, Paediatric Nursing, 17(4): 14–18

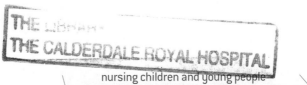
3

Lowes, L (2007) Impact upon the child and family, in F Valentine and L Lowes (eds), *Nursing Care of Children and Young People with Chronic Illness*, Oxford: Blackwell

Luce, T (2003) *Death Certification and Investigation in England, Wales and Northern Ireland: The Report of a Fundamental Review 2003*, London: TSO

McAlister, W (2010) Anaesthesia in children, in L Shields (ed.), *Perioperative Care of the Child: A Nursing Manual*, Oxford: Wiley-Blackwell

McSherry, W and Jolley, S (2009) Meeting the spiritual needs of children and families, in J Price and P McNeilly (eds), *Palliative Care for Children and Families*, Basingstoke: Palgrave Macmillan

Maughan, B, Brock, A and Ladva, G (2004) Mental health, in Office for National Statistics, *The Health of Children and Young People*, London: ONS

May-Chahal, C, Hicks, S and Tomlinson, J (2004) *The Relationship between Child Death and Child Maltreatment: A Research Study on the Attribution of Cause of Death in Hospital Settings*, London: NSPCC

Meltzer, H, Gatward, R, Corbin, T et al. (2003) *The Mental Health of Young People Looked After by Local Authorities in England*, London: TSO

Mental Capacity Act (2005) Office of Public Sector Information, London, available online at http://www.opsi.gov.uk/ACTS/acts2005/ukpga_20050009_en_1, accessed 30/01/2010

Mental Health Foundation (2005) *Childhood and Adolescent Mental Health: Understanding the Lifetime Impacts*, London: MHF

Mental Health Foundation (2006) *Truth Hurts: Report of the National Inquiry into Self Harm among Young People*, London: MHF

Ministry of Health (1959) *Committee of the Central Health Services Council: Report of the Committee on the Welfare of Children in Hospital* (The Platt Report), London: HMSO

Morse, T (2007) Day care surgery, in MA Chambers and S Jones (eds), *Surgical Nursing of Children*, London: Butterworth-Heinemann

Myers, J (2005) Community children's nursing services in the 21st century, *Paediatric Nursing*, **17**(2): 31–4.

NAO (National Audit Office) (2007) *Caring for Vulnerable Babies: The Reorganisation of Neonatal Services in England*, London: TSO

National Association of Hospital Play Staff (2000) *About NAHPS*, available online at http://www.nahps.org.uk/default.htm, accessed 19/1/2010

National Treatment Agency for Substance Misuse (2009) *Substance Misuse among Young People: The Data 2008-09*, available online at www.nta.nhs.uk/publications/documents/nta_substance_misuse, accessed 12/1/2010

Nessa, N (2004) Disability, in Office of National Statistics, *The Health of Children and Young People*, London: ONS

NHS (National Health Service) (2010) *Change 4Life*, available online at http://www.nhs.uk/change4life/Pages/Default.aspx, accessed 19/1/2010

NHS Confederation (2009) *Aiming High for Disabled Children: Delivering Improved Health Services*, London: NHS Confederation

NICE (National Institute for Health and Clinical Excellence) (2004a) *Eating Disorders: Core Interventions in the Treatment and Management of Anorexia Nervosa, Bulimia Nervosa and Related Eating Disorders*, Clinical Guideline 9, London: NICE

NICE (2004b) *The Epilepsies: The Diagnosis and Management of the Epilepsies in adults and Children in Primary and Secondary Care*, London: NICE

NICE (2005) *Depression in Children and Young People: Identification and Management in Primary, Community and Secondary Care,* Clinical Guideline 28, London: NICE

NICE (2006) *Postnatal Care: Routine Postnatal Care for Women and their Babies,* London: NICE

NMC (Nursing and Midwifery Council) (2008) *The Code: Standards of Conduct, Performance and Ethics for Nurses and Midwives,* London: NMC

NPSA (National Patient Safety Agency) (2004) *Understanding the Patient Safety Issues for People with Learning Disabilities,* available online at www.npsa.nhs.uk/admin/publications/docs/learningdisabilities_issues.pdf, accessed 19/1/2010

NPSA (2005a) *How to Confirm the Correct Position of Nasogastric Feeding Tubes in Infants, Children and Adults,* London: NPSA

NPSA (2005b) *How to Confirm the Correct Position of Naso and Orogastric Feeding Tubes in Babies under the Care of Neonatal Units,* London: NPSA

NSPCC (National Society for the Prevention of Cruelty to Children) (2008) *NSPCC Evidence to Lord Laming's Review of Child Protection,* available online at http://www.nspcc.org.uk/Inform/policyandpublicaffairs/Consultations/2008/Lamingresponse_wdf62413.pdf, accessed 12/1/2010

Office of National Statistics (2008) *Childhood Stress Linked to Emotional Disorders,* available online at www.statistics.gov.uk/pdfdir/cpm1008.pdf, accessed 12/1/2010

Parry-Langdon, N (ed.) (2008) *Three Years On: Survey of the Development and Emotional Wellbeing of Children and Young People,* London: ONS

Payne, D, Martin, C, Viner, R and Skinner, R (2005) Adolescent medicine in paediatric practice, *Archives of Disease in Childhood,* 90: 1133–7

Phaire, T (1545) *The Boke of Chyldren,* London: Reprinted by the Royal College of Child Health and Paediatrics, 1955

Price, J and McNeilly, P (2009) *Palliative Care for Children and Families,* Basingstoke: Palgrave Macmillan

RCN (Royal College of Nursing) (2004a) *Adolescent Transition Care,* London: RCN

RCN (2004b) *Child Protection: Every Nurse's Responsibility,* guidance for nursing staff, London: RCN

RCN (2009)*The Recognition and Assessment of Acute Pain in Children,* London: RCN

RCPCH (Royal College of Paediatrics and Child Health) (2003) *Bridging the Gaps: Health Care for Adolescents,* London: RCPCH

RCPCH (2004) *Duties of Doctors in Child Protection Cases with Regard to Confidentiality,* RCPCH: London

RNIB (Royal National Institute for the Blind) (2000) *Stereotypical Behaviour in People with Visual and Learning Disabilities,* London: RNIB

Scanlon, K and Sorrentino, AL (2006) Health problems during infancy, in A Glasper and J Richardson (eds), *A Textbook of Children's and Young People's Nursing,* Edinburgh: Churchill Livingstone

Shields, L (1999) A comparative study of the care of hospitalized children in developed and developing countries, PhD thesis, University of Queensland, available online at http://library.uq.edu.au/search/ashields+l/ashields+l/1,3,4,B/frameset&F=ashields+linda&1,2, accessed 18/6/2006

Shields, L and Tanner, A (2010) Care of the child in the operating room, in L Shields (ed.), *Perioperative Care of the Child: A Nursing Manual,* Oxford: Wiley-Blackwell

3

Shields, L and Waterman, L (2002) Psychosocial care of children in the perioperative area, in L Shields and H Werder (eds), *Perioperative Nursing,* London: Greenwich Medical Media

Shields, L, Pratt, J and Hunter, J (2006) Family-centred care: a review of qualitative studies, *Journal of Clinical Nursing,* **15**(10): 1317–23

Shields, L, Kristensson-Hallström, I, Kristjánsdóttir, G and Hunter, J (2003) Who owns the child admitted to hospital: a preliminary discussion, *Journal of Advanced Nursing,* **41**(3): 213–22.

Towner (2002) *The Prevention of Childhood Injury,* background paper prepared for the Accidental Injury Task Force, University of Newcastle upon Tyne, available online at http://www.dh.gov.uk/assetRoot/04/07/22/15/04072215.pdf,accessed 19/1/2010

UNICEF (United Nations International Children's Emergency Fund) (1989) *UN Convention on the Rights of the Child,* UNICEF, available online at http://www2.ohchr.org/english/law/crc.htm, accessed 20/1/2010

UNICEF UK (2009) *An Introduction to the Baby Friendly Initiative,* available online at http://www.babyfriendly.org.uk/pdfs/infosheets/introduction_infosheet.pdf, accessed 20/1/2010

Viner, R and Keane, M (1998) *Youth Matters: Evidence-based Best Practice for the Care of Young People in Hospital,* London: Caring for Children in the Health Services

Wake, E (2009a) Communicating with children; the legal dimensions, in A Dunhill, B Elliott and A Shaw (eds), *Effective Communication and Engagement with Children, Young People, their Families and Carers*, Exeter: Learning Matters

Wake, E (2009b) Children's voices: working with children and young people with additional needs, in A Dunhill, B Elliott and A Shaw (eds), *Effective Communication and Engagement with Children, Young People, their Families and Carers*, Exeter: Learning Matters

Warner, HK (2006) *Meeting the Needs of Children with Disabilities: Families and Professionals Facing the Challenge Together,* London: Routledge

Wheeler, R (2006) Gillick or Fraser? A plea for consistency over competence in children, *British Medical Journal,* 332: 807, doi:10.1136/bmj.332.7545.807

WHO (World Health Organization) (2009) *Infant and Young Child Feeding: Model Chapter for Textbooks for Medical Students And Allied Health Professionals*, available online at http://whqlibdoc.who.int/publications/2009/9789241597494_eng.pdf, accessed 20/1/2010

Wood, C (1888) The training of nurses for sick children, *Nursing Record,* 1: 507–10.

Woodward, VA, Webb, C and Prowse, M (2006) Nurse consultants: organizational influences on role achievement, *Journal of Clinical Nursing,* **15**(3): 272–80

Young Minds (2003) *Children and Young People Get Depressed Too,* London: Young Minds

14 caring for people with learning disability

Peter Birchenall and Susan Baldwin

In this chapter we will explore:

> What learning disability is
> Normalisation and social role valorisation
> Community care
> Challenging behaviour
> Dual diagnosis
> Person-centred planning
> Genetics

Introduction

This chapter will take you through historical perspectives and terminology into a more enlightened modern approach to understanding and caring for people with learning disabilities. Traditional concepts surrounding normalisation are explored as a means of illustrating how thinking has moved on from the world of rigid institutional care to a wider understanding of care in the community, including the importance of advocacy and the role of the community learning disability nurse. As learning disability may be an area of nursing you are unfamiliar with, this chapter contains a case study that offers you an insight into this area of practice. Through a case study approach, you will engage with the lives of two people with learning disability. You are invited to compare their lifestyle with your own.

What is learning disability?

In the UK alone there are approximately one and a half million people with **learning disability**, so perhaps we should begin by addressing several misconceptions about people with this form of disability. First, a learning disability is not the same as dyslexia, neither is it a mental illness, although people with a learning disability can develop a mental illness in much the same way as anyone else. Its actual meaning is that the person experiences difficulty in learning and problem solving, which explains why internationally it is known as 'intellectual disability'. Sometimes there are serious problems with social functioning and adaptive behaviour, that is, communication and personal relationships, and for people who have profound learning disability, the basic activities of daily living often have to be provided for them, such as help with personal hygiene, sexuality, health needs, feeding and dressing.

Historically, there have been various ways of describing people who have a learning disability. Archaic labels such as 'oligophrenia', 'amentia', 'idiot', 'imbecile', 'feeble-minded', 'mental deficiency', 'mental subnormality' and 'mental handicap' have, at one time or another, been applied and enshrined in legislation (Spencer 1997). In the early 1990s, the Department of Health introduced the term 'learning disability' as this seemed to be preferable to 'handicap', but, for some, it was still a label (Clarke 2000). The initial presentation of learning disability usually occurs in childhood, although not always. In most instances, the cause is genetically determined. Other causes can be linked to postnatal injury or prenatal or postnatal infection such as German measles (rubella embryopathy), which can affect an embryo during early pregnancy, causing severe damage and leading to a learning disability. In a minority of cases, the cause (aetiology) remains unknown. Learning disability is no respecter of family status, social class, religion or ethnic background. Although there is evidence to suggest that certain syndromes associated with learning disability appear more regularly in some cultures than others, the consequences remain the same for the individual and their family. In some cases, learning disability is accompanied by a related physical disability. For example, Craft et al. (1985) make reference to Tay–Sachs disease, which is a proven cause of learning disability and associated blindness within the Ashkenazi Jewish community. People with Down's syndrome may develop cardiovascular problems. **Tourette's syndrome**, also known as Gilles de Tourette's syndrome, is another disorder linked to learning disability as well as other conditions. It is a childhood-onset neurological disorder characterized by repetitive muscle movements and spontaneous vocal outbursts, some of which may be obscene. The condition involves small, repetitive movements, usually presented as facial tics with grimacing and blinking.

To have a learning disability means that the person will experience difficulty in learning at the same rate or to the same depth as a person who is not disabled in this way. This difficulty in learning varies considerably. There is a marked difference between people with profound and multiple learning disabilities (PMLD), who exhibit severe limitations in self-care, continence, communication and academic skills (WHO 1992), and those with moderate or mild learning disability who can live with much less support. People with PMLD have some of the highest support needs and are most reliant on services, whereas a person with a moderate or mild learning disability will always require some degree of specialist help to learn and retain the knowledge and basic skills necessary for living as an independent person in a supportive climate.

Contrary to certain beliefs, a learning disability is not the same as having a mental health problem but, as in the general population, mental illness can affect individuals with learning disabilities, and where this happens the term dual diagnosis is sometimes used. Each person is unique and it is important to recognise that people with learning disabilities are not all the same. Nurses, teachers and social workers who work with learning disabled people and their families fully respect this but historical labels are difficult to erase. Many of the earlier labels carried the prefix 'mental', which still retains its negative connotations. It is not unusual to find members of the general community who have difficulty realising that even though certain people may share similar anatomical features and behavior patterns, they are individual in all other respects.

Normalisation and social role valorisation

When the concept of **normalisation** was introduced, it represented a turning point in the evolution of care and support for people with a learning disability. It first came to prominence in the Danish Mental Retardation Act 1959. Niels Bank-Mikkelson (1969), the originator of normalisation, described it as a means of bringing normal living conditions, educational opportunities, the right to work and enjoyment of leisure facilities within the lifestyle of people with a learning disability. Bank-Mikkelson included those who were living in long-stay accommodation. Later, this description was extended to include the full spectrum of legal and human rights being available to people with a learning disability. Bengt Nirje (1969), then executive director of the Swedish Association for Retarded Children, wrote: 'The normalization principle means making available to the mentally retarded patterns and conditions of everyday life which are as close as possible to the norms and patterns of the mainstream of society.' Nirje applied normalisation theories to the way people progress through each stage of the life cycle. These theories embraced self-determination, equal rights at work and living standards. In his work, Nirje (1969) refers to 'the rhythm of the day, the week and the year'. By doing this, he focused attention on the negative effects of institutionalisation and how this way of life deprived people of the right to determine their own rhythm of life. This early work was powerful because of the insights it gave regarding the normality of daily living. It paved the way for improved conditions within the institutional philosophy of care, eventually leading to the demise, within Western civilisation, of this method of caring for people with a learning disability.

In 1976, the President's Committee on Mental Retardation adopted normalisation in the USA. The most common misunderstanding about the concept of normalisation is that it attempts to force normal expectations onto those who, by virtue of their disability, cannot meet them. Sinason, echoing the sentiments of Bank-Mikkelson and Nirje, suggested that, in its most basic form, normalisation is a process which 'uses means as culturally normative as possible in order to establish, maintain and support patterns of behaviour which are as near normal as possible' (Sinason 1992, p. 256).

Perhaps the most influential figure in the field of normalisation is US sociologist Wolf Wolfensberger (1972). He took the original concept to a higher

3

level by demanding that those with mental disabilities should be treated within the community and that their social roles should be valued. He moved away from rhetoric about normalisation to suggesting how a major shift in emphasis could be achieved through creating socially valued roles for disadvantaged groups of people. Wolfensberger's work in the area of 'social role valorisation' became a major influence within the community care movement. He argued that enhancement of the social role of persons at risk of social devaluation should focus on their social image and the enhancement of personal competences. Social image is a construct of where we live, the people we mix with, personal possessions and appearance. It is about the label that society applies to people. Social role valorisation underlines the notion that everyone has a life worth living and that no one should be excluded from opportunities to enhance their personal competence and status in society.

Community care

Background to modern concepts

To understand modern concepts of community care for people with learning disabilities, it is useful to have some knowledge of its historical background. The notion of community care for this group of people is rooted in the *Report of the Royal Commission on the Law Relating to Mental Illness and Mental Deficiency* (1957). A principal recommendation for a move from institutional care to community care began what proved to be far-reaching changes in social policy. Views on what community care should encompass broadened to include not only local domiciliary services and day centres as recommended by the commission, but also sheltered housing and special housing, hostels and respite care (Willmott 1989). The key word is 'local', and community care expanded to take into account local private residential and domiciliary services, voluntary services, self-help groups and the often hidden contribution of informal carers. In 1971, the government White Paper *Better Services for the Mentally Handicapped* (DHSS 1971) continued the agenda for change. Primarily, this document focused on reducing the number of beds in long-stay hospitals with a subsequent increase in community provision. In 1981, as community care became more established, the government signalled its recognition of the contribution made by informal carers and locally based voluntary organisations. The then Department of Health and Social Security redefined community care in its evidence to the House of Commons Social Services Select Committee (1985). The objectives of community care were directed towards inclusiveness. This meant giving people with learning disabilities opportunities and options regarding their individual lifestyles, something that had been denied them within the limited scope of institutional care. It meant supporting people to live in their own home where appropriate, to give support and relief to informal carers, to develop and deliver cost-effective individualised packages of care and to integrate resources within specific geographical areas. In cases where it was deemed impracticable to provide care within the person's home, small group homes or nonhospital residential accommodation would become available. As with many centrally funded initiatives, arguments regarding the allocation of resources often occur between government departments and agencies responsible for the delivery of services. According to Sir Roy Griffiths (1988), in his report *Community Care: Agenda for Action*, this form of care, while the ideal solution to the inadequacies of institutional care, had become the subject of rhetoric rather than action and the different bodies responsible for the delivery of care were in disarray. In recommending change to the way services were delivered, Griffiths (1988) identified three principles:

> Services should be provided early enough
> Clients should have a greater choice of providers
> People should be cared for in their homes if possible.

The Griffiths Report was a precursor to the NHS and Community Care Act 1990, which adopted these principles, the third of which would have enormous repercussions for informal carers. In 1995, the Carers (Recognition and Services) Act reached the statute book. This Act is concerned with specific groups of informal carers, including:

> people over 18, who provide or intend to provide a substantial amount of care on a regular basis
> children and young people (under 18), who provide or intend to provide a substantial amount of care on a regular basis
> parents who provide or intend to provide a substantial amount of care on a regular basis for a disabled child (DH 1996).

Valuing People

In 2001, the government published a White Paper outlining a new strategy for learning disability for the twenty-first century entitled *Valuing People* (DH 2001). This strategy set out a new vision, the principal factors being:

> Safeguarding human, legal and civil rights
> Promoting independence
> Enabling personal choice
> Promoting social inclusion within the local community.

The White Paper had eleven objectives that addressed issues relating to the essential components of community care for people with learning disabilities. These were:

1 To ensure that disabled children and young people are identified early and their needs assessed to enable full access to educational opportunities, health care and social care

2 To assist in the transition into adult life and ensure continuity of care and support for the young person and their family

3 To promote choice and control over personal lifestyles through access to advocacy and a person-centred approach to service planning and provision

4 To help and support carers to maintain their effectiveness

5 To provide effective health services

6 To enable greater choice and control over where people live and to promote independent living with appropriate support

7 To encourage people to lead full and purposeful lives

8 To encourage participation in all forms of employment, paid or otherwise

9 To ensure that care agencies provide high-quality, evidence-based services

10 To ensure that social and healthcare staff are properly trained and qualified to work as team members within a multiagency approach to workforce planning

11 To promote effective partnership working between relevant local agencies.

Collectively, these objectives offered a platform for a modern approach to community care and should, if fully realised, improve the quality of life for people with learning disabilities.

Challenges to *Valuing People*

Set against the above, it is important to recognise that the vulnerability of people with a learning disability can place them at risk. Indeed, Blair (cited in DH 2001) commented that while some people with a learning disability lead fulfilling lives, some experience bullying, prejudice and poor treatment.

The *Valuing People* White Paper (DH 2001) highlighted the impact of negative attitudes, values and beliefs towards this group. One area it highlighted as a particular problem in the life of people with a learning disability was the discriminatory care they received in mainstream health services. It is well established in the literature that people with a learning disability experience a higher prevalence of physical and mental health needs than the general population. It is also well established that people with a learning disability are less likely to receive equal access to healthcare as the general population (DH 2001; Mencap 2004a; NPSA 2004; DRC 2006).

Van Schrojenstein Lantaman-De Valk et al. (2000) have highlighted that people with a learning disability are two and a half times more likely to experience major health problems than those individuals who do not have a learning disability. Indeed, the *Health of the Nation* (DH 1992) identified these major health problems to be centred on heart disease and stroke, cancer, sexual health, accidental injury and mental illness. The Department of Health (1999) reported similar issues affecting people with a learning disability and stated that:

> Physical disability affects up to one-third of the population of people with learning disabilities. The associated health problems arise from the consequences of postural deformities, hip dislocations, chest infections, eating and drinking difficulties and gastrointestinal problems

> Sensory impairment of varying degrees affects over 40% of people with a learning disability, with potentially a high rate of undetected visual and hearing problems in the remainder

> Epilepsy was identified as a major health issue, with approximately one-third of people with a learning disability also having one or more types of seizure

> People who have a known genetic cause of their learning disability, for example Down's syndrome, are at greater risk of physical problems to their cardiac, respiratory and endocrine systems and senses

> Mental health problems are said to occur in approximately 50% of people with a learning disability, and it is important to recognise that dementia, occurring as a complication of increasing age, affects people with a learning disability. For example, there is a particular association between Down's syndrome and Alzheimer's disease.

We have shown that *Valuing People* (DH 2001) clearly set out the government's commitment to improving life chances and opportunities and streamlined services to ensure that people with a learning disability feel included and valued within society. Indeed, it has been instrumental in changing the lives of many people with a learning disability. However, concerns about access to healthcare and appropriate treatment regimes are still highlighted in a number of reports since the publication of *Valuing People*. At the forefront of these concerns are those expressed by people with a learning disability in their first national survey (Emerson et al. 2005). People with a learning disability perceived that they were disadvantaged when compared to the general population, citing poorer health, social isolation and poor finances.

Mencap (2004a) launched the Treat Me Right campaign to highlight the issues faced by people with a learning disability when accessing appropriate and good quality healthcare. Mencap argued that this campaign was a wake-up call to the NHS, calling for urgent action to be taken to improve the health of people with a learning disability. Areas of concern primarily focused on a lack of knowledge and understanding on the part of healthcare practitioners, leaving them to feel ill equipped to care for or assess the needs of people with a learning disability. Healthcare practitioners very often believe that the health problems of this client group are a result of their learning disability, and, as a consequence, this leads to 'diagnostic overshadowing' (Mencap 2004a). More alarming, however, is the discrimination that Mencap refers to in the body of opinion involving value judgements by healthcare staff about the worth of people with a learning disability.

Mencap's follow-up report *Death by Indifference* (2007) explored some quite fundamental flaws in the way six individuals were treated in mainstream health services, who subsequently died needlessly. In this report, Mencap points to a number of factors leading to these untimely deaths, including discrimination, indifference, lack of training and a poor understanding of the needs of people with a learning disability.

A parliamentary ombudsman and a local government ombudsman investigated the complaints made by Mencap on behalf of the families of these six individuals (Abraham and White 2009). Although not upholding all the complaints made, their report inferred that the investigation illustrated some significant and distressing failures in service across both health and social care. The report established that this led to situations in which people with a learning disability experienced prolonged suffering and inappropriate care (Abraham and White 2009).

The report gives detailed accounts of the care received by each of these six individuals. These in themselves are distressing to read, but serve to instruct the health and social care practitioners who are required to provide a good quality of care to all individuals, which include people with a learning disability. The report demonstrates how negative or indifferent attitudes, lack of knowledge and lack of skill can impact on human suffering and inappropriate care.

The lack of knowledge, skills, positive attitudes and beliefs could be argued to be factors that led to a failure to 'offer good care to individuals in very vulnerable situations' (Abraham and White 2009). Practitioners need to be continually vigilant that the care they offer is based on recognition of their area of expertise, a willingness to work in partnership with other professionals and the client and/or their carers and with the utmost dignity and respect.

Community learning disability team

Successful community care for people with learning disabilities is dependent on the way in which locally based professional groups work together as a team when meeting the needs of their clients. Although they can be organised differently, usually a community learning disability team will contain members from the nursing, social work, psychology and psychiatry professions. Most teams will also incorporate other professions such as physiotherapy, occupational therapy, speech and language therapy and behavioural therapy. The team will generally work on a referral basis when providing an assessment and management service aimed at supporting people with learning disabilities and their carers. This support is often required when issues arise that militate against the client enjoying a good quality of life. These issues are discussed within the confidential environment of a case conference where each member of the team enjoys equal standing.

The role of the community learning disability nurse

Community nurses working in the field of learning disability are specially trained and are registered with the UK's Nursing and Midwifery Council. Predominantly, their role is to work in partnership with colleagues on the community learning disability team from a health perspective, where the emphasis is on health gain through surveillance and positive health promotion. In addition to common health problems such as coughs and colds, people with learning disabilities may experience physical, social and psychological problems that require specialist nursing intervention. For example, the person may have epilepsy or display emotional disorders that require specialist management. In some cases, positive action to prevent accidental injury in the home may be required. As well as in the home, community nurses can often be seen supporting staff within small residential care facilities where their broad spectrum of skills are put to good use in many different situations. The following case study illustrates this.

Case study 1

David, a teenage boy with profound and multiple learning disabilities, lives with several other people with learning disabilities in a social services residential facility. In addition to his learning disabilities, he also has a spectrum of physical disabilities that restricts his movement. David experiences problems with his swallowing reflex, resulting in regurgitation of food. Ensuring that David received adequate nutrition had become a serious concern for the care staff and his parents began to express their concern at his deteriorating condition.

For many months John, a visiting learning disability nurse, had been working with the staff in developing a feeding regime for David but had to finally admit that, in order for the deterioration to be reversed, surgical intervention was the only remaining option. All surgery carries risks but in David's case these risks would be amplified. His parents were unhappy about their son being given a general anaesthetic, therefore the decision was made to carry out the procedure under sedation but they understood that, without the treatment, his prognosis was poor.

John spent time listening to David's parents, sharing their concerns. He reassured them that he would be working closely with the care staff to ensure that David received the best possible aftercare.

A surgical procedure, called a percutaneous endoscopic gastrostomy (PEG), was carried out, which inserted a feeding tube into David's abdomen. Recovery from the surgery was uncomplicated and David began to receive his nutrition through this artificial route. His physical condition improved. The brightness returned to his eyes and a ready smile greeted everyone who spoke to him. David's parents were amazed at how alert and responsive he had become.

Two years have passed since the PEG was inserted and David is now at his correct weight. He enjoys an enhanced quality of life and his parents remain convinced that, without specialist nursing and surgical intervention, David would no longer be with them. Through regular visits John remains in contact with David and his parents.

Bereavement and relationship intervention

The community nurse could be called upon to support a client who is bereaved or, in the case of relationship problems, to exercise counselling skills. Nurses, by nature of their profession, have a clinical responsibility but their skills and experience will enable them to discharge that responsibility within a team framework. Consequently, they will be expected to understand the professional standpoint of other colleagues when discussing the best strategy for a client who has suffered loss or is coming to terms with other complex personal difficulties.

Community care: a different approach

From the philosophy of inclusiveness grew a unique organisation that enjoined the notion of community ideology with one that supported the right of people with learning disabilities to live alongside their peers. L'Arche is such a place and people with learning disabilities are at its heart. It is of interest to note that much of the philosophy evident within *Valuing People* (DH 2001) is evident within the L'Arche philosophy. Here, people live in ordinary houses, sharing in the responsibilities and decision making necessary for a successful, harmonious coexistence. Patterns of living within the L'Arche organisation take the form of small family-like clusters supported by live-in assistants who contribute towards creating and maintaining an atmosphere of friendship, companionship and trust.

L'Arche welcomes men and women aged 18 and over who have a wide-ranging profile of disabilities and abilities. These include people with differing levels of independence related to physical, social and emotional needs. Residents of this community are from varied backgrounds and reflect a wide age range, including those who seek a less demanding existence in retirement. Some of the younger members have adopted the L'Arche way of life as part of their move towards gaining independence from the family home. For them, it is a halfway house to full community integration.

Jean Vanier founded L'Arche in 1964. Prior to this he had visited a small institution in northern France for men with learning disabilities. Here, Father Thomas Philippe, the chaplain, encouraged Jean Vanier to think about how the care of people with learning disabilities could be improved. Famously, Father Thomas suggested that Jean Vanier should begin 'something' – it was that vague. At this time, Jean Vanier was teaching moral philosophy in Toronto, Canada, but being a devout Christian, he always felt that God had another purpose in mind for him. When he next visited France, Father Thomas made the same suggestion to him and Jean Vanier began to visit other places where people with learning disabilities existed, including asylums. He decided to do something, initially on a small scale, and the idea of L'Arche, the French for ark, after Noah's vessel of salvation, was born. Jean Vanier purchased a small house in Trosly-Breuil, to the north of Paris, and cleared the way, legally and practically, to use the property for the purpose of creating a home where people with learning disabilities could learn to live together as friends. Raphael Simi and Philippe Seux were the first to join Jean Vanier in his new venture and from somewhat primitive beginnings, L'Arche grew into what it is today. There are now 130 L'Arche communities in 30 countries on five continents, including nine in the UK, with a further two planned. Within these communities, 2,700 people with learning disabilities are cared for (for more information, see Spink 1990).

Case study 2: a lifetime of care

Michael is 50 years old and lives as part of a small group of people with learning disabilities in a purpose-built bungalow. This accommodation is situated near the centre of a small market town and the residents enjoy a full social life, doing everyday things such as shopping, eating out, going to the theatre and visiting local public houses.

However, this way of life has not always been Michael's experience. In 1966, as a boy of 10, he was admitted to the children's ward of a long-stay hospital. Initially, this admission was for a few weeks to give his parents a break as Michael had severe behavioural difficulties that would now be termed 'challenging behaviour'. He also had the occasional epileptic seizure. It was the first time he had been away from home and he did not settle. His abusive behaviour to other children and staff resulted in him being heavily tranquilised, which at the time was a way of managing this type of behaviour.

His parents returned from their holiday saying how much they had enjoyed the break but were looking forward to having Michael home. Before leaving with their son, Michael's parents were seen by a consultant psychiatrist who suggested they should consider placing Michael in long-term care. Initially, they rejected the idea but a few months later Michael was admitted to the hospital on a permanent basis.

At home he had his own room; here in the hospital he was allocated a bed in a dormitory. Approximately 40 other children, all with severe learning disabilities, shared the same living and sleeping accommodation. At home, he would eat his meals sat at a table with his parents. In the hospital, he would sit with others at a long table in a dining area that doubled as a day room. At home, his meals were cooked and served by his mother. In the hospital, all meals came from a central kitchen and were served by people wearing white coats or traditional nurses' uniforms. At home, Michael was part of a family. In the hospital, he was just another patient whose behaviour and epilepsy were treated from a clinical standpoint. At home, he would dress in his own clothes. In the hospital, nursing staff would select clothing for all the patients from a central storage area. Footwear was usually a pair of regulation baseball boots.

During the week, he attended a hospital school staffed by teachers who were not well versed in managing his challenging behaviour. On numerous occasions he was brought back to the ward as his disruptive behaviour constantly interfered with the education of other children. Eventually he was excluded from school.

Michael soon became institutionalised and when he eventually entered adolescence, he was transferred to an adult male ward in another part of the hospital. There he was assessed by the medical staff as being suitable for work in the occupational therapy department, which became his life. Over a period of time, his behaviour improved. The only real connection he had with the world outside came from weekly visits by his parents, occasional trips out in the hospital minibus and an annual summer camp at the seaside organised by the hospital management.

Eventually, the hospital was earmarked for closure and Michael, nearing 30 years of age, was assessed for transfer to a community facility a few miles from the hospital. The facility was staffed by nurses from the hospital who had to get used to working in a different way without the protection of a uniform. Despite reservations, Michael took to his new way of life and was soon helping out in the bungalow with small tasks such as cleaning and washing up. It seemed that he had come full circle. From originally living at home where he had a certain amount of privacy, he'd spent 20 years in the closed institution of a long-stay hospital where he had no privacy, before moving into accommodation where he could became an individual again.

In time, Michael's parents requested that he be moved closer to them, as travelling had become difficult. A multidisciplinary team of professionals from health and social services met to consider the request. Within a short time, Michael was moved to his current place of residence, which is staffed entirely by social carers and where he has made new friends. He sees his parents each week and sometimes spends weekends at home.

Activity 14.2

Reflect on Michael's story. Regarding opportunities, choices, motivation and direction, how does Michael's life compare with your own? To what extent are these differences related to social factors rather than intellectual impairment?

If possible, visit a modern local residential unit for people with learning disabilities and discover as much as you can about the lifestyles of people who live there.

Advocacy

In the field of learning disabilities, **advocacy** is about helping individuals to get their wishes and rights respected. In a formal way, advocacy can be described as a means of influencing local and national decisions that impinge directly or indirectly on the lives of individuals. According to Teasdale (1998), it is about power. This particularly applies when trying to influence public policy and resource allocation. A less formal description of advocacy is giving a voice to someone who otherwise may not be heard. Mallik (1995) suggests that advocacy, in its most usual form, is 'triadic', meaning that advocacy involves three parties, the client, the advocate and another person or organisation that the advocate and client seek to influence.

There are different styles of advocacy that can be applied to people with learning disability. Each of these, in its own way, is valuable and should not be placed in any order of importance. The values and principles underpinning all forms of advocacy are the same.

Citizen advocacy

Citizen advocacy relies on a long-term partnership between a person with learning disabilities and a volunteer worker. The thing to remember is that an advocate in this sense is unpaid and will be carefully matched to the person being helped. The role of the citizen advocate is to form a positive relationship within the partnership, resulting in a deeper understanding of the person's needs than would be possible within a short-term arrangement. In most instances, this relationship will enable the advocate to offer emotional support.

Case/crisis/short-term advocacy

Case/crisis/short-term advocacy is provided only for a short period of time. It is single-issue advocacy, put in place to solve a particular problem or meet a specific individual need. Because of the many potential difficulties facing people with learning disabilities, advocates with specialist knowledge and understanding of the issues are sought. An example would be to assist someone who is experiencing problems obtaining a winter fuel allowance or a pension supplement.

Professional advocacy

Professional advocates do their work as part of paid employment, which may be as a social worker, nurse or care worker. Teamwork is at the core of this style of advocacy, with each advocate supporting a number of people. Again, professional advocacy is usually for a short period of time and is focused on achieving clear objectives or targets. In this sense, it is task oriented. One of the main strands of this type of advocacy is that the advocate will work in the best interests of the person. What that person actually wants or feels is not always taken into account.

Self-advocacy

Self-advocacy is led or organised by people with a learning disability. Self-advocacy is carried out alone or from within a group where, acting collectively to build each other's confidence, an effective personal challenge against discrimination at local or national level can be made.

Peer advocacy

Peer advocacy is not as usual as other styles of advocacy and may be carried out on an informal unplanned basis. It is where two people with learning disabilities share things that are common to each of them. For example, they may attend the same day centre or share living accommodation. Peer advocacy is aimed at empowering the other person to own and resolve problem situations.

A peer advocate may work with more than one person, providing they share similar experiences.

Family and friends advocacy

Family and friends advocacy is carried out from within a circle of family or friends and is used mainly for children and people with profound and multiple disabilities. Because of its focus, family and friend advocacy is not usually as visible as other forms of advocacy.

Legal advocacy

Legal advocacy is based on legal issues and not on the wishes or needs of the person with a learning disability. Because of the nature of legal advocacy, it usually has to be paid for. The advocate will work with individual clients or groups, using specialist knowledge of the law, to bring about change.

Collective or class advocacy

Collective or class advocacy is where a group or a collection of groups join forces to address a common issue. For example, a change in the system for allocating formal carers may be causing difficulties or there may be plans to close a local amenity that people with a learning disability use on a regular basis. Collective or class advocacy can also extend to confront national issues. Sometimes, circumstances may call for paid representation to be made.

See Mencap 2004b for a detailed explanation of these styles of advocacy.

Challenging behaviour

Challenging behaviour has been described as behaviour of such an intensity, frequency or duration that the physical safety of the person or others is likely to be placed in serious jeopardy. This kind of behaviour is likely to seriously limit or delay access to and use of ordinary community facilities (DH 1993). In this case, prefixing behaviour with the adjective 'challenging' describes behaviour that is extreme to the point where it challenges available services to provide person-centred resources to support the individual and their carers. Slevin (1999, p. 242) has suggested that challenging behaviour is an umbrella term embracing forms of behaviour that are:

> inappropriate for the person's age
> harmful to self and others
> antagonistic to learning
> capable of causing significant stress to others.

Challenging behaviour, as a term, will resist efforts to define it with any degree of accuracy. Behaviour of this kind can involve violent episodes, antisocial behaviour, hyperactivity, uncontrolled personal habits and psychological disturbances that are sometimes exhibited in bizarre ways. Challenging behaviour often results from more than one cause. The effect it can have on the individual, those in a caring role and the immediate living environment can be devastating. It can destroy any attempt at community or educational integration, isolating the person within a restrictive caring environment, which is in direct opposition to government policy of care in the community. It also has serious disruptive effects on the lives of carers, who can experience similar isolation from the community they live in. It has been said that one of the positive things about the long-stay hospital system was that it offered respite care facilities, giving carers a much needed rest from the stress of living with challenging behaviour (Slevin 1999).

In attempting to understand and explain challenging behaviour, it is relevant to consider several avenues of thought:

> *Organic brain injury:* Self-injurious behaviour is a relatively common condition associated with severe learning disability, which in turn indicates a relationship between this form of behaviour and diverse organic brain dysfunction
> *Mental health problems:* In cases where the dual effect of learning disability and mental illness is present, there is a possibility that some form of challenging behaviour will become manifest (Quinn and Mathieson 1993)
> *Influences from within the environment:* Overcrowded or unsuitable living conditions can exacerbate challenging behaviour. Destructive behaviour towards the fabric of the living accommodation can be particularly distressing to others who reside there
> *Attention-seeking behaviour:* There is a theory that people with learning disabilities will use forms of challenging behaviour as a means of nonverbal communication. Thorndike's law of effect suggests that when behaviour is rewarded, it is usually repeated; therefore, taking a behavioural psychologist's viewpoint, it could be argued that challenging behaviour is used as a means of achieving reinforcing stimuli.

Gentle teaching

Gentle teaching is a strategy built upon four main primary goals of care giving. It is nonviolent in origin and is focused particularly on helping people with learning disabilities and, when appropriate, those with challenging behaviour. The four primary goals of care giving are to teach the person:

> how to feel safe in society
> how to feel engaged with society
> to feel unconditionally loved by significant others
> to feel loving towards significant others.

Gentle teaching is principally based on a psychology of interdependence. This approach proffers a view that all change within human circumstances is mutual and should bring about a feeling of companionship and community that symbolically embraces justice and nonviolence. The psychology of interdependence is based on three assumptions:

> Each of us has a mind, a body and a spirit
> Each of us has a basic need for companionship
> Bonded relations are the fundamental building blocks of those basic human values deemed to be essential for living a moral life and developing personal life goals.

Advocates of gentle teaching argue that it is not a behavioural or behaviour modification technique relying on a reward and punishment approach. Neither is it a fast or easy pathway towards helping others. To acquire gentle teaching skills is demanding of time and dedication – the carer has to be committed to this approach because it is more than just a way of changing someone else's view of reality. To understand how gentle teaching works, carers must first be prepared to undergo a personal reality change aimed at becoming more open, welcoming and nonjudgemental towards the people they care for. The central tenet of gentle teaching is to define what we, as carers, want the person with a learning disability or challenging behaviour to become. It is about recognising those elements of a person's life that undermine emotional wellbeing and then to create an environment that fosters feelings of companionship and safety. Within the school of thought guiding gentle teaching, it is argued that feelings of companionship can be taught.

These feelings are created through the related notions of belonging and inclusiveness. Practitioners in this field argue that companionship is essential as a means of preventing people with learning disabilities becoming lost and isolated. The argument also includes a view that people with challenging behaviour have learned not to trust others and, indeed, have developed a fear of others.

Gentle teaching is strongly linked to the quality of life debate and there is a loosely structured hierarchy of basic values that guide practitioners who work with people with learning disabilities. These are as follows:

> *Bodily integrity* – promoting health gain through good nutrition, cleanliness and being well dressed
> *Feeling safe* – not being afraid of others or of going outside. Feeling relaxed in the presence of others
> *Feeling self-worth* – viewing oneself as a good person. Being able to express personal gifts and talents for the benefit of other people
> *Having a life structure* – developing a daily routine; having personal rituals and beliefs
> *Having a sense of belonging* – enjoying the company of close friends, having a home and being loved by others as well as loving others. Feeling the warmth of companionship
> *Social participation* – enjoying what the community has to offer
> *Having meaningful daily activities* – enjoying life and engaging in activities that fit a life plan

> *Inner contentment* – experiencing freedom from psychological trauma, and having a feeling of inner contentment.

It could be said that this hierarchy encompasses all the elements of effective caring, and that gentle teaching is one way of developing a strategy of care based on good practice. Within the hierarchy, there are covert references to Maslow's (1970) hierarchy of needs and Roper et al.'s (1996) activities of daily living. However, exponents of gentle teaching would argue that theirs is a unique approach, mainly through its focus on companionship.

Dual diagnosis

In the event of a person with a learning disability developing a mental illness, the term 'dual diagnosis' is applied. However, there are complexities associated with this diagnosis because the terminology can also be applied to people with mental illness who misuse alcohol or drugs. Learning disability is often equated with mental illness but it is important to recognise that the two conditions are completely different. Learning disability is often diagnosed at birth or during childhood, whereas it is unusual for a diagnosis of mental illness to be made during this early stage of a person's life. It is when an individual has left childhood and entered adolescence or adulthood that mental health problems such as schizophrenia and depression can occur. Because of the involvement of brain dysfunction, the effects and consequences of learning disability are permanent, unlike the varying types of mental illness that, in many cases, can be treated and cured. However, it is not unusual for people with learning disabilities to experience mental health problems; indeed, there is evidence to suggest that mental illness is more common among this group than it is among the general population (Hunt and Tarleton-Lord 1998). People with learning disabilities can find it difficult to articulate their feelings and this may result in mental illness becoming manifest through actions rather than words, with a consequence that it may remain undetected during the early stages. Episodic behaviour changes or mood swings are not uncommon and the signs of an encroaching mental health problem could be misconstrued as just another phase. This is particularly so when the person is said to display patterns of challenging behaviour. More recently, nurses and other service providers have come to realise that people with learning disabilities who develop mental health problems have a complexity of need that demands expert care. Support services in the area of dual diagnosis are still developing and the national picture regarding their availability remains patchy. This can result in difficulties being experienced by professional carers when attempting to refer people with a learning disability who have a dual diagnosis involving a mental illness (Mind 2003).

Person-centred planning

Person-centred planning for people with learning disabilities is part of an empowerment process that seeks to turn ambition, hopes and personal dreams for the future into reality. As a framework for understanding the notion of person-centred planning, work undertaken by the Joseph Rowntree Foundation (2000, p. 1) reported: 'There is a growing consensus that daytime opportunities for people with learning difficulties and disabled people need to be improved.' As part of this consensus, the Joseph Rowntree Foundation suggests that people should be supported to achieve new lifestyles that include work, learning new skills, enjoying leisure activities and spending time with friends, old and new, in ordinary community settings.

When considering approaches to person-centred planning, the King's Fund Changing Days project (Wertheimer 1996) is considered to be a good place to start. This project explores opportunities for developing new lifestyles when moving from segregated day services to a service based on individual needs. Person-centred planning is usually focused on residents living in small group residential accommodation, beginning with an initial consultation day when each person is given the time and space to say what they want from their lives. This individual approach is essential because otherwise there is a possibility that the overall needs of the group could usurp the needs of the individual. Once the consultation stage has been undertaken, each person is allocated a 'planning circle' comprising a group of people from inside and outside the service. The planning circle will, at all times, keep the individual's needs central to its discussion. This is achieved by including the disabled person at all times, ensuring that all views and opinions are given equal consideration and the development of goals and actions are not dictated by service considerations. Each planning circle has a trained facilitator who will encourage and support members to remain involved. Committed staff members are an essential part of the process. Person-centred planning is challenging because it takes members of the planning circle beyond their personal comfort zones into the world of the resident whose lifestyle priorities may not always match their own. This form of planning empowers people to be open about personal ambition with a consequence of developing greater control over their lives. Person-centred planning within a residential home calls for a balance between the welfare of the residents as a group and supporting the individual in developing a personal and fulfilling lifestyle.

Genetics

Genetics is the scientific study of inheritance. It looks at how the many traits that make each human being unique are passed down from their parents and the effect this has on physical and psychological development. Recently, through the work of the International Human Genome Sequencing Consortium, it is confirmed that the sequence variations of the human genome can play a major part in identifying the aetiology of certain diseases or disabling conditions (Burton and Stewart 2003). From this understanding, new treatments and therapies will be developed to reduce the effect of these conditions or eliminate them altogether.

The study of genetics is founded on the work of Gregor Mendel (1822–84), an Austrian monk. Mendel developed a certain expertise in biology but it wasn't until long after his death that the full implications of his experimental work on variations, heredity and evolution in plants became fully recognised. So important was his work that Mendel's findings are now considered to be the bedrock upon which modern genetics and evolutionary theory are founded. While in holy orders, he became particularly interested in the common garden pea, *Pisum*, which he cultivated in the monastery garden. Between the years 1856 and 1863, Mendel cultivated and tested 28,000 pea plants. From his painstaking experiments, he identified seven pairs of seeds that he carefully analysed for comparison. For example, he compared shape, colour, tall or short stemmed and tall or short plants. His work was meticulous. He even wrapped each individual plant to prevent accidental pollination by bees and other insects. Seeds harvested from the plants were replanted and the offspring observed for familial traits. He discovered that some plants bred true and others did not. By crossing tall plants with short ones, he noticed they inadvertently produced hybrids that resembled the tall plant rather than being of a medium or short variety. His explanation of this suggested the presence of hereditary units, which we now refer to as 'genes'. Mendel's laws of heredity are formed around the existence of dominant traits that show up in the offspring and recessive traits, masked by a dominant gene, that remain subordinate. This basic understanding of inherited traits is still used today.

The science of genetics begins with the premise that every living organism consists of cells. Normally, in the human being, each cell contains 23 pairs of chromosomes that carry inherited genetic material. From conception, when only one cell exists, the zygote will grow and develop through a process of cell duplication (mitosis) that determines the sex and physical make-up of the individual. It is also considered that some mental illnesses, such as schizophrenia, have a genetic link. More recently, through the work of Watson and Crick, the discovery of deoxyribonucleic acid (DNA) revolutionised our understanding of the genetic code of inheritance. Genes are made up of DNA, which in turn consists of a combination of four chemicals (adenine, thymine, cytosine and guanine). As human beings, we have approximately 30,000 genes, each of which has a specific part to play in our individual make-up. The human genome project is dedicated to identifying each of these genes and the role they play in our existence.

Faulty genes cause disorders and because of their inherited nature, it is possible to identify genetically linked disorders that run in families. The aetiology of some learning disabilities can often be linked to genetic inheritance. Several syndromes have been identified where inheritance factors play a part, the most common being Down's syndrome and Fragile X syndrome. Other, less common syndromes include Cri du chat syndrome, Prada–Willi syndrome and phenylketonuria. (For a full description of these and other syndromes, see Clarke 2000, Ch. 3.)

Autism is one of the pervasive development disorders of the brain for which there is no known cure. This group of disorders is characterised by a delay in socialising and communication functions. Symptoms can present themselves in early infancy but usually not before a child has reached three years of age but they do continue through life. Principally, these symptoms can include difficulties in understanding language and relationship development; the person may have restricted or severely restricted social skills and may not recognise routines associated with normal rhythms of the day. People with autism can display unnatural responses to sensory stimulation including sound or touch and display strongly held narrow obsessional traits. However, it would be wrong to suggest that people with autism never show emotion or make eye contact or communicate through speech or laughter. There are many people with this disorder who communicate extremely effectively.

Studies into the aetiology of autism strongly suggest a multiple genetic predisposition to the disorder. However, ongoing studies are investigating other possible factors that could have a bearing on the development of autistic behaviour. For example, environmental factors such as the use of certain childhood vaccines are thought by some scientific experts to play a role. Despite this, it is generally accepted in the scientific community that autism results from a disruption in early fetal brain development and that it affects boys rather than girls at an approximate ratio of four to one.

As stated above, there is no known cure for autism but through educational and behavioural programmes a person with this disorder can develop and enhance interpersonal relationships while reducing inappropriate patterns of behaviour. Schools that specialise in educating children with autism and other special needs provide highly structured, child-centred interventions aimed at socialising the individual. As in all young people, adolescence is a time of major change, physically, socially and psychologically. Behaviours can become inwardly focused and teenagers may appear to be selfish and awkward in dealings with others. When reaching this milestone in their development, children with autism often exhibit amplified behavioural traits, which are extremely challenging. Sensitive teachers and parents will adjust their responses to take account of the child's changing needs.

Although no two people with autism are alike, there are certain behavioural traits that are common to many of them and may be displayed in various combinations. These are:

> Remaining detached – seeming to prefer their own company to that of others
> Resisting any form of change – sameness becomes important
> Crying or laughing for no obvious reason
> Echolalia – repeating words or phrases back rather than responding in a normal conversational way

- › Extremes of underactivity or overactivity
- › Aggressive responses to occurrences that would not normally evoke extreme behaviour
- › Self-injury
- › Frustration at not being able to adequately express personal needs and wants. This expression can be in the form of a verbal or nonverbal response
- › Motor skills and coordination can vary between individuals. For example, some can finger-spin objects with great skill and dexterity
- › Fearlessness in the face of potential danger
- › Response to pain or discomfort can be exaggerated or ignored
- › Difficulty in interacting with others. This can take the form of nonresponse to verbal cues, avoiding eye contact, resisting physical contact (although it is not unusual for there to be a strong attachment to an inanimate object) and having tantrums
- › Failure to respond to normal methods of teaching
- › Playing in a way that seems strange or different from the norm.

People with autism have a normal life expectancy, although some will develop various disorders not common in the general community, such as epilepsy. In a minority of individuals, the effects of autism will be reduced to the point where many ordinary life experiences can be enjoyed.

Learning Disability Task Force

The Learning Disability Task Force is made up of people who work with the government to check and ensure that recommendations within the document *Valuing People* are being taken forward. Members of the task force offer a wide cross-section of expertise relating to learning disability. For example, there are members who can offer an authoritative input on:

- › Advocacy
- › Benefits
- › Health
- › Disability rights
- › Housing.

An important element of the work of the task force is to ensure that people with a learning disability enjoy an improvement in their lives, particularly those with high individual support needs. For example, the task force takes steps to ensure that the needs of people with a dual diagnosis, that is, an additional disability such as hearing or eyesight loss, are appreciated. In addition, a main focus of the task force's work revolves around community safety. This requires the maintenance of a close working relationship with the police and judiciary. In taking a sensitive approach to community safety, it is now realised that the sight of a uniform can frighten people with a learning disability, particularly when that uniform represents authority such as a police officer. Some officers experience difficulty when attempting to communicate with people who have a learning disability. Indeed, because of this, it is possible for police officers not to believe a learning disabled person. The police and other community agencies may employ educational resources such as instructional DVDs to illuminate essential factors that should be considered when called upon to deal with people who have a learning disability. Dr Colin Dale provides an informed profile of problems and issues facing government and the judiciary where the care and treatment of offenders with learning disabilities is concerned (http://www.ldoffenders.co.uk/). He highlights factors that have a direct bearing on this, including:

> The lack of appropriate alternative routes when considering diverting people from the criminal justice system
> Some people learn how to disguise their learning disability, which is sometimes referred to as a 'cloaking device'
> The need for stronger ties with schools for early detection and intervention of maladaptive behaviour patterns.

Conclusion

This chapter provides an overview of the complexities associated with learning disabilities. A study of the history of this branch of nursing shows how much it has changed from its beginnings in the long-stay hospital to its present position in a modern community-based service. This has happened over a relatively short timescale, resulting in several reappraisals of the nursing role in a community setting. Change is never far away from this dynamic branch of nursing and it says much for the resilience of nurses in learning disability that they have consolidated and built upon their professional knowledge and skill base to an extent that they are now an essential part of the caring team.

Further reading and resources

Clarke, D (2006) What is intellectual disability?, in A Roy, M Roy and D Clarke (eds), *The Psychiatry of Intellectual Disability*, Oxford: Radcliffe

For an introduction to genetics, go to www.genetics.org.uk

For more information on Tourette's syndrome, go to www.mentalhealth.com

For an overview of the philosophy and work of L'Arche, go to www.larche.org.uk/disability

For a discussion on the work of Gregor Mendel, go to www.zephyrus.co.uk/gregormendel.html

References

Abraham, A and White, J (2009) *Six Lives: The Provision of Public Services to People with Learning Disability*, HC 203-1, London: TSO

Bank-Mikkelsen, NE (1969) A metropolitan area in Denmark: Copenhagen, in RB Kugel and W Wolfensberger (eds), *Changing Patterns in Residential Services for the Mentally Retarded*, Washington DC: President's Committee on Mental Retardation

Burton, H and Stewart, A (2003) From Mendel to the human genome project: the implication for nurse education, *Nurse Education Today*, **23**(5): 380–5

Clarke, D (2000) What is learning disability?, in M Roy, D Clarke and A Roy (eds), *An Introduction to Learning Disability Psychiatry*, Oxford: Radcliffe

Craft, M, Bicknell, J and Hollins, S (1985) *Mental Handicap: A Multidisciplinary Approach*, London: Baillière Tindall

DH (Department of Health) (1992)*The Health of the Nation: A Strategy for Health in England*, London: TSO

DH (1993) *Services for People with Learning Disabilities and Challenging Behaviour or Mental Health Needs* (Mansell Report), London: HMSO

DH (1996) *The Carers (Recognition and Services) Act 1995: Policy Guidance*, London: HMSO

DH (1999) *Once a day: one or more people with learning disabilities are likely to be in contact with your primary healthcare team. How can you help them?,* London: HMSO

DH (2001) *Valuing People: A New Strategy for Learning Disability for the 21st Century,* Cmnd 5086, London: HMSO

DHSS (Department of Health and Social Security) (1971) *Better Services for the Mentally Handicapped*, Cmnd 4683, London: HMSO

DRC (Disability Rights Commission) (2006) *Equal Treatment: Closing the Gap*, London: DRC

Emerson, E, Malam, S, Davies, I and Spencer, K (2005) *Adults with Learning Difficulties in England 2003/4*, Leeds: Health and Social Care Information Centre

Griffiths Report (1988) *Community Care: Agenda for Action.* A Report to the Secretary of State for Social Services by Sir Roy Griffiths, London: HMSO

House of Commons Social Services Select Committee (1985) *Community Care with Special Reference to Adult Mentally Ill and Mentally Handicapped People,* London: HMSO

Hunt, G and Tarleton-Lord, T (1998) Snapshots of the mind, *Nursing Times*, 94: 16

Joseph Rowntree Foundation (2000) *Developing New Lifestyles with Disabled People, Findings,* 19 September, available online at http://www.jrf.org.uk/publications/developing-new-lifestyles-with-disabled-people, accessed 9/6/2010

Mallik, MA (1995) Advocacy in nursing, MPhil thesis, Nottingham University

Maslow, AH (1970) *Motivation and Personality*, New York: Harper & Row

Mencap (2004a) *Treat Me Right: Better Healthcare for People with a Learning Disability*, London: Mencap

Mencap (2004b) *Advocacy Strategy*, available online at http://www.aqvx59.dsl.pipex.com/MencapAdvocacystrategy.pdf, accessed 9/6/2010

Mencap (2007) *Death by Indifference: Following up the Treat Me Right Report*, London: Mencap

Mind (2003) *Learning Disabilities and Mental Health Problems*, available online at http://www.mind.org.uk/help/people_groups_and_communities/learning_disabilities_and_mental_health_problems, accessed 8/6/2010

Nirje, B (1969) The normalization principle and its human management implications, *The International Social Role Valorisation Journal,* **1**(2): 1994

NPSA (National Patient Safety Agency) (2004) *Understanding the Patient Safety Issues for People with Learning Disabilities*, London: NPSA

Quinn, F and Mathieson, A (1993) Associated conditions, in E Shanley and T Starrs (eds), *Learning Disabilities: A Handbook of Care*, London: Churchill Livingstone

3

Report of the Royal Commission on the Law Relating to Mental Illness and Mental Deficiency 1954–1957 (Percy Commission), Cmnd 169, London: HMSO

Roper, N, Logan, WW and Tierney, AJ (1996) *The Elements of Nursing* (4th edn), London: Churchill Livingstone

Sinason, V (1992) *Mental Handicap and the Human Condition: New Approaches from the Tavistock*, London: Free Association Books

Slevin, E (1999) Challenging behaviour in people with learning disabilities, *Mental Health Care*, **2**(7): 242–5

Spencer, DA (1997) Concept of learning disability: historical background, in SG Reed (ed.), *Psychiatry in Learning Disability*, Edinburgh: WB Saunders, available at www.questia.com

Spink, K (1990) *Jean Vanier and L'Arche: A Communion of Love*, London: Darton, Longman & Todd

Teasdale, K (1998) *Advocacy in Health Care*, London: Blackwell

Van Schrojenstein Lantaman-De Valk, H, Metsemakers, JF, Haveman, MJ and Crebolder, HF (2000) Health problems in people with intellectual disability in general practice: a comparative study, *Family Practice*, 5: 405–7

Wertheimer, A (ed.) (1996) *Changing Days: Developing New Opportunities with People Who Have Learning Difficulties*, London: King's Fund

WHO (World Health Organization) (1992) *The ICD-10 Classification of Mental and Behavioural Disorders: Clinical Descriptions and Diagnostic Guidelines*, WHO: Geneva

Willmott, P (1989) *Community Initiatives: Patterns and Prospects*, London: Policy Studies Institute

Wolfensberger, W (1972) *The Principle of Normalization in Human Services*, Toronto: National Institute on Mental Retardation

3

15 mental health nursing

Jacquie White, Tim Welbourn, Michael Howe,
Neil Burton, Hugh Palmer, Tracy Flanagan,
Carl Slee, David Glenster and Ian Barkley

In this chapter we will explore:

> The recovery approach
> Social inclusion
> Services
> Working systemically
> Family therapy
> Self-awareness and emotional intelligence
> Working within boundaries
> Mental health nursing education

Introduction

Mental health has been defined as:

> a state of well-being in which the individual realizes his or her own abilities, can cope with the normal stresses of life, can work productively and fruitfully, and is able to make a contribution to his or her community. (WHO 2001, p.1)

Many internal and external events can threaten this equilibrium, leading to the experience of mental distress. For example, work problems such as redundancy, relationship breakdown or physical ill health can all lead to low mood and a lack of optimism about the future. In some people, such experiences will result in a change in their ability to cope with day-to-day living and achieving their potential over time.

The six most common presenting mental health problems in primary care are depression, **anxiety**, alcohol use problems, chronic tiredness, sleep problems and symptoms where an underlying physical cause cannot be identified. One-quarter of routine general practice consultations are for these types of problems and one in four of us will visit our GP complaining of symptoms like these in the course of the next year (WHO 2000).

The vast majority of people will only need to be seen in primary care but 10% will be referred to mental health services for a specialist assessment, usually because there are concerns about increasing disability, risk (most often about suicide or self-neglect) or the correct diagnosis and treatment. Mental illness is the other end of the spectrum of mental health. It has been defined as: 'an inability to adjust to and respond accordingly to the demands of social and emotional life' (Harbottle and Mudd 2004, p. 68).

Secondary mental health services are focused on the care of people with mental illnesses, such as severe depression and anxiety, dementia, **personality disorders**, **schizophrenia** or **bipolar disorder**. Tertiary services provide ongoing support for individuals who have long-term needs, for example rehabilitation and support.

Mental health nurses (MHNs) are the largest group of professionals working in mental health services today. In 2004, there were 47,000 qualified MHNs working throughout the NHS (DH 2005a) in both inpatient and community settings, in primary, secondary and tertiary care. MHNs have the most contact time with mental health service users of any health professional and this provides a unique opportunity for the nurse to form a relationship with the service user and promote positive change within the context and support of this relationship. The role of the MHN is, therefore, to support the service user with mental illness, or at risk of mental illness, to effect positive change and achieve their potential (McCabe 2002). In this chapter we will explore the key themes of recovery, social inclusion, mental health service structure, engagement in positive change, relationship boundaries and education and support.

The recovery approach

The most recent review of mental health nursing *From Values to Action* (DH 2006a, p. 4) recommended that MHNs should 'incorporate the broad principles of the Recovery Approach into every aspect of their practice'. Recovery is a normal rather than an abnormal concept (Anthony 1993). The recovery approach is based on the key principles of social inclusion, the rights of individuals to strive towards life goals and aspirations that are meaningful to them, and the maintenance of hope and optimism for the future. Recovery does not necessarily mean that the person will return to being how they were before they experienced distress and illness. Importantly, **recovery** is seen as living a meaningful and satisfying life with, rather than in spite of, illness and disability. Indeed, the experience of mental distress is seen as a positive force towards change, rather than a negative limitation to be hidden and stigmatised. It is the role of the MHN to support and enable the service user and their carer(s) in this positive change journey.

The development of mental health problems is a huge event in someone's life but they are not necessarily a tragedy. Indeed, many people who have experienced mental health problems, including severe and enduring mental health problems, say that ultimately their lives have been richer because of their experiences. They have become wiser and kinder to themselves and others as a result of their own experiences of mental health problems. This is not at all to minimise the very real emotional distress that is at the centre of mental health problems, because, at the time, such distress can be terrifying, not only to the individual, but to their family and friends. However, in the depths of emotional distress, treasures can be found that afterwards can make life so much more worthwhile.

The problem many people face is the lack of hope of others. In the depths of distress, when individuals are experiencing voices and visions and are unable to even keep themselves clean without prompting or actual help, it simply does not help if those around you tell you that you might never get better, that you will never work again, that no one will want you again. Families and friends sometimes say such things because all they may know about is the old 'mental hospital' but not about contemporary mental health services. However, it's not just families and friends who do not help. Sometimes professionals say unhelpful things. And just as often they omit to say helpful things.

When an individual is feeling utterly hopeless for their future, it is important that someone holds hope for them, reminding them that they have looked at life in a different way in the past, and that their future may be full of opportunities that they cannot imagine at the moment. It doesn't help when professionals forget to find out if someone is in employment, or omit to explore what skills someone has used in the past. People can lose their job during a crisis because of poor communication between employee and employer, or by the professional ignoring someone's past skills, giving out the message: 'With that diagnosis, you'll never get another job.'

What is said and what is done, and what is not said and not done by an MHN when someone is in crisis, or starting out on the path of recovery, is of vital importance to someone's future. It's important to get it right to help the client towards recovery, even though in the past professionals have not always done this. The result is that people have never recovered not only from their original mental health problem, but also never recovered from the contact with mental health services. This is the problem for mental health services today – getting it right for recovery.

Social inclusion

Stigma is a ubiquitous and universal experience of pain, discrimination and marginalisation cutting across all cultures and societies. While an attitude change is critical, this may be difficult to fashion. Planning better mental health services, improving access and encouraging more positive attitudes in the professionals manning them may be steps towards this goal. (Thara 2003, p. 96)

Negative attitudes can reinforce someone's isolation and impede their recovery. In a 2004 campaign called 'One in Four' run by Mind Out for Mental Health, a number of well-known people agreed to have their photographs taken and spoke openly about their experiences of mental health. Paul Merton, a comedian known for his quick wittedness on TV programmes such as the BBC's *Have I Got News For You*, offered this insight:

> Such is the taboo of mental illness that I was reluctant for many years to talk about my stay in the Maudsley. What saddened me was that my visitors felt so uncomfortable. They thought the doors were going to slam shut behind them ... Most of all people shouldn't feel ashamed for having a mental illness. We don't feel ashamed for having a broken leg, so why a mental illness? (quoted in the Mind Out for Mental Health campaign material)

According to Mind (2004a), four out of five people experiencing a mental health problem believe themselves to be alienated and state that their isolation is a real barrier to recovery:

> I find I'm isolated because of people's reaction to me having a mental health problem, I get mocked, pushed and stared at, so feel isolated and I can't go out much or make friends so I get more depressed as a result. (Mind 2004a, p. 5)

So what are some of the problems? The UK government's Social Exclusion Unit (SEU 2004) highlights the following:

> Severe mental health problems such as schizophrenia are relatively rare, affecting one in 200 adults each year. But depression and anxiety can affect up to one in six of the population at any one time, with the highest rates in the most deprived neighbourhoods.
> Only 24% of adults with mental health problems are in work – the lowest employment rate for any of the main groups of disabled people.
> Fewer than four in ten employers say they would recruit someone with a mental health problem.
> People with mental health problems are at more than double the risk of losing their job than those without.
> Many people experience their first episode of mental health problems in their late teens or early twenties, which can have serious consequences for their education and employment prospects.
> A person with a diagnosis of schizophrenia can expect a significantly shorter life expectancy than people in the general population.
> People with severe mental health problems are three times more likely to be divorced than those without.
> People with mental health problems are three times as likely to be in debt as those without.
> People with mental health problems are four times more likely to say their health has been damaged by the quality of their housing.

People with mental health problems are often excluded from what most of us accept as the basic necessities of ordinary life. There is increasing evidence that the physical health needs of people with mental health problems are not being met and they are dying 20–25 years earlier than people in the general population, largely from cardiovascular disease and preventable cancers (Robson and Gray 2007; Shuel et al. 2009). The fact that experiences of exclusion encountered by individuals and groups of people can sometimes be a precursor to mental health problems is also well recognised. For example, *Mental Health and Deafness: Towards Equity and Access* (DH 2005b) indicated the high incidence of mental health problems among deaf people compared to the hearing population. Citing studies showing that 40% of deaf children have mental health problems, compared to 25% of hearing children, this report goes on to say that many deaf people suffer from social exclusion and reduced educational and employment opportunities and are overrepresented in prisons and the criminal justice system.

The problems of social exclusion and mental health are not unique to the UK, nor are they unique to those born in the UK. Schulze and Angermeyer (2003), working in Germany, also found that people with schizophrenia believe that they are stigmatised at work and in the community. For those coming to the UK, such as refugees, the Social Exclusion Unit has identified that approximately two-thirds experience anxiety and depression. Rates of **psychosis** among white people migrating to predominantly white communities are twice as high as the general population and four times as high among black people migrating to predominantly white communities (Graae and Selten 2004).

There are, of course, many strong advocates within the general public, both individuals and groups, who speak out and challenge **stigma**, discrimination and exclusion. In 2003, *The Sun* newspaper carried a front-page story about former world heavyweight boxing champion Frank Bruno headlined 'Bonkers Bruno locked up'. As the result of an enormous and immediate public outcry, the headline in later editions was changed to 'Sad Bruno in mental home'. The following day the newspaper launched a fund for the former boxer and the editor subsequently spent a day with the mental health charity Sane, learning about mental health issues in an endeavour to bring about more responsible reporting. This change of heart from the newspaper was widely welcomed, but its treatment of someone generally perceived to be a fondly regarded national hero emphasises just how difficult life can be, purely on the basis of discrimination and social exclusion, for those experiencing a mental health problem.

A vital role of those involved in mental health is to actively promote a more positive and inclusive view of mental health. The following points have been highlighted as ways to enhance social inclusion (SEU 2004):

> *Inclusive communities* – working to reduce stigma and discrimination in local communities, support reintegration and acceptance of people with mental health problems as equal citizens
> *Early intervention* – offer easily accessible nonstigmatising support and help before people reach crisis situations

> *Focus on employment and meaningful activity* – recognise that jobs provide a sense of worth and identity as well as financial security. Working is associated with better health and a reduced need for services

> *Promoting broader social participation* – education, volunteering or training, particularly in mainstream settings, can enhance job prospects as well as being valuable in their own right. They can help build self-esteem, confidence and social networks, as can sports, particularly benefiting physical health, and arts activities

> *Securing basic entitlements* – decent housing, education, finance and transport

> *Acknowledging people's social networks and family relationships* – recognising the central role that family members and friends can play in reintegration into communities

> *Building confidence and trust* – making services more welcoming and promoting understanding of different needs to encourage people who may mistrust services, such as some ethnic minorities or parents for example, to engage readily.

MHNs are well placed to engage in a range of activity to promote social inclusion and fundamentally change attitudes. Nurses can examine local policy and practice and ensure that it matches national policy and initiatives such as *New Horizons* (DH 2009), a cross-government programme of action with the twin aims of improving the mental health and wellbeing of the population across the life span. Now read the following introduction to Kevin. You will pick up on this young man later in the chapter.

Case study: introducing Kevin

Kevin, who is 19 years old, currently lives with his mother Jayne, stepfather Peter and his five-year-old sister Katy. They live in a semi-detached house on a new-build estate in the suburbs of a medium-sized city. Jayne is a manager in a local call centre and Peter has recently been made redundant after 14 years in a local engineering company. Kevin attends the city's further education college and is in his first year of a media studies foundation degree.

All the activities in this chapter ask you to reflect on the information presented in Kevin's story and are proposed to help you think about some of the skills and attributes required by today's mental health nurse.

Activity 15.1

Thinking about the changes being experienced by the members of Kevin's family at this time and reflecting on families you know (including your own), identify three possible causes of stress from the above scenario.

Services

For many, psychiatric care is still associated with the Victorian asylums that inhabited the isolated outskirts of our towns and cities and where the 'men in white coats' would take you away if you were deemed 'mental'. Indeed, many nurses still in practice today will have trained and worked in these large institutions. The institutions were largely established during the nineteenth century and flourished well into the twentieth century. However, by the middle of the last century, alternative ways of caring for people with mental illness were beginning to be considered and developed. The advent of the NHS in 1948 and the development of the modern welfare state meant that unwaged people suffering from mental illness could be cared for in public housing without the need for them to be removed to the institutions. Greater access to drug treatments came through better GP services and improved supervision and support was provided through social services and primary care. Outpatient clinics and community psychiatric nursing began to emerge alongside new psychiatric units located in district general hospital sites (Boardman 2005).

By the 1980s, mental health services were routinely being delivered in primary care either through GP practices or by community psychiatric nurses in people's own homes. Secondary care, that is, shorter term inpatient care, was still being provided by the institutions but now also within district hospital settings and specialist localised services. Tertiary care, that is, long-term care, was also still provided within the old asylums but a significant proportion of the patients who had spent many years in an institutional setting were 'rehabilitated' and moved into the community via hostels, sheltered housing or their own accommodation. Other patients still requiring continuing care were moved into private or voluntary nursing and residential homes. Slowly, the old asylums began to empty and close.

By the end of the twentieth century, institutional care had been replaced by a range of services delivered in both residential and community settings. In the latter, services were delivered largely by community mental health teams (CMHTs), comprising a range of specialist mental health professionals, including nurses, psychiatrists, social workers, occupational therapists and psychologists. The number of psychiatric inpatient beds in England has decreased dramatically from its peak of 150,000 in 1955 to around 40,000 today. However, despite the increased range and comprehensiveness of community care, there has still been a steady rise in the numbers of people being admitted to inpatient care (NIMHE 2003). The impact on inpatient services has been highlighted in several reports that chronicle the poor environments, increasing numbers of disturbed patients with a greater proportion detained under the **Mental Health Act**, increased levels of violence and aggression and decreased staff morale (SCMH 1998; SNMAC 1999; Rethink et al. 2004; Mind 2004b).

The reasons behind the increased admission rates are multifaceted. It may

3

simply be that there is an increased level of mental illness being experienced in society. There is evidence to show that the patient population is changing and that more people are being admitted with multiple issues as well as their mental health concerns, including drug and alcohol misuse, poverty, homelessness, relational and family problems (SCMH 1998). The re-emphasis of the risk presented by those who have mental illness, as portrayed through high-profile cases such as Christopher Clunis, who had been diagnosed with paranoid schizophrenia and stabbed and killed Jonathan Zito in an unprovoked attack, may also have led to an increase in 'defensive practice'. Thus psychiatrists and other mental health professionals will use admission to hospital as a means of reducing the risk a person presents and avoiding the possibility of an untoward event occurring even if it may not be the most appropriate or beneficial course of action for the person. They are not only protecting the wider public and the person themselves from the consequences of any perceived risk but also defending themselves from the risk of blame and potential litigation.

Part of the reason for the increasing demand and pressure on inpatient beds could be seen as a failure of community services to provide people with an alternative to admission or to facilitate people being discharged from hospital at the earliest possible opportunity. CMHTs operate on a 'nine-to-five' basis and are expected to deal with a wide range of problems and needs. As such, CMHTs have been expected to:

> pick up emergency referrals from GPs
> offer a service to people with 'common mental health problems' such as depression and anxiety
> monitor and support people with serious and enduring mental illnesses such as chronic schizophrenia (NIMHE 2003).

The breadth of expectation experienced by the CMHTs has placed an ever increasing burden on their limited resources. It has also meant that mental health services have failed to provide service users and their carers with sufficient access to community-based services in a crisis, or specialised and intensive treatment outside the hospital setting.

In 1998, the government set out its intention to modernise mental health services in the White Paper *Modernising Mental Health Services: Safe, Sound and Supportive* (DH 1998), which was followed in 1999 by the *National Service Framework for Mental Health* (NSFMH). The NSFMH (DH 1999) outlined seven standards across five main areas, which were to be delivered over 10 years (Figure 15.1).

In order to meet these standards, providers of mental health care have had to restructure and reconfigure their services. Within primary care, there has been an increased focus on effective screening and provision of psychological approaches for common mental health problems such as depression and anxiety. Early intervention teams have been developed to pick up younger people who show signs of developing schizophrenia or who are experiencing

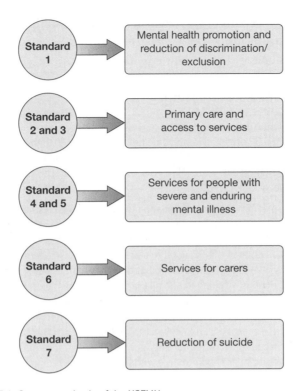

Figure 15.1 Seven standards of the NSFMH
Source: Adapted from Boardman and Parsonage 2005

their first or second episode of the illness. By catching them early in the progression of the illness and treating them with the appropriate medication and psychological approaches, they are much less likely to develop an enduring and chronic illness. To ensure that patients and carers can access help at any time, 24-hour community-based services including crisis and intensive home treatment teams have been developed that operate seven days a week. People who have severe and enduring mental illnesses or who have a history of 'opting out' of care are referred to specialist assertive outreach teams. They have small caseloads and work flexibly with their service users to maintain contact and engagement with services.

The overall structure within which these new services function is described as a whole system. Each part of the service should be integrated with the others, while also working closely with other organisations and the wider community. This should allow ease of access and 'seamless' care for the service user, regardless of where they are or the state of their mental health (NIMHE 2003).

We now return to Kevin and see how these new services can positively influence a person's experience of care as a consequence of mental distress and illness. Kevin's case study demonstrates how the whole system approach facilitates integration, adaptability and continuity throughout the person's journey through different parts of the system. It also shows how the principles of recovery and social inclusion can be incorporated into service configuration and delivery.

Case study cont'd: Kevin's journey

Kevin's mother Jayne decides to encourage Kevin to go to see his GP. Kevin refuses, so she goes to see the GP on her own for some help. She tells the GP that Kevin has been behaving strangely, isolating himself in his room, muttering to himself and has become obsessed with watching old videos of Dr Who. Kevin's GP is concerned enough to make a referral to the local CMHT.

Kevin is seen by a community mental health nurse from the local CMHT. Following assessment, it is thought that Kevin may be experiencing psychotic phenomena and suggested that he is referred to see the consultant psychiatrist. He refuses and two weeks later Jayne contacts the GP again to say that Kevin has become increasingly disturbed and frightened and has told her that he believes he is being watched by Daleks and can hear them talking to him all the time. Kevin is then referred to a specialist early intervention team (EIT) who work exclusively with 16–25-year-olds. He is initially reluctant to see anyone from the team but one of their young male workers offers to take him to a local gig and Kevin tentatively begins to build a relationship with him. He is encouraged to talk a bit more about his thoughts and experiences, but while he is happy to keep regular appointments with his worker, he remains quite guarded about what is going on in his head.

Over the summer, Kevin goes to a festival with some friends and consumes a significant amount of cannabis. He becomes floridly psychotic and is subsequently admitted to hospital under Section 2 of the Mental Health Act. He is given medication that appears to take away his distressing psychotic symptoms and, after three weeks, the team decide he can go home. While in hospital, his worker from the EIT sees him regularly and is able to establish more clearly with Kevin some of the things he has been thinking and believing. On discharge, he continues to see his worker but becomes increasingly reluctant to take his medication, and it also becomes clear that he is periodically using cannabis.

Over the next two years, Kevin has three more admissions to hospital, his relationship with his family deteriorates significantly and following his latest admission, his mother Jayne says that she does not want him home again. His worker from the EIT continues to have regular contact with Kevin but reports that he is inconsistent in taking his medication. He suggests that Kevin moves into a local Mind hostel with nine other young people with mental health problems.

Kevin remains in hostel accommodation for 18 months and is seen regularly by his worker. However, he does not take his medication, is unwilling to attend a day hospital and is generally isolative and uncooperative with staff, spending most of his time in his room. He says that he wants to live in his own place and not with a load of other 'nutters'. He is offered the opportunity to move into a council flat with the support of a housing support officer and workers from the assertive outreach team who take over his care as he is now 25. He enrols at the local college on a photography course and starts seeing his family again after a year of no contact.

Engagement in change

Mental distress is, by its nature, disturbing for the person experiencing it, as well as family members and carers. The experience of feeling distressed can lead to a vicious circle in which the symptoms of mental illness become more intense. Imagine what your thoughts would be if you heard voices when no one was present. You might believe that someone is watching you or that someone has control over your mind. If the comments made were critical and offensive, this is likely to produce feelings of distress and loss of control. The distress will influence how you behave. You might attack those around you as you feel threatened, or, contrastingly, withdraw and isolate yourself to avoid the threat. You may take cannabis or excessive amounts of alcohol for their pleasurable effects or in an attempt to feel better. However, the intoxicating or withdrawal effects of these substances may make your symptoms worse. You may become so preoccupied by your thoughts that your usual activities such as undertaking work or caring for yourself are neglected. Our case study illustrates how the initial symptom of hearing voices can lead to secondary problems. Although many people hear voices without a negative outcome, in our example, the person can lose track of who they are and where they are going. A cycle of despair with a loss of hope can be created, with death as the only escape: indeed 10–13% of people experiencing the above symptoms commit suicide (Caldwell and Gottesman 1990). A significant number also experience premature death from physical illness or accident. It is, therefore, important for MHNs to find ways to engage people in positive change to help them fulfil their potential.

Core skills

Engagement of the service user in a **therapeutic relationship** is the first and most important role of the mental health nurse. This process is underpinned by the humanistic concept that every individual person is responsible for their own destiny and everyone has the potential for growth and self-development (Rogers 1959). Positive 'therapeutic' change occurs in a climate of warmth, respect and acceptance. If these core conditions can be established and maintained within the MHN–service user relationship, the service user can come to realise that someone else believes that they have the potential to cope and change. Feeling valued and accepted and prepared to trust the nurse, they can then be facilitated to explore, understand and take action.

The tidal model

Although models of nursing have been around for many years, Phil Barker's tidal model is one of the first to focus on mental health (Barker 2000). One of the great strengths of the tidal model is its accessibility to all through the use of metaphor, incredibly useful when trying to explain, share and understand personal experiences. Using the metaphor of the 'movement of water as life' and the individual's journey as they navigate through all sorts of weather at sea, a positive focus on the individual's strengths and challenges is enabled, rather than a focus on problems and illness (Barker 2001). Change is rarely experienced as a straightforward linear process, more often change is experienced as a circular process, with a number of setbacks as well as positive steps forwards before a steady state of change (or safe harbour) is reached. Interestingly, in the change management literature as well as the scientific literature, there is now an increasing recognition of how change most often seems to occur at the edge of chaos (for example Ackerman 1997; Bak 1997).

When planning to change a behaviour or pattern of behaviour, it is common to experience ambivalence about the proposed change. For example, when thinking about stopping smoking, most people will describe a tension between wanting to prevent the health risks of smoking for themselves and their families and a resistance to giving up the pleasure they experience from cigarettes at points throughout their day. In addition, most ex-smokers will tell you that they experienced many attempts at stopping before they were able to fully kick the habit. This pattern has been identified as a cycle, where the person passes through different stages (including relapse) before solving the problem and maintaining the change (Prochaska and DiClemente 1982).

Motivational interviewing

Motivational interviewing is a collaborative style of helping, which facilitates people to explore and resolve their ambivalence to change, choose what to do, take action and maximise recovery (Miller and Rollnick 1991). Originally developed in the 1980s by psychologists as an approach towards alcohol and drug addiction, motivational interviewing strategies are now being applied by MHNs to a range of change needs, including promoting self-management of long-term conditions, reducing risk behaviours and medication management.

Principles of the approach include the use of active listening skills alongside a questioning style, known as Socratic questioning, which helps the person to explore any discrepancy between their words, beliefs and actions. Padesky (1993, p. 7) defines this as asking the person questions that:

> They have the knowledge to answer
> Draw their attention to information that is relevant to the issue being discussed but which may be outside their current focus
> Generally move from the concrete to the more abstract so that the person

can, in the end, apply the new information to either re-evaluate a previous conclusion or construct a new idea.

Later on in the change cycle, the person will be supported to set future goals and contingency plan for times when relapse may occur. In this approach, the helper has the role of enabling the person to take responsibility for their own change, rather than telling the person what they need to do. An important goal of this approach is to avoid resistance, for example by not giving 'expert' advice or getting into a debate. Both ambivalence and relapse are considered normal, rather than due to any personal failure or illness. If resistance is experienced, this is considered to be a sign that the incorrect technique is being used by the helper for the stage of change for that person. For example, it is not appropriate to help someone choose future goals if they are not ready to accept the need to change at that time. At this stage, it is more appropriate to raise awareness of the need to change by promoting reflection on personal experience and exchanging information.

Cognitive behavioural therapy

Hope is fundamental to a person's wellbeing and enables them to begin their journey towards recovery. Recovery, however, is not necessarily about being symptom free; Anthony (1993) defines it as living a valued and valuable life with difficulties; finding ways of understanding and coping with problems, as much as getting rid of them.

While hope has to come from within the person experiencing mental distress, carers, including healthcare professionals such as MHNs, have an important part to play in its development. Nurses need to have a positive attitude and ability to see the person and their potential. A positive attitude towards a person experiencing mental distress is therefore an essential prerequisite in engaging with the person and forming a therapeutic relationship. One way of enabling carers to see the person rather than the illness involves viewing symptoms of mental distress as an exaggeration and extension of normal responses.

Everyone has variations in mood or felt anxious. Even hearing voices is a common experience, for example you may have been alone then heard a noise and believed that someone had called out your name. When one talks about one's own experiences in a matter-of-fact way, it can reduce barriers and helps to normalise the symptoms associated with mental illness. This process encourages the person to open up and talk more extensively about their experiences. Very often people feel embarrassed and ashamed about mental illness, particularly if they hear voices. They often feel isolated and that they are the only ones having these experiences – ultimately, they feel they are 'going crazy'. Encouraging a person to talk about their voice-hearing experiences enables the person to put them into perspective, and reduce associated anxiety. For example, when a person talks about how they feel threatened by voices they regard as powerful, the actual power and authority of the voices can now be challenged. Open discussion about voice-hearing experiences enables people to realise that others also hear voices, which also reduces associated anxiety. Reducing anxiety very often reduces the intensity of the voices. The approaches described above are examples of cognitive behavioural therapy (CBT).

CBT is a structured, collaborative approach. It takes a fresh approach to mental health problems regarding thoughts, emotions and behaviours. These are considered to be interactive and interlinking processes, so that a change in one brings about a change in the other. People with mental distress are prone to negative automatic thoughts, a depressed person may ruminate about failures, thinking 'I'm useless, I never do anything right', then avoiding activities, losing confidence and remaining depressed. CBT seeks to break this vicious circle. CBT involves a joint exploration of how a person's thoughts, emotions and behaviours are linked. This approach invites the person to adopt a more objective view of themselves, their relationships and world. In addition to examining beliefs, CBT uses behavioural approaches, for example desensitisation programmes, whereby a person is gradually introduced to an object or situation they feared such as social situations. The introduction to the feared situation demonstrates to the person that there is nothing to fear, so that they change their beliefs about the feared object.

CBT has traditionally been viewed as a treatment for people with anxiety and depressive disorders. It can, however, be used more extensively, for example in severe disorders such as schizophrenia. The process of actively listening to the person, recognising their concerns, questioning and collaboratively testing their beliefs enables people to examine the evidence for and against their conclusions in a more objective way.

Case study cont'd: CBT and Kevin

Kevin disclosed to the nurse from the assertive outreach team his voice-hearing experiences. The nurse undertook further assessment using the Belief About Voices Questionnaire (Chadwick and Birchwood 1995). The assessment revealed that Kevin's voices usually occurred when he was alone in his room at the hostel in the afternoon. During this time, he would be feeling fed up and upset thinking about his stepfather's comments that he would never amount to much. The voices he heard made critical abusive comments that both scared Kevin and reinforced his negative beliefs about himself; the intensity of the voices would then increase. Working collaboratively, Kevin and the nurse identified some distraction techniques to reduce the intensity of the voices. Kevin felt that listening to music on his MP3 player reduced the intensity of the voices. The other area that Kevin and the nurse worked on was his negative self-perception. Using a Socratic questioning approach, the nurse was able to explore with Kevin his negative beliefs. Socratic questioning enabled Kevin to objectively evaluate his own negative thoughts by questioning how logical they were. For example, the nurse helped Kevin to identify his positive qualities such as his photographic work. The above work resulted in the voices occurring less frequently.

Working systemically

Systemic practice enables practitioners within health and social settings to explore connections and communication patterns between individuals, couples, families and organisations, and help people with difficulties discover their own solutions.

To work systemically means to begin to be aware of and take account of the broader contexts which you and the person you are trying to help occupy. For example, most service users have families and social networks that have a huge impact on their lives. As professionals, we too work in context; there are the structures and rules of the organisation we work in, the physical environment, whether it be a ward or people's own homes, and our own professional rules and regulations. We bring our own stories to our work; our own family history, our experiences and beliefs all impact on the work we do.

One of the main objects of working systemically is for us to think about, reflect upon and bring into the open as much as possible all the things that might impact on service users and us. The breadth of working systemically along a continuum can involve consulting with family members when someone is ill through to concepts like open dialogue (Seikkula and Olson 2003), where *all* contact with the therapeutic team takes place with the service user and their network, which could include family, friends and colleagues. In this dialogic approach, everyone has an equal voice and all treatment decisions are made openly within these meetings.

Working this way is a stark contrast to what was known as the 'medical model', where practitioners focused all their attention on symptoms, in other words, treating the symptoms out of context. On the other hand, working systemically could be considered the most holistic approach to care. Mental health systems are beginning to change to reflect the principles of recovery (Anthony and Ashcraft 2005).

Family therapy

The orientation of a modern family therapist is to discard the 'expert' position in favour of a position of curiosity, where the focus of work is in creating a dialogue and a conversational space where everyone involved has an equal voice.

As a form of treatment, family therapy has undergone a huge amount of change in the 50 or so years it has been around. It has a rich history, and some of the personalities involved in developing new ideas have been very charismatic, making family therapy quite an exciting and challenging area to work in.

In the early days, family therapy was heavily influenced by the revolution in 'cybernetics' – the multidisciplinary field of study that was concerned with feedback mechanisms in both mechanical and societal organisations and systems. Later developments recognised that rather than the therapist being an outside observer of a family system (therapist) + (family), the therapist was in fact part of a new system (therapist + family) and that the therapist needed to recognise and think about their own role within the therapy. This significant move is often referred to as 'second-order cybernetics'. More recently, family therapy has been influenced by more postmodern ideas, especially social constructionism, and many therapists work collaboratively with their service users (Anderson and Burney 1997), working alongside them to create new meanings and understandings of their difficulties. Other therapists have embraced the narrative ideas developed by Michael White and David Epston (1990) and work with families to create alternative stories.

Nowadays, family therapy services provide support to lots of different families, some affected by problems relating to difficulties with young children or adolescents, some with young adults with severe mental illness, with learning disabilities or an older relative with health problems, for example dementia.

The evidence base for family therapy is beginning to grow (Stratton 2005), and organisations such as the National Institute for Health and Excellence (NICE) are beginning to recommend family interventions as part of the recommended treatment options for mental health problems, including depression and schizophrenia (NCCMH 2002, 2005).

Training in family therapy is available across the UK, with a range of courses from introductory levels through to qualifying training as a family therapist, which is usually at Masters level.

Self-awareness and emotional intelligence

Jenny, who had been admitted to the ward this morning, was crying in the lounge. Mary, the staff nurse on duty that afternoon, knelt down and took hold of her hand. 'Don't cry,' she said, 'it will be all right, you'll see.' Mary stood up and patted Jane's shoulder once more. 'Cheer up,' she said, as she walked away.

When experienced mental health nurses talk about 'levels' of self-awareness or of 'being self-aware', they mean that they are aware of their own emotions or feelings – their strengths, limitations and motives and, overall, the effect they are having on others and the effect others are having on them *as they occur*. This is the concept of 'emotional intelligence': 'the capacity for recognising our own feelings and those of others, for motivating ourselves, and for managing emotions well in ourselves and in our relationships' (Goleman 1998, p. 317).

So if the nurse above had reflected a little more on her own responses to Jenny before she had acted, she might have realised that seeing people in distress made her feel uncomfortable and so, while appearing to offer comfort to Jenny, Mary was, in fact, asking her to stop crying.

The development of this kind of personal awareness is encouraged in nurse education and sometimes specific exercises are used in order to explore thoughts, feelings and attitudes; for example, how uncomfortable might a nurse be if they had to intervene where a service user was expressing loud anger, particularly if they had experienced angry outbursts as a child who was distressed and helpless to intervene.

It is to work more effectively with service users and other people in a care team that nurses are helped to explore the influences on their own ability to experience feelings such as trust or anxiety as well as maintain self-esteem and self-confidence. Working sometimes with service users that challenge us or with those from a different culture, the nurse will need to be aware of their own values or prejudices in order to put these aside (bracket) and be open to encouraging and initiating a therapeutic relationship within which meaningful communication can take place.

Working within boundaries

Legislation such as the Mental Health Act 1983 necessarily tries to offer clear dos and don'ts in the interest of protecting the rights and safety of people experiencing vulnerability through their mental health status. Recent attempts by the government to refocus this legislation on public safety highlight a paradox in the role of MHNs to both care and protect the individual while acting to control risk. As well as working within these difficult external boundaries, MHNs must examine their internal processes to keep service users safe.

The ability of MHNs to manage their emotional responses and needs within the therapeutic relationship is an important skill which can only be developed over time, with experience and an accompanying development of self-awareness. Sharing the experience of the individual through empathic understanding of their distress, coupled with the nurse's own emotional investment in the person's recovery, may come at a cost that the nurse must be prepared to manage if they are to remain both effective and 'whole'. At one end of the care continuum, there is a risk that the nurse 'overly invests' in the person's recovery, in that they may become unhealthily attached and overly reliant on the person making progress and moving forward. All too often, the path towards recovery is faced with pauses and even relapses and the nurse must be prepared for these events. Similarly, the frustrations and demands of the role may lead to a nurse distancing themselves from that very risk to a point where the 'relationship' is a stilted and defensive one, which aims to protect the nurse from the emotional cost of caring.

Managing personal/professional boundaries is a skill that demands of the professional an ability to manage possible risks such as overdependence and inappropriate attachment to the nurse and even vice versa and inappropriate attachment to the individual. On the safest emotional level for the nurse, the role becomes a formalised and procedural one in which the nurse simply meets the person's minimum needs clearly evident in the nature of their role and responsibility to the individual. This may, for instance, take the form of engaging in visiting the person in order to 'check on them' but not usefully engaging in specific therapeutic actions to enhance recovery. There are many constraints that may lead to this approach, both in terms of organisational demands, such as the size of the nurse's caseload limiting the amount of time that can be spent with each individual, to cultural demands in which there is an expectation from colleagues that their failings are not exposed by significantly different behaviours from others within the team. Sometimes, nurses may actively avoid 'investing' in the relationship and limit themselves to a more formal and procedural role because they find it difficult to establish and maintain the therapeutic engagement with a service user, either for personal reasons pertinent at the time or through a lack of confidence in their abilities to meet the needs of the individual.

Contemporary language in discussing this issue is also important in how the concepts are perceived, in that to talk in terms of 'setting boundaries' tends to engender a sense of a rigid and fixed limitation aiming to 'manage' the individual, whereas the effective therapeutic agent (nurse) acknowledges the fluidity and flexibility of boundaries, in that they move and 'breathe' with the different presentations of behaviour and needs during the relationship. Setting boundaries is also required, in that the frequent involvement of more than one health or social care agency requires that all people involved need to present a consistency in approaching the needs of the individual if they are going to be effective in supporting their recovery.

Known as 'the mother of mental health nursing', Hildegard Peplau (1952) suggests that professionals may have various unconscious expectations of how an individual in their care should behave. If these expectations, such as the individual seeing the professional as a caring person, as knowledgeable and confirming their intentions as well meant, are not acknowledged, it is likely to affect the quality of the relationship. If the nurse remains unaware that they carry these expectations and the expectations are not met by the person, it is more likely the relationship will be less effective or break down completely, without the nurse or individual recognising why.

Overinvolvement between an MHN and an individual might be said to be the most commonly acknowledged boundary violation, the most severe of which is sexual involvement with the person being cared for. Levels of overinvolvement in the therapeutic relationship do, however, cover a whole range of behaviours that might be considered to cross the boundary of caring. The difficulty in identifying any specific action as inappropriate or 'boundary crossing' invalidates the idea of holistic and individualised care and risks stifling the quality of support offered and potentially offered by services. Discussion above regarding withdrawal from or avoidance of a purposeful and progressive

key concepts: branches of nursing

therapeutic relationship represents an underinvolvement in care, which is perhaps, in light of demands on the practitioner, the most frequently occurring form of boundary violation. In the absence of opportunity to clearly identify the extent and nature of behaviours expected of the professional and the individual, the choice of what is appropriate and what is not is left to the professional to decide at any given time in the course of the relationship, and to manage this effectively, it must be based on the knowledge and awareness of both the individual seeking support and the self-awareness of the nurse.

Often MHNs are told that they must ensure they have the appropriate attitude. This does not help very much because it is difficult to see an attitude like a barcode on someone's forehead. What the nurse must ensure is that everything they do and everything they say is helping someone, and not hindering them. This is not just about verbal communication, that is, the words used, but also vocal communication, that is, the tone of voice, and nonverbal communication, that is, how arms and legs are held, the angle of the head on the shoulders, and even the warmth of one's eyes. In a sense, attitudes are written on the forehead, because frowning and half-closed eyes can easily be seen as unfriendly.

The nurse might not be aware of the details of their communication, and maybe others will not be able to state very clearly how they communicate. But afterwards, they will say to their family and friends, 'Don't speak to nurse John, he always ignores you, and if you persist he gets snappy', so it's important that communication is a help and not a hindrance to others.

Becoming aware of your own communication and that of others can be difficult. Also, being kind to someone who is rude to you when they are in crisis, even though you will know that persistent kindness is essential, can be difficult. So self-awareness moment to moment is essential. However, it is important that this self-awareness does not result in you becoming stilted and lacking spontaneity. However, the reality of mental health nursing is that it is hard work, and it will take many years to learn. Indeed, if ever it transpires that you feel there is nothing more to learn, then it is probably time to leave and find another job. Don't expect to get it right straightaway; you have three years to reach a minimum level of practice before you can register with the Nursing and Midwifery Council (NMC), but that minimum level will be continuously built upon during the many years that stretch ahead you.

Mental health nursing education

As professor of Nursing Studies at Edinburgh University from 1976 until 1983, Annie Altschul played a leading role in gaining academic recognition for mental health nursing in Britain. Her research and profile promoted the notion that mental health education should provide both knowledge and skills from a wide range of sources and promote efficacy of the nurse–patient relationship.

Over the past decade, mental health nurse education faced many challenges as it transferred from its traditional home within the NHS, via a collegiate system, into its current incarnation within the higher education sector. During this time, educational providers have had to recognise the changing role of the modern mental health nurse and develop educational and training programmes that provide newly qualified MHNs with the academic and practice skills that enable them to work effectively within the ever shifting world of clinical practice (NMC 2009).

In order to achieve these goals, all full-time pre-registration educational programmes have a requirement for students to spend 50% of their time in clinical practice environments and 50% in the classroom. In addition to this full-time option, the Open University offers part-time pre-registration programmes spanning four to six years. These courses are aimed at experienced health workers who meet NMC requirements for entry to nurse training. The NMC is the professional body responsible for the maintenance of professional standards and requires all nurses to keep up to date in terms of their practice and theory base. It oversees the delivery of all pre-registration courses and verifies the 'lifelong learning' of qualified nurses through mandatory re-registration.

After qualification and professional registration, MHNs are able to access many post-registration education programmes, the type and focus of which depends upon the career pathway chosen by the individual MHN. Such **continuing professional development** enhances academic and clinical skills and opens the door to professional progression and career enhancement.

Clinical supervision

To some nurses, clinical supervision sounds a bit like it might involve Big Brother looking over your shoulder checking up on you. The reality is far from that. Clinical supervision is about the development of the nurse's skills, and according to Butterworth and Faugier (1992), it is an exchange between practising professionals to enable development of professional skills. In other words, clinical supervision is a venue for nurses to talk about their nursing practice in order to help improve what they do.

Nursing can be quite stressful at times, especially when we work with people who are showing a lot of emotion; they may be frightened, angry or very sad. Clinical supervision also has the function of enabling nurses to talk about the stresses of their work, and this can really help us be more able to cope and develop our own strategies for managing our own feelings.

Sometimes we might recognise areas where we need to develop our skills, and, again, clinical supervision can provide a good opportunity to discuss these issues.

There is an aspect of ensuring that we work to professional and organisational standards implicit in clinical supervision; Bishop (1994) felt that supervision can help to support the delivery of optimum care by safeguarding standards and developing professional expertise. These three domains of clinical supervision are sometimes referred to as 'formative', 'normative' and 'restorative' (Proctor 1986), where:

> the *formative* aspect represents meeting the learning needs of the supervisee
> the *normative* aspect helps to ensure that the organisational and professional requirements of the supervisee are met
> the *restorative* function of supervision enables the ventilation of feelings, coping with emotional labour and stress.

Ideally, clinical supervision should be considered an integral part of the nurse's work, with a formal arrangement to meet regularly (at least once a month) for supervision provided by someone who has relevant expertise in the same type of clinical work, but also, importantly, has the skills of being a supervisor. A good clinical supervisor will appreciate the importance of good listening skills and use some kind of framework or model to guide the process.

Ultimately, clinical supervision offers a process for nurses to reflect on what they do, to talk through some of the difficulties they face and enhance the quality of their care.

Case study cont'd: clinical supervision to support Kevin's care

Although Kevin's nurse from the assertive outreach team was feeling pleased with the results of the last session, she wondered what else she might be able to do to help him. She decided that talking to her clinical supervisor about her work with Kevin would be useful, and made some brief notes to take to her next clinical supervision meeting.

At the beginning of the clinical supervision meeting, the supervisor asked the nurse what issues she would like to bring to the session, and she told him about her work with Kevin. Before focusing on the interventions she had made, the supervisor asked the nurse about her relationship with Kevin, and about what thoughts Kevin might have about her. Being able to talk about her feelings about Kevin, and thinking about how he might perceive her, enabled the nurse to develop a broader appreciation of the therapeutic relationship, and helped her to recognise that Kevin probably saw her as a helpful and caring person. She thought about how she was able to empathise with Kevin, and how she appreciated the difficulties he was having in managing his voices, and how scary it could be for him at times. She also was able to talk about the sadness she felt about the situation with Kevin's family and her hopes that if he was better able to manage the voices he heard and have a more positive self-perception, this might help improve his relationship with his family.

The supervisor, who was an experienced nurse, asked about the interventions she had used, including the distraction techniques that she and Kevin had talked about (for example listening to his MP3 player), and together they also explored the techniques that had been used in thinking together about Kevin's self-perception. The nurse realised that, with her help, Kevin had made some significant improvement; Socratic questions had enabled Kevin to discover his own answers to some of the problems he was facing, but also this collaboration had helped to forge their therapeutic relationship.

◥

She then began to think of other techniques she could use with Kevin to enhance his recovery, and discussed these with the supervisor. She felt that using role play with Kevin might help him develop strategies for dealing with difficult situations in the future, and the supervisor agreed that this might enhance his self-perception too. At the end of the clinical supervision session, the nurse felt satisfied with the collaborative work she had done, and felt equipped to carry on working in collaboration with Kevin to assist his recovery.

Activity 15.4

How comfortable are you in talking about your feelings about people and your perceptions of how they may feel about you?

What do you need the person who is listening to these personal thoughts of yours to be like to enable you to feel safe enough to have these sorts of conversation?

Conclusion

In this chapter, we have explored the key themes of social inclusion, mental health service structure, engagement in positive change, relationship boundaries and education and support for MHNs within a recovery-oriented approach. As mental health nurses, we need to be aware that the consequences of illness can sometimes be more distressing than the illness itself. Recovery is normal and can happen without professional intervention but some people need assistance with their own recovery process. Recovery is not a linear process and interventions should reflect this by acknowledging where the person is in their change cycle. To achieve this in mental health services, we need well-educated, emotionally intelligent, supported and positive mental health nurses who work in systems that facilitate their desire to get it right for recovery.

References

Ackerman, L (1997) Development, transition or transformation: the question of change in organisations, in D van Eynde, J Hoy and D van Eynde (eds), *Organization Development Classics: The Practice and Theory of Change – The Best of the OD Practitioner,* San Francisco: Jossey Bass

Anderson, H and Burney, P (1997) Collaborative inquiry: a postmodern approach to organizational consultation, *Human Systems: The Journal of Systemic Consultation and Management,* **7**(2/3): 177–88

Anthony, WA (1993) Recovery from mental illness: the guiding vision of the mental health service system in the 1990s, *Psychosocial Rehabilitation Journal,* **16**(4): 11–23

Anthony, WA and Ashcraft, L (2005) Creating an environment that supports recovery, *Behavior Healthcare Tomorrow,* **14**(6): 6–7

Bak, P (1997) *How Nature Works: The Science of Self-organised Criticality,* Oxford: Oxford University Press

Barker, P (2000) The tidal model of mental health care: personal caring within the chaos paradigm, *Mental Health Care*, **4**(2): 59–63

Barker, P (2001) The tidal model: developing an empowering, person-centred approach to recovery within psychiatric and mental health nursing, *Journal of Psychiatric and Mental Health Nursing*, **8**(3): 233–40

Butterworth, T and Faugier, J (1992) *Clinical Supervision and Mentorship in Nursing*, London: Chapman & Hall

Bishop, V (1994) Clinical supervision for an accountable profession, *Nursing Times*, **90**(24): 35–9

Boardman, J (2005) New services for old: an overview of mental health policy, in A Bell and P Lindley (eds), *Beyond the Water Towers: The Unfinished Revolution in Mental Health Services 1985-2005*, London: Sainsbury Centre for Mental Health

Boardman, J and Parsonage M (2005) *Defining a Good Mental Health Service: A Discussion Paper*, London: Sainsbury Centre for Mental Health

Caldwell, CB and Gottesman II (1990) Schizophrenics kill themselves too: a review of risk factors for suicide, *Schizophrenia Bulletin*, **16**(4): 571–89.

Chadwick, P and Birchwood, M (1995) The omnipotence of voices II: The Beliefs About Voices Questionnaire (BAVQ), *British Journal of Psychiatry*, 166: 773–6

DH (Department of Health) (1998) *Modernising Mental Health Services: Safe, Sound and Supportive*, London: HMSO

DH (1999) *The National Service Framework for Mental Health*, London: HMSO

DH (2004) *The Ten Essential Shared Capabilities: A Framework for the Whole of the Mental Health Workforce*, London: DH

DH (2005a) *NHS Hospital and Community Health Services: Non-medical Staff in England: 1994–2004*, London: DH

DH (2005b) *Mental Health and Deafness: Towards Equity and Access, Best Practice Guidelines*, London: DH

DH (2006a) *From Values to Action: The Chief Nursing Officer's Review of Mental Health Nursing*, London, DH

DH (2009) *New Horizons: A Shared Vision for Mental Health*, available online at http://www.newhorizons.dh.gov.uk/assets/Reports/299060_NewHorizons_acc.pdf, accessed 08/1/2010

Goleman, D (1998) *Working with Emotional Intelligence*, London: Bloomsbury

Graae, EC and Selten, JP (2004) Schizophrenia and migration: a meta-analysis, *Schizophrenia Research*, **67**(1): 63

Harbottle, C and Mudd, D (2004) Working with people who have special needs and disabilities and mental health problems, in S Kirby, DA Hart, D Cross and G Mitchell (eds), *Mental Health Nursing: Competencies for Practice*, Basingstoke: Palgrave Macmillan

McCabe, S (2002) The nature of psychiatric nursing: the intersection of paradigm, evolution and history, *Archives of Psychiatric Nursing*, **16**(2): 51–60

Miller, WR and Rollnick, S (1991) *Motivational Interviewing: Preparing People to Change Addictive Behaviour*, New York: Guilford Press

Mind (2004a) *Not Alone?: Isolation and Mental Distress*, London: Mind

Mind (2004b) *Ward Watch*, London: Mind

NCCMH (National Collaborating Centre for Mental Health) (2002) *Schizophrenia: Core Interventions in the Treatment and Management of Schizophrenia in Primary and Secondary Care*, London: NICE

3

NCCMH (2005) *Depression in Children and Young People: Identification and Management in Primary, Community and Secondary Care*, London: NICE

NIMHE (National Institute for Mental Health for England) (2003) *Cases for Change: A Review of the Foundations of Mental Health Policy and Practice 1997-2002*, Leeds: DH

NMC (Nursing and Midwifery Council) (2009) *Standards of Proficiency for Pre-registration Nursing Education*, London: NMC

Padesky, C (1993) Socratic questioning: changing minds or guiding discovery? A keynote address delivered at the European Congress of Behavioural and Cognitive Therapies, 24 September, London

Peplau, HE (1952) *Interpersonal Relations in Nursing*, New York: GP Putnam & Sons

Prochaska, JO and DiClemente, CC (1982) Transtheoretical therapy: toward a more integrative model of change, *Psychotherapy: Theory, Research & Practice*, 19: 276–88

Proctor, B (1986) Supervision: a co-operative exercise in accountability, in M Marken and M Payne (eds), *Enabling and Ensuring*, Leicester: National Youth Bureau

Rethink, Sane, the Zito Trust and the National Association of Psychiatric Intensive Care Units (2004) *Behind Closed Doors: The Current State of Acute Mental Health Care in the UK*, available online at http://www.mentalhealthshop.org/document.rm?id=140, accessed 8/1/2010

Robson, D and Gray, R (2007) Serious mental illness and physical health problems: a discussion paper, *International Journal of Nursing Studies*, 44: 457–66

Rogers, CR (1959) A theory of therapy, personality and interpersonal relationships, as developed in the client-centered framework, in S Koch (ed.), *Psychology: A Study of Science*, New York: McGraw-Hill

Schulze, B and Angermeyer, MC (2003) Subjective experiences of stigma: a focus group study of schizophrenic patients, their relatives and mental health professionals, *Social Sciences and Medicine*, 56: 299–312

SCMH (Sainsbury Centre for Mental Health) (1998) *Acute Problems*, London: SCMH

Seikkula, J and Olson, M (2003) The open dialogue approach to acute psychosis: its poetics and micropolitics, *Family Process*, 42: 403–18

Shuel, F, White, J, Jones, M and Gray, R (2009) Using the serious mental illness health improvement profile [HIP] to identify physical problems in a cohort of community patients: a pragmatic case series evaluation, *International Journal of Nursing Studies*, doi:10.1016/j.ijnurstu.2009.06.003

SNMAC (Standing Nursing and Midwifery Advisory Committee) (1999) *Mental Health Nursing: Addressing Acute Concerns,* London: HMSO

Social Exclusion Unit (2004) *Mental Health and Social Exclusion: Social Exclusion Unit Report*, London: Office of the Deputy Prime Minister

Stratton, P (2005) *Report on the Evidence Base of Systemic Family Therapy*, Warrington: Association for Family Therapy

Thara, R (2003) People with schizophrenia believe that they are stigmatised at work and in the community, *Evidence Based Mental Health,* 6: 96, available online at http://ebmh.bmj.com/cgi/reprint/6/3/96.pdf, accessed 8/1/2010

White, M and Epston, D (1990) *Narrative Means to Therapeutic Ends,* New York: WW Norton

WHO (World Health Organization) (2001) *Strengthening Mental Health Promotion*, fact sheet no. 220, Geneva: WHO

WHO (2000) *WHO Guide to Mental Health Disorders in Primary Care*, London: Royal Society of Medicine Press

16 caring for older people

Fiona Irvine and Colin Jones

In this chapter we will explore:

> The physiological context of ageing
> The psychosocial context of ageing
> Recognising and dealing with abuse

Introduction

Working with older people brings challenges and rewards for nurses. As we work in an ageing society, it is inevitable that whatever speciality we are involved in, be it primary, **acute care** or critical care, we will be offering our services to older people. Although older people can face challenges in their lives, they have the benefit of life experience, and many live long, rich and active lives.

The first part of this chapter is focused on the physiological changes that occur as we get older. Although initially, our focus turns to physiology, it is important to recognise that we do not look at ageing in an entirely physiological way. To do this would be reductionist and insensitive. Remember that **holistic nursing practice** is based on body/mind/spirit elements, as well as the many complex social, financial and environmental dimensions of care. Also keep in mind the many cultural variations involved in becoming an older person in society. We turn to these sociological and psychological elements of ageing later in the chapter.

Growing old is inevitable, growing up is optional

We really like this expression because it helps keep the *person* in focus, amid myriad physiological changes. It is easy to concentrate on the dysfunctional parts of the body as we get older, and in doing this, we perhaps overlook some of the more positive and human-centred issues that are to be celebrated in the older person.

In this chapter, there are a number of short activities for you to complete. They are intended to help you to understand some of the key issues and will not take up much of your time. It might be a good idea to have a notepad and pen to hand as you may wish to write down thoughts and ideas, which can then be organised as evidence of what you have learned.

Physiological context of ageing

The physiology of ageing is an anxiety-producing topic. Most of us are frightened of becoming old, infirm, losing our independence or having to leave our loved ones because we have become a burden to society. It is easy to see that these physiological factors are shaped by the others we mentioned earlier. For example, if you were to develop increasingly severe arthritis and it became difficult for you to mobilise, this may be made more difficult by the type of housing you lived in, for example a house or a block of flats.

All of us have seen how the body changes as we age. Physical changes such as greying hair, lines and wrinkles in the skin, and reduced mobility, and problems with memory and cognition are perhaps the most familiar to us. But all these changes cannot be seen in isolation. The changes are part of a complex link between physiological issues affecting almost all body systems.

Activity 16.1

Make a list of changes that occur in the body as we get older.

From this activity you will be able to identify that all body systems are affected by the ageing process. Your list will probably include words that are often associated with a series of physiological changes, for example:

> stiffening
> thickening
> **degenerating**
> slowing

> decreasing
> calcifying
> fibrosing
> narrowing.

While many of these changes affect multiple systems in the body, the exact mechanism of why the changes occur remains unclear. There are a number of theories of the ageing process that can help us in our quest for understanding.

Theories of ageing

Theories on how our bodies are thought to change as we get older can be helpful when we come to treat diseases or consider nursing interventions. While there are accepted theories, there is widespread acknowledgement that there is interplay, connection and exchange across all of them, given the great complexity in the many biological factors involved. For the purpose of this chapter, we will explore three theories, although there are many more for you to consider, so have a look at the Further reading at the end of the chapter.

Hayflick limit theory

As with many medical terms, the name comes from the person who discovered it. In the early 1960s, Dr Hayflick theorised that human cells have a limited number of times they can divide before becoming exhausted and then dying; in a similar way to a photocopy being photocopied again and again until it becomes so faded that it almost disappears. Hayflick identified that each time a cell divides, it loses some deoxyribonucleic acid (DNA), which is the cellular 'blueprint information'. It was theorised that after about 50 divisions, there would be no more DNA left to divide again, so the cell would die. Hayflick proposed that if we want to live longer, we need to slow down the rate of cell division.

Activity 16.2

How could we slow down the rate of cell division?

Slowing down the rate of cellular division is an interesting thought. When thinking about this, you may have thought of the claims of some amazing new facial moisturiser, which promises to make you look 25 years younger with just one application. Interestingly, we turn to look at the nutrition and hydration of cells in the slowing down/division process, which is where the Hayflick theory begins to interface with many other theories.

Cellular nutrition is thought to be influential in optimising function and dispensing with excessive division, known to contribute to the ageing process. Diet and lifestyle changes are now considered important, as is the damage caused to cells by the attack of free radicals, insulin and high glucose levels.

Ribonucleic acids (RNAs) are a critical component of DNA and there is a suggestion that supplements of RNAs have a number of positive biological benefits for elderly people.

Neuroendocrine theory

Neuroendocrine theory appears to take a more 'master control' perspective, by proposing that the hypothalamus plays a critical part in the ageing process.

Activity 16.3

Write down what you remember about the hypothalamus (hint – it is sometimes referred to as the 'master gland').

We know that the hypothalamus is responsible for orchestrating the complex chain reactions and hormone-releasing activities within the body. The hypothalamus gives instructions to other glands and monitors levels of circulating hormones and makes fine-tuning adjustments so everything remains in balance.

Neuroendocrine theory proposes that, as we get older, the hypothalamus fails to regulate activities as precisely as it used to. This loss of precision is thought to be caused by the long-term exposure of the hypothalamus to the stress hormone cortisol. The theory proposes that as the hypothalamus is damaged, more cortisol is produced, which in turn damages the hypothalamus even more – a vicious circle of continuing damage and continued disordered hormone production and regulation.

Free radical theory dates back to 1956, where it was first developed by Harman at the University of Nebraska. Free radicals are essentially 'rogue' molecules with an extra electron attached to them. This makes them highly reactive, oxidative and unstable as they bind to other molecules and take their electrons. In addition to cellular activity and respiration, free radicals are produced from our diet especially from tobacco and alcoholic drinks. This theory believes that cells are attacked by free radicals and that cell membranes are damaged during the process, leading to waste products being produced. The accumulations of these waste products interfere with DNA, RNA and other substances, thereby damaging normal cellular functions. You may have heard of 'antioxidants' such as beta carotene, which are helpful in blocking cellular attack from free radicals.

Physical changes in later life

In this section we will review some of the major systems of the body and explore some of the physical changes that may occur as we grow older. As we discussed before, even though we are exploring physical changes, remember the psychological and social factors that accompany all health-related issues.

It is easy to focus on matters like mobility problems, incontinence, cognitive problems, memory loss and personality changes, but these are only part of the whole story. No matter what physiological consequence there is of ageing, the person remains an individual and should be holistically cared for with sensitivity and dignity. Refer to the established models of nursing, which may help guide you in structuring care for the older person (Roper et al. 1980).

Activity 16.4

Complete the table below, which will help you identify some of the changes that can occur in body systems as we grow older. (One has been completed for you to start your ideas.)

Age-related disorder	Body system affected	Specific change in function
Cataract	Ophthalmic system: lens of the eye	The lens becomes opaque, causing progressive loss of vision
Arthritis		
Osteoporosis		
Pressure sores		
Reduced blood flow		
Loss of balance/ unsteady on feet		
Loss of hearing		
Loss of appetite		
Poor memory, forgetfulness		

Let's take a look at some of the common physiological changes that occur with ageing from a systems perspective. It is beyond the scope of this chapter to review all the possible changes that could occur, so use this as a starting point.

Ophthalmic system

There are many changes that can affect the eye in later life, and one of the more common ones is a condition called 'cataracts'. Inside the eye is a transparent lens that helps to focus light onto the retina, which is essentially nervous tissue transmitting light into vision. In order to focus light on the retina, the lens must be crystal clear. With cataracts, the lens becomes cloudy and opaque, causing vision to become blurred and reduced. The cause of this is believed to be a hardening of the substance of the lens, which leads to changes in its density, making it more and more opaque as we get older. Figure 16.1 shows how vision may be affected in a person with a cataract.

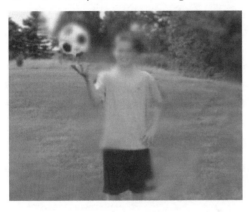

Figure 16.1 How cataracts affect vision
Source: Austin County Eye Associates (www.austincountyeye.com/understanding-cataracts.html)

3

Activity 16.5

What impact could this type of visual loss have on daily life for an older person?

Skin

As we age, the skin tends to become drier and thinner and more wrinkled. Importantly, other changes in the blood supply to the layers of the skin can mean that it is more susceptible to breakdown or take longer to heal. You may have noticed that some elderly patients have 'paper thin' or 'tissue paper-like' skin, which can tear or break very easily, especially if the patient is left in one position in a bed or chair for a long period of time. This can lead to a 'pressure sore' or pressure ulcer causing a great deal of discomfort to the patient. The key management is regular observation of the major pressure areas of the body, remembering that relief of pressure is the treatment goal.

Joints

Activity 16.6

Think about how joints normally work. What types of joints do we have in the body?

Joints can be extensively affected as we age, arthritis being a good example of this. As we become less mobile, joints tend to stiffen and with less movement, ligaments can contract, causing even further loss of joint mobility. Blood flow to joints can also be reduced, which in turn reduces the flow of the lubricant fluid (synovial fluid) our joints need for free movement. These factors, coupled with the depositing of calcium salts at joints, can lead to a generalised reduction in the way joints move, further restricting mobility.

Bones

Bone density generally decreases with age, leading to disorders like **osteoporosis**. This also has implications for the older person who may fracture bones, as the healing process takes a much longer period of time. Additionally, blood cell production may also be affected by changes in the bones seen in later life. Bear in mind also that if bone density and character changes, there may also be implications for the attachment of other structures such as muscles and ligaments.

Vascular system

As we know, the major function of the vascular system is the transport of oxygen and nutrients.

Activity 16.7

What problems could arise from changes in the way blood is transported around the body?

Vascular changes such as arteriosclerosis can interfere with delivery of blood and nutrients to various systems and organs of the body. Reduced blood flow can lead to **ischaemic changes** throughout the body, leading to microinfarcts, clot formation and changes in pressure within blood vessels.

The psychosocial context of ageing

People are living longer in Western society, leading to a growing population of older people. Many live long, healthy, productive and happy lives. They reach their goals and ambitions, develop new relationships, care for others, lead and influence events in their community, thereby achieving their full potential. However, as people age, they also have to deal with living in a changing society, loneliness, poverty, loss and bereavement and medical problems. These life transitions require that healthcare professionals develop a range of knowledge, skills and expertise to be able to provide the quality services that older people need within a framework that promotes optimal health and favours dignity and respect.

Growing old in the UK today

Overall, the UK population is ageing. According to the recently formed Age UK (a result of the merger of Age Concern and Help the Aged), almost 1 in 5 of the UK's total population are of state pension age, which at this moment in time – 2010 – is 60 for women and 65 for men (Age UK 2010). There are now more over 65s than under 16s living in the UK and this is set to rise: in the next 30 years, the population over 75 is projected to double. What's more, women live longer than men; current UK life expectancy at 65 is 85.0% for women and 82.4% for men.

Activity 16.8

Write down what you think may be the reasons why people are living longer.

There are many reasons why people are living longer and these include:

> better medical care
> increased average wealth
> better living conditions.

Tabernacle et al. (2009) explain that women's longer life expectancy is due to factors such as:

> fewer women dying during childbirth
> women having a greater capacity to care for themselves
> women have increased financial and political power.

Older people find themselves living in a world that is constantly changing and they need to adapt to keep up with all the changes. The technological advances that have taken place in the life of an 80-year-old are phenomenal. In their earlier years, there would have been few cars, no electricity and certainly no mobile phones, computers and televisions. Imagine what it must have felt like before the technology that we accept as a normal part of life came into existence and think what it must be like trying to keep up with all this new technology. Many parents laugh about the fact that they have to rely on their children to operate the TV, DVD and other technical gadgetry. In other words, younger adults are struggling to keep up with new technology and this challenge is more pronounced for older people. This phenomenon, known as **digital exclusion** where people are excluded from using technology, has been shown to increase with age. For example, according to Age UK (2010), only 36% of people aged 65 and over have ever used the internet and while 81% of households in the UK had a mobile phone in 2007, mobile phones were used by only 50% of one-adult households aged 60 or over. One important use of technology is to keep in touch with family and friends.

Activity 16.9

Think of the methods you use to maintain contact with your loved ones and jot them down.

Your list probably includes using texts, email and instant messaging as a means of communication. These channels of communication are not open to the older people who are digitally excluded and therefore their means of keeping in touch are constrained, which may be a factor that contributes to the high levels of loneliness experienced by older people.

Loneliness

Loneliness is a real part of many older people's lives. Age UK (2010) states that more than half (51%) of all people aged 75 and over live alone, and just over 1 million (11%) people aged 65 or over in the UK say they always or often feel lonely. Loneliness means that you have fewer relationships than you want and these relationships are less satisfying than you would like.

The social circles of older people can become restricted due to factors such as reduced mobility, disability and ill health and bereavement, so for many older people, TV is their main form of company. Loneliness can lead to unhappiness, anxiety and depression and poor physical health; and in recognition of this, social services and charities offer a range of services and activities that aim to help older people meet new people, make new friends and combat loneliness.

Activity 16.10

Think of the services and initiatives available in your area that help to prevent loneliness and make a note of them.

The sort of things that are on offer include home visiting and befriending, 'adopt a granny' schemes, daycare services, meals on wheels, transport and social activities. Nurses need to know what services are available in their area and ensure that this information is available to older people so that they can be properly supported to overcome loneliness.

One of the main contributors to loneliness is the loss of a spouse or partner; losing a close companion with whom you may have shared many years of your life is an isolating experience.

Bereavement

As people get older, it is inevitable that they face the loss of friends and loved ones; for example, Age UK (2010) tells us that 62% of women aged 75 and over are widowed. Bereavement can be emotionally devastating; every aspect of a person's life changes and coming to terms with this requires that older people draw on their personal resilience and, of course, their support networks. It is not only emotional stability that is affected by bereavement; there are often many practical issues that older people have to consider when they lose a partner, such as reduced income, managing money, getting out and about, managing household chores and home maintenance. Activities that were once shared easily with a partner can become burdensome when they all fall to one person.

Although it can be a long and painful struggle, many older people are able to work through bereavement and adjust to life without the deceased. It has been shown that a good recovery from bereavement is influenced by older people's social networks, gender (women do better than men), the way the partner died and the relationship they had with the partner. If it is not managed properly, bereavement can lead to increased morbidity (ill health) and mortality (death), anxiety and depression, alcohol abuse and an increased suicide risk.

Activity 16.11

Write down what you think we can do to help bereaved older people.

Practical and emotional help probably featured in your list. The sort of thing that can be helpful include being there, listening, encouraging them to talk about the deceased, offering advice about the normal patterns of grief, giving information on the bereavement support services (often voluntary) that are available, encouraging people to take on new roles and develop new friendships, recognising when grief is complicated and referring the person for additional help.

One of the consequences of bereavement can be a loss of financial security as a partner's income or pension may stop or be reduced.

Poverty

> Poverty is defined relative to the standards of living in a society at a specific time. People live in poverty when they are denied an income sufficient for their material needs and when these circumstances exclude them from taking part in activities that are an accepted part of daily life in that society. (Scottish Poverty Information Unit, n.d.)

In the UK, 2.0 million pensioners (18%) live below the poverty line and older women are poorer than older men, in fact there are four times as many poor older women than poor older men.

Activity 16.12

List five reasons why older women have less money than older men.

Men have far higher pensions and more savings than women. When they were of employable age, it was less usual for older women to work or to work full time and so they contributed less money towards pensions and had little spare money to save. A widow may not be entitled to her husband's pension after his death and divorced women cannot make up for the loss of their ex-husband's income.

Many older people who are entitled to additional benefits do not claim them; Age UK (2010) says that a staggering £3.6–5.4bn of means-tested benefits that should rightfully go to older people in Great Britain went unclaimed in 2007–08. Often the reason given for this underclaiming is that pensioners are too proud to claim benefits. This may be true in some cases but many older people do not claim because they do not realise they are entitled to the money or because the claims process is too complicated. Help the Aged (2008) think that the government should simplify the process and pay older people the money they deserve directly rather than waiting for them to make a claim.

The *average* disposable weekly income for single pensioners is around £144, although, of course, a great many pensioners live on less than this – the basic state pension is around £95 a week. Disposable income is the amount of income left to an individual after taxes have been paid, to spend on goods and services (like fuel, handymen, transport) or to save.

Activity 16.13

Take a minute to think about your weekly outgoings. Include all the essentials that you have to spend money on (include any assistance made by parents or relatives) and the money you spend on leisure, such as going out, buying clothes and so on. Are you spending more than £144 per week? What do you think you would have to do without to live within this weekly budget?

Often pensioners sacrifice their leisure activities so they stop going out and meeting people, thus exacerbating the social isolation and loneliness we discussed earlier. Some older people make the decision to continue to work beyond pension age to meet the shortfall between their income and their outgoings. We know that people of pensionable age are still working, for example in retail and leisure services. This of course can be a very positive experience, as not only does it mean more income but it also keeps older people physically, mentally and socially active.

However, many older people can't afford to pay for essential commodities such as fuel and are not able to heat their homes sufficiently during cold weather. This problem, known as **fuel poverty,** is now well recognised: Age UK (2010) estimates that there are 3.5 million older people in fuel poverty and says that 36% of people aged 60 or over in the UK sometimes stay or live in just one heated room of their home to save money.

Given these figures, it is not surprising that there are links between poverty and poor health but it has also been shown that poverty is linked to falls and to elder abuse.

Recognising and dealing with abuse

According to Age UK (2010), **elder abuse** affects roughly 5% of the older population, which amounts to some 50,000 individuals. Elder abuse is defined by Action on Elder Abuse (2004) as:

A single or repeated act, or lack of appropriate action, occurring within any relationship where there is an expectation of trust, which causes harm or distress to an older person.

Activity 16.14

With this definition in mind, think about the types of abuse that older people are subjected to.

Elder abuse has been categorised into five different forms, namely physical, psychological, sexual, financial and neglect. It is important that nurses are able to recognise some of the signs of abuse so that it can be reported and dealt with appropriately. Table 16.1 gives an overview of the main indicators of abuse.

Table 16.1 Main indicators of abuse by category

Category	Main indicators
Physical	Bruising, cuts, burns and fractures that are not consistent with the explanation Bruising that is in various stages of healing Bruising with unusual shapes or patterns, for example finger marks Nervousness and flinching Covering up with clothing Cigarette burns Hair loss Skin damage and wounds Use of furniture and equipment as a means of restraint Failure of carer to report obvious injuries Unusually sleepy or docile
Psychological	Fearfulness, avoiding eye contact, or flinching on approach Ambivalence to a carer or unwillingness to be left with another person Loss of appetite or overeating Deference, dependency, resignation and passivity Emotional withdrawal Sleep disturbance Low self-esteem Acute changes in mood or behaviour when certain people are around Observed shouting, swearing or belittling behaviour by another person
Sexual	Disclosure or hints of sexual abuse Unusual difficulty in walking and sitting Torn or stained underclothing Excessive washing Pain, itching, bruising and/or bleeding in genital or rectal area Bite marks, bruises or finger marks Changes in sexual behaviour or language Unexplained faecal or urinary incontinence Sexually transmitted infection or urinary tract infections

3

Category	Main indicators
Financial	Unusual or inappropriate bank account activity
	Recent change of deeds or title of house
	Person lacks belongings or services they can afford
	Unpaid bills
	Possessions going missing
	Acquaintances being unusually affectionate towards older person with money or property
	Individuals taking an unusual interest in financial issues
	Withholding money
	Refusal of care services
	Lack of cooperation or evasiveness from person managing financial affairs
Neglect	Poor personal hygiene
	Poor physical condition of person, for example ulcers, bed sores, untreated incontinence
	Dehydration, malnutrition and loss of weight
	Clothing in poor condition or unsuitable for weather
	Inadequate heating and/or lighting
	Failure to give prescribed medication
	Failure to seek appropriate medical or social care
	Lack of privacy and dignity
	Lack of stimulation
	Lack of necessary safety equipment

It is essential that nurses are able to recognise elder abuse and take appropriate action if it is suspected. In 2000, *No Secrets* (DH/Home Office 2000) was produced, which provided clear guidance on protecting vulnerable adults. This was followed in 2009 by *Safeguarding Adults* (DH 2009), a review of the guidance, and the government is now preparing a response to this review. Guidance has also been published by the Nursing and Midwifery Council (NMC 2009) on preventing, identifying and managing abuse, *Guidance for the Care of Older People*.

Activity 16.15

Using the web links given in the References, access *No Secrets* (DH/Home Office), *Safeguarding Adults* (DH) and *Guidance for the Care of Older People* (NMC). Familiarise yourself with the main messages that you should take on board from these documents.

The key steps that need to be taken if abuse is suspected or disclosed involve:

> Identifying and documenting indicators of abuse
> Reporting the details to your manager straightaway and if the situation is urgent, calling the emergency services
> Contacting the police (or ensuring that your manager does so) if you believe that the law has been broken
> Attending case conferences if needed
> Giving evidence in court if needed.

It is important, however, that you remember where the boundaries lie; you need to protect yourself and the victim, so it is not appropriate to confront the suspected abuser, question witnesses, question the alleged victim or hunt for evidence.

Although the extent and seriousness of elder abuse has only been recognised in more recent years, the publication of clear guidelines and the subsequent establishment of safeguarding procedures in health and social care services go some way to ensure that abuse is prevented, identified and dealt with appropriately. It is important to acknowledge that the vast majority of older people live their lives free of neglect and abuse. While recognising the devastating effect that abuse can have on older people, we should also to celebrate the positive aspects of old age.

Celebrating old age

Ill health, poverty and social isolation are not inevitable parts of growing old; there are many positive aspects to ageing.

Activity 16.16

Make a list of all the positive aspects of old age that you can think of.

Retirement from work means that older people have more leisure time and many take up new hobbies, activities and sports, engage in education and learning, take on volunteering work and use their newfound freedom to travel. These ventures help to broaden social worlds by fostering existing friendships and developing new ones. Getting out and about and keeping active helps to maintain and improve physical health; and engaging in education helps to develop intellectual abilities and prevent cognitive decline.

Three-quarters of all adults will become grandparents and many enjoy the experience of being a great-grandparent. The availability of more leisure time allows grandparents the opportunity to develop close relationships with their grandchildren and as people live longer, there is the additional benefit of maintaining a long-term relationship with grandchildren. Age UK (2010) reveals that many grandparents take on caring roles among families where the mother is in work. It is reported that 31% of lone parents and 32% of parent couples rely on grandparents for informal childcare. Grandparenting offers positive outcomes for older people:

> it helps them to stay connected with a changing and developing society
> it keeps them in touch with youth culture
> it prevents isolation and loneliness.

Moreover, children, grandchildren and society in general all benefit from close relationships across the generations; grandparents help to maintain strong family bonds, they can share their wisdom and life experiences and, when they take on caring responsibilities, they enable parents to work and contribute to the economy.

As people age, they can become more confident, more comfortable within themselves, more content and more satisfied with their achievements. There is less pressure to conform to rules and regulations, thus allowing older people more freedom of expression and to live the way they wish to. Many older people also take the opportunity to give something back to society by caring, volunteering and befriending the more vulnerable. For example, 21% of those aged 75 plus in England participate in formal volunteering at least once a month (Age UK 2010). These altruistic roles help to give older people a sense of self-worth as they make a valuable contribution to society.

Older people may also become more politically aware or politically active, thereby actively influencing the shape of society. In the last general election, 75% of older people voted, whereas only 37% of people in the 18–24 age group chose to vote. Political parties are beginning to acknowledge the power of 'grey voters' and are taking account of older people's needs and concerns.

Growing old is a mandatory process and, as Maurice Chevalier said: 'Old age isn't so bad when you consider the alternative.'

In this chapter we have shown that ageing brings challenges and provides great rewards. We have explored some of the physiological, psychological and social issues that come to the fore in old age and we have identified some of the measures we can take to improve the quality of older people's lives and make a difference to their physical, psychological and social wellbeing. You are now invited to consider the following case studies and follow the associated activity.

Case study 1: Martha

Martha is 76 today and wonders how she will continue coping with her life. She lives in a two-bedroom local authority-owned bungalow with her 40-year-old son Artie. Artie has Down's syndrome and has a tendency to be overweight for his height of 5ft 3ins. He is mostly happy, goes to the local college two days a week, and spends the rest of his time at home watching TV or playing games on his computer. He loves his mum and expects to be fully cared for by her.

Martha is starting to feel the pressure of caring for a somewhat demanding permanent teenager. She knows her eyesight is failing but cannot find the time to do something about this. She feels that new glasses are outside her budget, but is frightened that there is something more wrong. Lately she has been having trouble with her knees and experiences shortness of breath when walking up the short hill from the local supermarket. She has made an appointment to discuss this with her GP. She has never learned to drive and has no other children. Her husband died 12 years ago. Her only support is a neighbour of a similar age to herself and the local church group, although nowadays she finds getting to church difficult.

Case study 2: John and Vera

John and Vera are typical of many people in their eighties. They live in a three-bedroomed house with fairly steep stairs and one bathroom. They brought up two children in this house and the mortgage was paid off once John retired from the local car factory where he fitted parts on a production line. Their son and daughter are married and live in different cities at least three hours drive from them. They have enjoyed a good retirement – bowling, dancing and taking holidays. Recently, John has experienced lucidity problems and, although he has no recollection of these moments, he is aware that his wife is worried. This has caused him to raise concerns about the future as he does not want to be 'put away'. He takes regular medication for 'blood pressure', as he puts it. They both have had cataract surgery in the past and Vera is recovering well from a successful knee operation three months previously.

Both case studies, although different, have one common denominator and that is the ageing process for the key people. They could expect to be given opportunities to talk about their difficulties and fears whenever they visit their GP. But set against this is the busy nature of general practice and the reticence of people from their generation to ask for help or, in their words, 'bother the doctor'. In relation to the two case studies, consider the following:

> To avoid the possibility of people 'falling through the net', how should health services support people like Martha, John and Vera?
> What might be happening to John? Given the range of possibilities, how can Vera be supported?
> Martha has an another difficulty added to her own health problems. She has to continue to care for her son who is dependent on her. This concern is preventing her from seeking help that will mean she has to spend time in hospital and recovering. How can health and social services liaise to ensure that she also receives positive continuing care?

Conclusion

This chapter will have given you insight into some of the main issues associated with caring for older people in hospital and throughout the wider community. Nursing and medical research continue to play a large part in our understanding and treatment of the physical, social and psychological disorders affecting people in the later stages of their lives. Through this research, we have come to recognise the importance of how nurses can contribute towards ensuring that older people enjoy a positive quality of life through empowerment, encouragement and comfort.

Further reading

Department of Health (2001) *National Service Framework for Older People*, London: DH. Sets out a programme of action and reform to address the needs of older people in England.

Squire, A (2002) *Health and Wellbeing for Older People: Foundations for Practice*, Edinburgh: Baillière Tindall. Comprehensive textbook that focuses on health promotion for older people.

Stanfield, C (2010) *Principles of Human Physiology* (4th edn), San Francisco: Pearson. Contemporary text that applies broad principles of physiology to clinical situations and conditions.

Tabernacle, B, Honey, M and Jinks, A (2009) *Oxford Handbook of Nursing Older People*, Oxford: OUP. Covers all aspects of nursing care for older people, from the sociological and psychological issues through to the common conditions experienced by older people.

Tortora, GJ and Derrickson, BH (2008) *Principles of Anatomy and Physiology*, Hoboken, NJ: John Wiley & Sons. Comprehensive and easy-to-follow text gives detailed information on normal physiology and anatomy.

References

Action on Elder Abuse (2004) *Hidden Voices: Older People's Experience of Abuse*, London: AEA

Age UK (2010) *Older People in the United Kingdom*, available online at http://policy.helptheaged.org.uk/NR/rdonlyres/29341400-5DF0-49B7-BD90-00CE05A0F46F/0/uk_facts.pdf, accessed 12/3/2010

Help the Aged (2008) *Lifting Pensioners out of Poverty*, available online at http://policy.helptheaged.org.uk/NR/rdonlyres/A01E3AC9-D204-443F-99BF-A8FC0E3932AF/0/liftpenspov190808.pdf, accessed 13/7/2010

DH (Department of Health) (2009) *Safeguarding Adults: A Consultation on the Review of the No Secrets Guidance*, available online at http://www.dh.gov.uk/en/Consultations/Liveconsultations/DH_089098, accessed 15/6/2010

DH/Home Office (2000) *No Secrets: Guidance on Developing and Implementing Multi-agency Policies and Procedures to Protect Vulnerable Adults from Abuse*, available online at http://www.dh.gov.uk/en/Publicationsandstatistics/Publications/PublicationsPolicyAndGuidance/DH_4008486, accessed 15/6/2010

NMC (Nursing and Midwifery Council) (2009) *Guidance for the Care of Older People*, available online at http://www.nmc-uk.org/Publications/Guidance/, accessed 15/6/2010

Tabernacle, B, Honey, M and Jinks, A (2009) *Oxford Handbook of Nursing Older People*, Oxford: OUP

3

part 3 glossary

Acute care A branch of tertiary healthcare where necessary treatment of a disease is given for a brief but severe episode of illness.

Advocacy Supporting people with a learning disability to have their voices heard, to say what they think and to make decisions about their own life.

Anxiety Physical symptoms, for example dry mouth, palpitations, overbreathing, and psychological symptoms, for example fear, poor concentration, poor memory, as a normal reaction to stress or a frightening situation.

Anxiety disorder Where anxiety symptoms continue for longer than expected and interfere with a person's ability to get on with their daily life.

Arthritis A group of conditions involving damage to the joints of the body.

Autism A neural disorder associated with children that can result in difficulties with social interaction.

Bipolar disorder A disorder where the person begins to lose the ability to carry out normal, everyday activities for themselves. Typically a disease of ageing but some types can occur in younger people.

Care-by-parent Model of delivering hospital care where children and their family members stay in a special area, furnished in a comfortable, home-like style and care is delivered by parents and supervised by nurses.

Casts Material such as plaster of Paris or Dynacast used to immobilise a limb.

Challenging behaviour Challenging behaviour can vary in its severity but generally it is of such an intensity, frequency or duration that the physical safety of the person or others is likely to be placed in serious jeopardy, or behaviour that is likely to seriously limit or delay access to and use of ordinary community facilities.

Community nurse A registered nurse (RN) who practises in the community.

Community psychiatric nurse A registered mental health nurse who practises in the community and who may have undergone further study to specialise in this area.

Continuing professional development (CPD) The Nursing and Midwifery Council has set a standard that requires all nurses to undertake at least 35 hours of learning in the previous three years. The learning must maintain and develop the nurse's professional competence and be recorded in a personal professional profile.

3

Critical care A branch of medicine concerned with the provision of life support or organ support systems in patients who are critically ill and who usually require intensive monitoring.

Cultural competence Behaviours and attitudes that enable practitioners to work effectively in cross-cultural situations.

Degenerating Deterioration in the medical sense. Generally, it is the change from a higher to a lower form.

Dementia The name for a group of diseases that affect the normal working of the brain. The changes in the brain slowly lead to memory loss and confusion, and affect people's personality and behaviour. They begin to lose the ability to carry out normal, everyday activities for themselves. Typically a disease of ageing but some types can occur in younger people.

Depression Depressed mood is just one of a number of symptoms of depression that can include psychological symptoms, for example depressed mood, loss of interest or pleasure, poor memory, being very quiet or agitated and possibly thoughts of death or suicide, and physical symptoms, for example poor sleep, mood swings, low appetite, tiredness or loss of energy. Symptoms carry on for longer than a low mood, which most people experience from time to time. A depressed mood can interfere with the person's ability to get on with their daily life.

Digital exclusion People are said to be 'digitally excluded' if they have no access to the internet. There is thought to be a link between digital exclusion and social exclusion. A fully documented report can be found at www.communities.gov.uk. Once in the site, type in Understanding Digital Exclusion – Research Report.

Disease prevention Primary prevention is reducing the number of new cases of a disease through activities such as immunisation, accident prevention, dental prophylaxis. Secondary prevention is shortening the duration or diminishing the impact of a disease or condition through early detection and prompt, effective intervention. Tertiary prevention is reducing impairments and disabilities and minimising suffering caused by existing health problems and promoting adjustment of child and family conditions that cannot be ameliorated.

Dual diagnosis A diagnosis of mental ill health in a person with learning disability. Also refers to someone with mental health problems who misuses drugs and/or alcohol.

Elder abuse 'A single or repeated act, or lack of appropriate action, occurring within any relationship where there is an expectation of trust, which causes harm or distress to an older person' (Action on Elder Abuse 2004, www.elderabuse.org.uk).

Elective Procedures applied to the patient, often surgical, that may not necessarily be life saving, but may be life enhancing. Either the doctor, patient or both may choose when to schedule the procedure.

Empathy Literally translates as 'in feeling', the capacity to share in another person's emotions and feelings.

Family-centred care Model of nursing which ensures that care is planned around the whole family, not just the individual child, and in which all the family members are recognised as care recipients.

Fuel poverty A term that applies to households that cannot afford to keep adequately warm at reasonable cost.

Genetics The scientific study of heredity embracing humans and all other organisms.

Health protection Strategies adopted to safeguard the health of the community as a whole such as clean water, good sanitation, safe roads and playgrounds.

Holistic nursing practice A concept in nursing practice upholding that all aspects of people's needs, psychological, physical and social, should be taken into account and seen as a whole.

Infant A child from birth to one year of age.

Integrated working Everyone supporting children and young people works together effectively to put the child at the centre, meet their needs and improve their lives.

Internal fixation The use of screws, nails and plates to hold a fracture in alignment to allow healing to take place.

Intraoperative During operation.

Ischaemic changes A restriction in blood supply.

Learning disability A state of arrested or incomplete development of mind, resulting in significant impairment of intellectual functioning and adaptive/social functioning.

Mental Health Act The law in England and Wales regarding the assessment, treatment and rights of people with mental health conditions. There are two Acts, Mental Health Act 1983 and Mental Health Act 2007, which amends the 1983 Act.

Neonate A baby in the first 28 days of life.

Nerve entrapment Entrapment of a nerve in soft or hard tissue.

Normalisation A set of principles supporting the idea that people with a learning disability should live in ordinary surroundings doing ordinary things, and through interacting with ordinary people on a daily basis, they will experience normal life patterns.

Osteoporosis A loss of bone density that can lead to fracture formation.

Partnership in care A nursing model where clinical nursing care for a sick child can be given by the parents with support and education from a nurse, and family care can be given by the nurse if the family is absent.

Patient-controlled analgesia A device that allows the patient to deliver a restricted dose of analgesia as a bolus, usually intravenously.

Personality disorder People with personality disorders find it difficult to make or keep relationships and control their feelings and actions. They may harm themselves or other people due to difficulty in learning how to control their patterns of behaviour over time.

Podiatrist A person who diagnoses and treats conditions and diseases of the feet.

Psychosis A general term for a mental state often said to be a 'loss of contact with reality'. People who suffer from psychosis may have hallucinations – seeing, hearing or feeling things that are not there – or delusions – believing something is true even though all the evidence shows that it is false – and may have personality changes and disorganised thinking. This may result in unusual or odd behaviour, as well as difficulty with normal social contact and not being able to carry out normal activities of daily living.

Recovery A personal journey that may involve developing hope, a secure base

3

and sense of self, supportive relationships, empowerment, social inclusion, coping skills, and meaning.

Schizophrenia A mental health disorder that affects thinking, feeling and behaviour where the person displays symptoms of psychosis (see above).

Splints An apparatus, usually rigid, to support, immobilise or protect an injured part, usually temporarily.

Stigma Severe social disapproval of personal characteristics or beliefs that are perceived to be against cultural norms. Stigma is often based on ignorance and results in social exclusion, damaging recovery.

Strapping The use of overlapping adhesive tape to support, cover or exert pressure on an injured part, for example for a sprained joint.

Synovium The connective tissue lining a joint cavity.

Therapeutic relationship The relationship between a mental health professional and a service user by which the professional hopes to engage with and effect change in the service user, thus supporting their recovery.

Tourette's syndrome A neurological disorder characterised by repetitive, stereotyped, involuntary movements and vocalisation called 'tics'. Early symptoms are almost always noticed first in childhood, with the average onset being between the ages of seven and ten years.

3

4 research and nursing

4

Introduction

In the fourth part of *The Nursing Companion* emphasis is placed on research and how this impacts on the quality of care. Research is now completely integrated within all programmes of nurse education because without it evidence-based practice would be unachievable. The relevance of research to nursing is explored through an overview of the concept of research, how it originated and how it has become a highly structured discipline. To begin with, only a few nurse researchers existed, much of what passed for nursing knowledge was either handed down from one generation of nurses to the next or dictated as part of the medical model. Research has liberated nurses and the relevance of systematic scientific enquiry is at the heart of progress, much of which has been quite rapid. The basic components underpinning research-based nursing are considered before moving on to the various designs employed in the collection, analysis and dissemination of data.

Nursing research has developed a sophistication derived from the initial utilisation of quantitative and qualitative design. Because advanced research design is the province of experienced nurse researchers, *The Nursing Companion* will focus on the essentials necessary for understanding and consolidating the basics. Part 4 offers insights into the main approaches involved in designing a quantitative study through descriptive, correlation, quasi-experimental and experimental design. Data collection is considered, for example the use of questionnaires, and various forms of data measurement are described.

4

17 the relevance of research to nursing

Elaine Ball

In this chapter we will explore:

> Research origins
> Research today
> A literature review
> Components of a research study

Introduction

Your nursing course is now, more than at any other time in history, equipped to offer you, as a man or woman, a variety of opportunities that should exceed expectation. The nurses who have gone before you have worked enduringly hard to professionalise the nursing fraternity to which you are now attached. Raising nurses' professional profile has been achieved in many ways, but principally through day-to-day practice and its development through the acquisition of knowledge and evidence. Since the 1850s and the innovative work of Florence Nightingale, the work of the nurse has become increasingly valued as a powerful force that directly affects the lives of clients. Thus, a rich tradition of knowledge and practice has evolved over the years, and will continue to grow. Perhaps the best part of this tradition is that we are all involved in its development in a multitude of ways. Different opportunities are always available to you, both in terms of clinical variety and through further studies, which will be of value to your clients, colleagues and the general nursing collective.

At some point in your learning experiences, both as a student and as a practising nurse, you will be exposed to the concept of research. Essentially, this is an investigative process by which current knowledge is expanded and refined by a thorough and structured enquiry into issues and problems that need an answer. The foundations upon which nursing is built have been steadily strengthened by nurses in the clinical and academic arena, who are writing up and publishing the projects, reports and studies they have undertaken to ensure that patient care is underpinned by the evidence those questions pose. In this way, the research done today becomes tomorrow's practice. In fact, the courses you undertake now and throughout your career will be strongly influenced by the latest evidence to support your practice. Your new abilities in

4

looking at this evidence with a critical eye will be the source of your power to change things.

Sometimes, nurses in the clinical arena face many challenges when it comes to familiarising themselves with the latest research. Lack of resources, especially time, lack of confidence or not knowing how to source material are just some of the barriers to utilising research (Funk et al. 1991). Yet, the fact remains, we are all affected by research. How can we justify this statement? Take a moment to think about a day on the ward – what would you do, see, use and tell. Examples could be:

> The internet or journal articles you read
> The clinical procedures that patients undergo
> The medicines you see being administered to people
> The information you tell patients, colleagues or family members.

These all stem from a research base – and may emanate from pure scientific research or a simple bit of searching, but all the information is based on evidence that can be seen, measured or tested. In short, all research is based upon what has gone before, and it is research that works.

Research origins

Over time, human civilisation has advanced into areas well beyond its own physical limits – curiosity has led to a pursuit of knowledge that, in turn, has led to understanding and wisdom. Initially, these investigations were focused on survival, yet as these needs were met, humans concentrated on making life easier for themselves. Enormous technological leaps have allowed human advancement to occur at an increasingly faster pace. One such innovation was the written word, which eventually led to the invention of the printing press. From that moment on, people could write ideas down and disseminate them to a wider audience.

In Western civilisation, the value and process of knowledge can be traced back to the writings of the Greek philosopher Plato. The written dialogues of Plato are examples of early records of the elements of structured enquiry that form the basis of research today: the art of definition, analysis and synthesis. A pupil of Plato, the philosopher Aristotle later refined these ideas and so created the foundation of the discipline of philosophy. Literally translated, philosophy means 'love of wisdom', which focused on the quest for true knowledge and the eradication of false opinions. Does this sound familiar? The same principles apply today in nursing practice and the appropriate use of evidence, although philosophers have continued the debate to the present day about the value and nature of knowledge. This, in turn, has led to the development of a whole array of research philosophies that inform the researcher in terms of how to look at the world. These different philosophical stances are beyond the scope of this text. For now, though, it is sufficient to know that they are there.

Before the written word, the practice of healthcare and medical science was an oral tradition, passed on from one person to another. Although people had ideas of what illness was and how the body worked, their knowledge was limited and, in most cases, misguided through superstition and spiritual beliefs. Therefore, medicine has always had a strong research and writerly tradition (evidencing research by writing it down). The earliest understanding of the body, and how it functioned, can be traced back to the ancient civilizations of Egypt, India, China, Persia and Greece. Western philosophical writings of Hippocrates date back to the 4th century BC, and represent the founding of medicine as a holistic and evidence-based science.

Hippocrates is viewed as the father of modern medicine, and is accredited with making the study of medicine a discipline in its own right, with specified training and a code of professional conduct, the Hippocratic Oath. What does he have to do with this research tradition? Well, unlike his predecessors, whose treatment of illness involved superstition and divine origin, Hippocrates used the philosophical principles of the day to define, analyse and synthesise knowledge to facilitate patient care. The *Hippocratic Corpus* is the collection of his works, recorded in minute detail. Although the principles were scientifically misguided (Hippocrates had almost no knowledge of anatomy and physiology as you or I understand it), his rejection of unfounded beliefs in conjunction with the use of treatment based on logical and critical observation was a huge turning point that is equally as vital today. Just as Hippocrates was the father of medicine, perhaps he also deserves the title of father of evidence-based practice.

Hippocrates' methods set the tone for the practice of medicine from then on: doctors became trained and professional persons throughout Greece. The trend continued later across Europe as the Roman Empire spread, giving students a commonality of practice and also language (Latin). This is a legacy still around today, as many medical terms have Latin or Greek origins. Thus, medicine can be traced through papers and books from the time of Hippocrates to today and can rightfully call itself a research-based profession.

The historical narratives that link present-day scientific research to a collection of writings that existed thousands of years ago is testimony to a written tradition that has spanned millennia. Philosophy, herbology, apothecary and alchemy are terms that predate the scientific rigour that we are assured of today. However, whenever philosophical rumination and intuition began, it was the start of our interest in the human body and the remedies to aid its healing. All eras use their own historical contexts and discourses to define the medicalisation of the human body, but one thing is certain: medicine has an identity that can be clearly profiled at each juncture in history. The same cannot be said for nursing. This is probably because nursing did not have the same writing tradition that medicine used to charter its advancement through research and its findings.

Consequently, nurses had little exposure to the research culture of academia, relying on a tradition of a more pragmatic approach to training.

Medicine has, therefore, had a 2,000 year head start as a research-based discipline. However, the past few decades have seen nursing take its place in the academic mainstream, and as a result, the culture and skills of legitimate research and enquiry have been embraced. In terms of nursing knowledge, Florence Nightingale (1820–1910) is generally acknowledged as the individual who constructed and first recorded an evidence-based profession with the publication of *Notes on Nursing* (Nightingale 1859). The postwar years saw the emergence of great nursing theorists, such as Virginia Henderson (1897–1996) and Dorothea Orem (1914–2007). Thankfully, nurses such as these have acknowledged the value of academic enquiry, and it is this legacy that has caused the shift of attitude towards research use and development. Hence, nurses have worked extremely hard towards producing a unique research base and enriching contemporary practice with good quality evidence, as rigorously obtained and equally as valid as that from any other academic discipline.

As time progressed, the practice of medical care became a specialised role in society. This role demanded a specialised training and knowledge and, as such, medicine emerged as a discipline for educated and professional persons. How the principles and concepts of good practice were known on a wider scale was due almost entirely to them being recorded and made available to an interested audience. Because nursing has relied more on an oral tradition, its bedrock is the nurse's close proximity to the patient and the communicative relationship the nurse has with their client. Communication underpins nursing and patients express their fears, expectations and feelings to nurses in a unique way. The nurse–patient relationship is constituted around a 24-hour contract of care. Nurses are best placed to identify and chart any changes that may take place in a patient's condition. The information they relay to a variety of other professionals within the multidisciplinary team relies heavily on this. Consequently, the nurse is in the strongest position to be the advocate for the patient.

Research today

Contemporary nurses sit at the confluence of theory and practice, and are constantly finding innovative ways to develop care for the benefit of the patient. As well as competent carers, nurses are also constantly generating and testing new evidence and ways of doing things in practice. They are not simply questioning the validity of how nursing operates, but identifying and applying current research in their own field.

Evidence-based practice

This ideological and political change has permeated through nursing with the development of evidence-based practice:

> Evidence-based practice (EBP) is an approach to health care wherein health professionals use the best evidence possible, i.e. the most appropriate information available, to make clinical decisions for individual patients. (McKibbon 1998, p. 397)

Evidence-based practice has led in strengthening the identity of the nursing profession. This approach to healthcare practice has increased autonomy among nurses and has provided a greater cross-dissemination of ideas inter-professionally. In part, this shift in role has given current nurses in practice the power to shape the destiny of the profession, and this is the baton that is now handed to you.

Sources of evidence

Activity 17.1

Research evidence can influence not only our professional lives but also the way in which we live generally.

Consider the claims made by advertisers as to the value of their products compared to other retailers. You may find it of interest to look at food brands and the way health-related claims are made.

How convincing are these claims?

Can you identify any problems with the way in which the data are gathered, interpreted and presented?

You could also look at potential bias in the source of funding for this research.

Taking into account the modern world approach to having evidence for common everyday products, we need to ask ourselves the question: 'Where do we get our evidence for clinical practice?' The answer is both complex and straightforward. In essence we get it from:

> published sources – journals, conference papers, practice protocols
> formal training and development – courses, study days, workshops
> expert opinion – multidisciplinary workforce.

Activity 17.2

Please respond honestly to the following statements. Give yourself a score out of 10 for each question and provide a rationale for your score:
1 I know where to look for information.
2 I know what types of information are available.
3 I know how to perform a computer literature search to find journal articles and abstracts.
4 I know what an abstract is.
5 I know what I can obtain from different databases.
6 I know how to organise my information once I have found it.

Activity 17.2 should highlight for you:

> the areas that you have confidence in using for research information
> those areas that you need to explore further.

An important task is to gain support and help if you are unfamiliar with this style of looking for knowledge. You will find it useful to record your findings from this activity in your learning journal/diary.

The need for evidence in practice was formalised by Archie Cochrane (1972) over three decades ago into what we now know as evidence-based practice; the role and function of which has evolved over time. Growing out of a medical model, it was adapted and utilised by many disciplines – evidence-based nursing is one such later permutation.

Examples of evidence-based practice in the clinical arena

Context

It is a busy Monday morning on a surgical ward – surgeons, junior doctors, specialist nurses, anaesthetists and other multidisciplinary professionals are all on the ward at the same time. Each employee has an agenda and schedule to be met and the ward-based staff have to help make things run smoothly. There is nothing unusual to this day; it is just another busy pre-theatre morning and Mrs Owen is being given initial information about her operation.

Evidence-based practice

In considering the two events described below, please remember that research provides us with enough information to show that patients who are given transparent and appropriate information before any procedure fare better afterwards. When risks are pointed out and calculated, the patient feels in greater control, able to assess any risk factor and move into healing more quickly. When the correct information is given to the patient, barriers between the patient and the healthcare team are broken down and they more likely to be seen as valuable and effective providers of care with the best interest of the patient in mind.

Event 1

Doctor Smith clerks-in his patient. He is extremely busy and after a very brief chat, he asks staff nurse Kate to give his patient, 29-year-old Mrs Owen, any ward-based literature regarding her ensuing operation. Mrs Owen is about to undergo bilateral prophylactic mastectomies and Kate gets the appropriate leaflets, which outline the place of incision, healing time and aftercare, complications, and further surgery for breast implants and nipple transplant. Kate takes one look at Mrs Owen and sees she is petrified. She draws the curtains round the bed and sits and chats for a few minutes about nothing in particular. Mrs Owen mumbles something about having too much information, so Kate agrees and tells Mrs Owen that, for now, the most important thing is to know she is in the hands of an expert team and her care on the ward will be equal to that of the surgeons. Kate discretely places the leaflets on the locker and tells Mrs Owen that if she wants to read them at some point or give them to her husband to read, they are there. Kate leaves Mrs Owen feeling as though she's

4

been treated in a good way – as an individual who is allowed to be afraid and who will unravel her life event in her own time.

Event 2

Doctor Smith clerks-in his patient. He is extremely busy and after a very brief chat, he asks the newly qualified staff nurse Rachel to give his patient, 29-year-old Mrs Owen, any ward-based literature regarding her ensuing operation. Mrs Owen is about to undergo bilateral prophylactic mastectomies and Rachel gets the appropriate leaflets, which outline the place of incision, healing time and aftercare, complications, and further surgery for breast implants and nipple transplant. Rachel does not see that Mrs Owen is petrified. Rachel is bright, knowledgeable and aware that patients fare better when they have all the appropriate information (as does Kate), and so she sits beside Mrs Owen, who mumbles that one can have too much information. Rachel agrees, and proceeds to outline the points listed in the leaflets. When Rachel has finished, she draws back the curtain, and Mrs Owen is left to feel like a tick in a tick-box list. Her anxiety has increased and she is left feeling helpless.

Activity 17.3

1 The evidence is clear, but how do we implement evidence-based practice in a safe way?
2 How do we ensure that evidence-based practice is contingent upon the individual patient's needs?
3 The most recent evidence-based practice literature states that there is still a surmountable theory–practice gap. How do we link experiential knowledge and theoretical knowledge?

Context

Two new theatre porters have joined the staff at your hospital. They are young, pleasant, good humoured and make the patients chuckle on the way down to theatre. You are the senior nurse in charge of the ward and, just recently, it has come to your attention that increasingly both new porters are chatting to the staff who accompany the patient to theatre, which means that the nurse is not spending this significant time with their patient. Consequently, the patient is not talked to en route to theatre and, hence, is not reassured or supported. Little credence is given to the fact that the patient is being pushed to perhaps a life-changing procedure.

Evidence-based practice

Evidence shows that communication is central to good nursing–patient care. Indeed, it is part of the basic nursing care process and is outlined in all recent government White Papers as an essential requisite for best practice. Good and effective communication is a 'tool' that enables structures, people and institutions to develop, evolve and share experiences. It is also the foundation on which all else is built.

As senior nurse, you take the opportunity to raise everyone's awareness in the monthly staff meeting regarding the above points, stating that the journey between the ward and the theatre is precious time that should be given over entirely to the patient. Everyone agrees and things not only return to normal, they are better. Staff who had never fully considered the ward–theatre transfer time as an opportunity to be fully present to their patient start to engage more actively. However, a reserved and inexperienced student called Brigid is asked to escort a patient to theatre and one of the above porters is pushing the bed. The porter starts as normal in his usual affable way to chat to the student; unable to direct the conversation to the patient and deflect conversation away from him, Brigid tells the porter she is not allowed to talk to him, only to the patient.

At first, the senior nurse thinks it is her imagination when she is ignored by a number of porters, but over the ensuing week, she begins to feel increasingly uncomfortable with the fact that she is snubbed by the portering staff entering the ward. Now it appears that the two porters are criticised for being pleasant and friendly.

Activity 17.4

1 The ward sister now has a compounded problem, what can she do to fix it?
2 Did she do anything wrong in the first place?
3 How, at this point, can she use evidence-based practice as an effective intervention?
4 In terms of current practice analysis, how can evidence-based practice highlight good practice and prepare the sister for any future management issues?
5 Are there any skill issues for the student nurses on the ward that need to be addressed?
6 Is there now evidence that a needs analysis for student communication could be carried out?
7 Does a literature review of the most current evidence need to be undertaken?

A literature review

Nursing research that successfully generates a sound empirical knowledge base for nursing practice ensures that safety and the right treatment is at the centre of patient care. The evidence to support best practice is located in the research process. A literature review is often the starting point of any research activity and should be included in your investigation; it meets a number of objectives and provides:

> background to the study
> a synthesis of relevant information such as previous work/research
> discussion of the clinical importance of the topic
> identification of gaps in current knowledge and research about the topic of interest
> justification for the need of the study.

An important point to remember is that the contextual setting of the problem will have an impact on the research and the findings. Ask yourself the following questions:

1 Can you safely and productively transfer the recommendations or findings of the study to your own clinical arena?
2 Can the study or any of its findings be applied to your area of practice?
3 Is the research useful or applicable? If not, go on to the next article or adapt the study to reflect your own requirements.
4 What evidence is used to support the research findings?

Box 17.1

A literature review is:

> a review of the literature, for example in the health sciences
> a classification and evaluation of what accredited scholars and researchers have written on a topic
> organised according to a guiding concept, such as your research objective, or the problem/issue you wish to address.

Look for bias within your literature search:

> a particular theoretical framework or model, for example a feminist examination of gender inequity in medical research
> the author's rhetorical purpose, for example a researcher's reasons for advocating the effectiveness of a certain drug
> an experience-based practical perspective, for example the belief that one approach to pain management is more effective than another.

We all value 'unbiased' scientific research, but no author is free from outside influence. To limit bias, we need to ensure that a systematic approach to research is taken so we can develop, expand and refine our knowledge – in fact, this is the research goal.

Nursing research is a systematic enquiry designed to develop knowledge and is a means through which questions can be answered by the application of certain investigative principles. There are a variety of research methods, which are discussed in greater detail in Chapters 18 and 19. However, in spite of different approaches, all research projects share some common features:

1 The hypothesis or question
2 The sample
3 A framework of investigation, for example qualitative or quantitative research
4 Analysis of data
5 Do the data answer the original research question?

6 Underpinning all this are ethical codes of behaviour that exist to protect participants from unscrupulous and unethical research.

Component parts of a research study

The components of a research study presented below are revisited in Chapters 18 and 19, each with a bias relevant to that chapter. But first an activity that will give insights into developing a research question. This is essential if you are serious about planning and carrying out your own research-based enquiry.

Activity 17.5 Developing a research question

When you become a qualified practitioner, you will be in a good position to see something that needs research, as you will be seeing things with fresh eyes.

Are there ways of doing things, 'practices', that do not seem to have a rationale?

From this observation, you can ask the question: 'Why does 'X' happen?'

It is important that your question is open and leads to a response that could begin with 'because'. Avoid asking a closed question with a one-word answer.

Your question may find that there is a reason for practice, but it is lost in time or you need to read up about it, and the first thing you will do in some research studies is explore the matter through the literature.

So as to ensure that you do not give yourself the whole library to read, you need to create a focused question. Such a research question should enable you to identify the areas of literature to read and also, through a literature search, inquire as to whether this question has been raised and answered.

In this internet savvy age, it is useful to think about the nature of search demands as these skills can be translated into research. There are similarities, in that precise demands provide the best responses from a search engine.

You may feel that there is no point to asking a question that has been answered. Carrying out such a task is far from pointless, because you will have practised the art of question development, read up and learned about the issue and know whether a puzzling aspect of practice is indeed research based.

So to the activity:

- Identify an aspect of practice that seems to have little or no explanation.
- Ask yourself the question: 'Why does 'X' happen?'
- Engage in a literature search. If nothing is found, reframe your question, ensuring that the key words are in the search criteria.

Still nothing? Then you may have found an example of outmoded practice or an area that requires further research. This could be useful later in your education when you will carry out some research, so make a note in your learning journal.

It is more likely, however, that you will find some reference to work in the area, but check the recency of the publication dates. Is further work required?

Research is an essential part of developing good practice and asking the right questions is an important part of this discipline. So start early and make those essential links between practice and theory as you develop your skills in research and nursing.

The hypothesis

Essentially, a **hypothesis** is a statement about something that the researcher identifies and poses at the beginning of the research process. The sole purpose of any research project is the subsequent proving or disproving (that is, confirming or rejecting the hypothesis) of your statement. An example hypothesis is:

Regular hand washing reduces the risk of cross-infection

If we were to pursue this statement and establish its truth, we would have to design a research approach that systematically examines each relevant variable. This would have to be done with a thoroughness that would withstand scrutiny and produce a result that can be reliably reported.

Reflecting back on the previous activity, you will see that supplementary to the hypothesis is the notion of the research question. This differs from the hypothesis, in that a question is something that needs to be answered, whereas a hypothesis is a conjecture that can either be proven or refuted. Research questions also share common features. Most can be formulated using the PICO framework:

> P – problem
> I – intervention
> C – context
> O – outcome.

If we apply the above statement to the PICO framework, we would have a question such as:

> P – cross-infection is the problem
> I – is there a link between hand washing and cross-infection?
> C – the context is hand washing in a certain clinical environment
> O – the outcome of this intervention (hand washing) when measured against the incidence of cross-infection.

Here is a similar question, divided into manageable parts. By highlighting key areas in italic, one can refer back to the PICO framework and see if each area has been addressed:

What *effect* does *improving hand-washing techniques* have in *reducing* the *incidence of hospital acquired infection* in *patients in hospital*?

We now have a starting point on which to set out our enquiry. In conducting this exercise, one can see from the application of this framework to a real problem that asking the right question is a fundamental stage in the process. The question has to be explicit enough to allow the reader exposure to all the essential elements of the study. In short, a proper research question is almost akin to a summary of the research itself. Research centres upon the effect of

4

one thing against another. A research project therefore needs a minimum of two elements that are compared to each other. For a moment, turn back to the key studies mentioned earlier, and come up with some questions that the researchers could have asked to tackle the issues.

Variables

Remember the earlier example of a hypothesis:

Hand washing reduces the risk of cross-infection

If we were to pursue this statement and establish its truth, we would have to design a research approach that systematically examines each element. In this instance, there are two elements that need comparison: hand washing and cross-infection. These elements are called variables and can be either dependent or independent:

> A **dependent variable** is something that is directly influenced by the actions of another element. For example, a patient's infection status is directly influenced by contact with a microorganism.
> An **independent variable** is something that directly influences another element. If we were to continue our hand-washing hypothesis, then the independent variable in this case would be the washing of one's hands (this variable can be identified and adjusted in terms of regularity, technique, soap product, drying methods and so on).

The essential aim of research, then, is to examine the interplay between these variables and look at the outcome in each instance. How this is done and the reliability of the findings relies on the other parts of the research project. These must be equally as robust as one another for a strong study to withstand critical examination. It would be safe to say, therefore, that a study is only as strong as its weakest part. These parts are discussed in more detail below.

The sample

Sampling is a process of selecting subjects who are representative of the **population** being studied. Good sampling is an essential part of research quality. Typically, the more rigorous the researcher has been at this stage will dictate:

> *How reliable the research is:* **Reliability** is, quite simply, how trustworthy a piece of research can be. Reliability is an indication of how much faith one has in the findings. A fundamental part of reliability (although not its sole component) is the **sample** quality.
> *To what extent it can be generalised:* This concept indicates to the reader how the findings of a paper apply to different situations or to wider populations. Smaller sampling or research carried out in specific groups can limit the relevance of the findings to just those groups or just that sample.

An example might be the recent evidence around the MMR vaccination, in which a specific sample was examined and conclusions were drawn that a combined vaccination was harmful (Wakefield 1999). However, the results were sensationalised by the media, causing widespread concern among parents. The major shortcoming of the study was that the sample of cases used was so small that generalisability was not realistic. It was a good paper subject to bad press because the findings were overgeneralised by the media (Goldacre 2005):

> Because of the *sample size* and *criteria*, the application of the findings to a wider population is not realistic. A far more comprehensive sampling strategy needs to be adopted before this research has any meaning to the population as a whole.
> The expectation that the *probability* of harm indicated would apply to everyone is *unreliable*. Consequently, the degree of statistical risk between combined and single vaccination is not significant.

Keeping these observations in mind, the researcher can perform a variety of processes to ensure that the sample and its formation can emulate the population at large while restricting errors. This can be done by:

> increasing the population size
> randomising the selection
> including or excluding individuals to construct an equitable range of people.

It would be safe to say that all good research studies should allow the reader to look at their sampling strategy and, at a minimum, address the above points when writing up their findings. This allows the research consumer (and yes, that means you) to assess whether the research has got anything to do with you in the first place, and if it does, to what degree you can rely on it.

One of the key aspects of rigorous sampling depends on findings that are transferable to a wider population and it is prudent to ensure that the sample is as representative as possible. Let's take another example. If a researcher, interested in studying the relationship between smoking cessation and gender, recruited 20 women and 1 man, it would be wrong to say that women are more successful at stopping smoking than men. This is because, in this instance, the sample is skewed, that is, the ratio of men to women is misrepresented. Ideally, the researcher would seek to recruit a sample that reflected the same distribution of men to women as the general population.

4

Framework of investigation

Researchers do not set out to solve problems on a whim. Any research study has to have a well-planned structure that will frame the investigation. In other words, the study must be framed in a way that is:

> workable
> realistic
> timely
> cost-effective
> logical
> measurable.

These six points are key aspects to explain how the researcher has set about tackling the identified problem and punctuate the research with markers that indicate aims, outcomes and **limitations** to the study. Any study has its limitations. The art of good research, though, is to draw a line somewhere and set some limitations. How does one decide where to set these limits? Obviously, research has finite resources such as time and money, but there should be some sort of limit, where doing any more work would yield little additional benefit. An example would be the study of hand washing by Ignaz Semmelweis in the late 1840s. He discovered that thorough hand washing was instrumental in the prevention of the spread of infection, specifically in maternity wards where puerperal fever was rife. His research resulted in a mandate for maternity staff to wash their hands before examining a patient, whereas prior to this research, it was quite common for medical students and physicians to work with cadavers then go directly to assist in the maternity delivery room, often without washing their hands. Semmelweis correctly hypothesised that the lack of efficient hand washing was the cause of the high mortality rate of women in the maternity delivery room. If he conclusively proved the link between cross-infection and hand washing, then what would be the point in continuing his study when the findings became obvious?

In the conduct of research, there are similarities between the nursing process and the execution of a study. A framework is outlined in Figure 17.1 that organises issues in practice and utilises the nursing process in research.

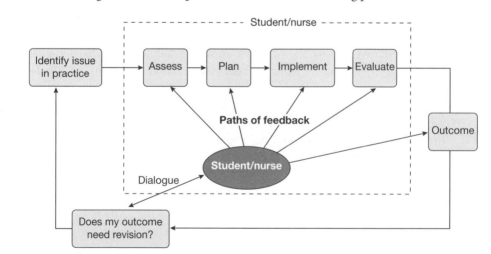

Figure 17.1 An example of the nursing process in research

research and nursing

Analysis of the data

Analysis is the detailed examination of phenomena, which we call **data**. The whole aim of doing research is to yield information, which can help the investigator to answer the questions they began with. All this information needs to be processed, organised and examined rigorously. Any departure from this intention may introduce errors, which could ultimately lead the researcher to the wrong answer. Indeed, when one examines research that has been published, it is a major part of the critical process to question how the researcher has dealt with the data. Typically, researchers use a variety of methods that can employ both numbers (statistics) and words to describe the findings.

Do the data answer the original question posed?

After analysing the data, the researcher must come full circle and revisit the original questions asked. If the previous steps have been completed correctly, the researcher will not only be in a position to answer these questions, but also to say to what degree they are proven or refuted. Whether or not the initial question or hypothesis is proven or not is, surprisingly, not the main priority. Principally, it is how these answers have been derived that is the most critical aspect of research. On this rests the possibility of applying the findings to a wider population with confidence and certainty.

Ethics

A preliminary but useful definition of ethics is that it is concerned with doing good and avoiding harm. All research should have undertaken ethical approval, and be conducted within an ethical framework. This includes:

> Doing no harm to participants
> Obtaining informed consent from participants
> Keeping data collected safe and confidential
> Using data properly.

Perhaps the best known example of ethically unsound health research is the Tuskegee syphilis study, which over a 40-year timescale managed to fall short in every one of the above categories. Readers are urged to access the excellent article by Susan Reverby (1998).

As an example, Gillon (1986) provides an overview of the ethical principle of autonomy. In summary, this is the capacity to think, decide and act on the basis of such thought and decision freely and independently and without let or hindrance. A problem for critical care nurses is that their clients may not always be in a position to think, decide and act. Morality requires that when we can, we treat persons autonomously, but that we also contribute to their welfare. Such beneficial actions fall under the heading of 'beneficence'. Beneficence refers to an action done to benefit others, and the moral principle of beneficence refers to a moral obligation to act for the benefit of others (Beauchamp

4

and Childress 2001). The ethical principle of 'nonmaleficence' asserts an obligation not to inflict harm on others. Critical care nurses often harm their clients when trying to act for the benefit of others. For example, a nurse may inadvertently cause pain to a patient in the process of passing tubes or injecting fluids and drugs (Bandman and Bandman 2002). When ethical principles conflict, the nurse must decide which takes precedence. Nurses are reminded that such decisions are not only the domain of doctors and politicians. Moral responsibility to clients demands involvement. In summary, nursing decisions affect people because nurses have the power to do good or harm to their client group. The potential for doing either of these depends partly on factual knowledge and partly on values. It is of vital importance that nurses do not rely solely upon their own values when making decisions about their clients. There are many ethical theories and principles that may help the nurse with ethical decision making.

Conclusion

This chapter has introduced you to the importance of research, its origins and relevance to nursing practice today. Furthermore, you should be able to recognise the important common elements in any research paper or study, and to assess their credibility and relevance to your practice. Increasingly, the modern nurse is expected to be an autonomous authority in practice. Although a significant part of this authority is provided through nurse education and experience, the credibility of the decisions made at the bedside rely increasingly on underpinning evidence to justify nurses' actions. The evidence upon which nurses base their decisions is not static and is constantly evolving, and one must keep pace with these changes.

Over the past few decades, the research output of leading nurse authors has shaped practice into what it is today. The output and quality of nursing research has increased year after year, and is showing no signs of slowing down. Add to this the output of nursing and government bodies, and one can see that there is a huge selection of evidence out there for the 'research-aware' nurse to use in practice for the benefit of others.

As a questioning attitude is now a prerequisite of the autonomous practitioner, the authors would argue that an understanding of the research process (and consequently the capability to critically examine research) is a progressively more important aspect of care in the twenty-first century. Indeed, as was said at the beginning of this chapter, a medical model subsumed nursing. However, in these competing discourses, nursing research is the inscribed narrative upon which its own future is shaped. This has given nurses the voice, capabilities and the power to question traditional hierarchies of healthcare delivery.

4

References

Bandman, E and Bandman, B (2002) *Nursing Ethics Through the Life Span* (4th edn), Upper Saddle River, NJ: Pearson Education

Beauchamp, TL and Childress, JF (2001) *Principles of Biomedical Ethics* (5th edn), New York: OUP

Cochrane, A (1972) *Effectiveness and Efficiency*, London: Nuffield Provincial Hospitals Trust

Funk, SG, Champagne, MT, Wiese, RA and Tornquist, EM (1991) BARRIERS: The Barriers to Research Utilisation Scale, *Applied Nursing Research*, **4**(1): 39–45

Gillon, R (1986) *Philosophical Medical Ethics,* John Wiley & Sons, Chichester

Goldacre, B (2005) Don't dumb me down, *The Guardian*, 8 September

McKibbon, KA (1998) Evidence based practice, *Bulletin of the Medical Library Association*, **86**(3): 396–401

Nightingale, F (1859) *Notes on Nursing: What Nursing Is, and What Nursing is Not*, London: Harrison & Sons

Reverby, SM (1998) History of an apology: from Tuskegee to the White House, *Research Nurse*, **3**(4): 1–9

Wakefield, AJ (1999) MMR vaccination and autism, *Lancet*, 354: 949–50

4

18 quantitative research

Susan Baldwin

In this chapter we will explore:

> Quantitative designs
> Methods of collecting data
> Organisation and analysis of data

Introduction

Previously we examined how research aims to expand the body of knowledge for the discipline in which it is conducted. As with any systematic approach, researchers must develop a detailed specification/design, in which the research problem can be developed or tested, while degrees of control are maintained. This degree of control is dependent upon the approach and methods that are employed by the researcher. The different approaches to research can be viewed as falling between two ends of a continuum. At one end, researchers apply methods designed to discover, explain or understand human emotional responses. Minimal or indeed no control is applied to this approach. Data from this approach are contextual, and presented in narrative format. This is known as qualitative research, which is explored fully in Chapter 19.

At the other end, the researcher uses methods that apply maximum control over the conditions of the study. This enables the researcher to test a particular theory and avoid any bias entering the research conditions. Data from this approach are quantifiable, in that the results can be presented statistically and establish a **cause and effect** relationship. This is known as **quantitative research** and the remainder of this chapter will focus on this aspect of research.

The methods used to collect and analyse data within the two approaches would be quite different. For example, if the researchers were trying to explain a cause and effect relationship between the administration of a new cancer drug on the size of a tumour, then the control applied to the study would be to ensure that no other variable could explain the reduction in the tumour. In healthcare, this approach can be seen in randomised controlled trials that test the effectiveness of an intervention, such as a new drug.

If, however, the researchers were trying to determine how a patient felt about their care while receiving treatment for a tumour, then they would adopt methods that enabled the researcher to ask the patient how they felt, and in doing so, understand the phenomena from the patient's perspective. The results would be analysed and presented as an explanation of the lived experience of the patient.

Quantitative designs

Quantitative designs, as the title suggests, collect, analyse and present data in numerical form, and as Mateo and Kirchoff (1999) suggest: 'seek facts or causes in a more objective and controlled way'.

While the literature differs in its way of classifying quantitative designs, four main classes can be identified. These are:

> quantitative descriptive designs
> correlation designs
> quasi-experimental designs
> experimental designs.

Each design can be classed by its purpose and the degree of control that it applies. Graziano and Raulin (2004) define **control** as any procedure used by the researcher to counter any potential threat to the **validity** of the research.

Graziano and Raulin (2004) discuss four types of control that can be applied to research:

1 The control that is applied over the general procedures of the research. This would include the environment and any measures that the researcher was using.
2 The control over the subject and researcher behaviour that would reduce any bias.
3 The selection of participants to a study is important and can be a threat to validity. This will be reduced significantly by the adoption of random sampling. A **random sample** applies much more control over a study than a **convenience sample** would.
4 Experimental designs use techniques to apply maximum control. These will be discussed later in the chapter.

Quantitative descriptive design

Quantitative descriptive designs can range in their methods from a simple **case study** to large population studies in which the researchers are attempting to explain or determine patterns in phenomena. Survey methods are an example of this method, in which the researchers document what is there, and do not attempt to manipulate variables. An example of the use of a descriptive design can be seen in the research conducted by Duncan and Dealey (2007). The researchers used a descriptive survey, employing a semi-structured questionnaire to explain patient opinion about asking healthcare professionals to wash their hands before contact with them. This piece of research provides an example of how the researchers sought opinion, and did indeed make some determination of patterns of behaviour within their discussion.

4

Correlation designs

Correlation studies are conducted when the researcher is trying to explore the significance of links between variables. The researcher can use results from this type of design to demonstrate that associations may occur between two or more variables. Ware et al. (2007) conducted a correlation study to determine the reliability and validity of selected pain intensity scales to an older and cognitively impaired minority sample. The researchers were able to conclude that there was an association to the degree of cognitive impairment and preference in pain scale to ethnic groupings.

Quasi-experimental design

Quasi-experimental designs test theory, but the level of control applied may not be maximised as it would be in a true experimental design. The level of control may be reduced in a number of areas. First, the researcher may not be able to randomise subjects into control or experimental groups. Additionally, the researcher may not be able to manipulate the environment, or the independent variable. An example of **quasi-experimental research** can be seen in the work of Lee et al. (2006). These researchers examined the effectiveness of implementing a bladder ultrasound programme in neurosurgical units. While most of the conditions for an experiment were present, the researchers did not randomly sample from the population – in this case, the population being the patients who potentially required catheterisation. Instead, they chose a convenience sample, which is sometimes referred to as an 'accidental sample'. This type of sampling, according to Burns and Grove (2005), is a weak approach to sampling and therefore does not allow the researchers to reduce bias that may be introduced into the research.

Experimental designs

The purpose of **experimental research** is to examine cause and effect relationships. This approach applies maximum control over the research conditions to enable an objective investigation. A number of conditions must exist:

1 *Randomisation:* in which the researcher randomly assigns subjects to either the control or experimental group.
2 *Control:* refers to the use of one or more constraints into the research. This is usually a control group in which participants are assigned randomly, measurements recorded, but no manipulation of the variable is applied. The control and experimental groups are then compared.
3 *Manipulation:* experimental research aims to explain cause and effect relationships. The cause element of the study is the element that the researcher attempts to manipulate. This is referred to as the independent variable. By manipulating the independent variable, the research can examine the effect it has within the study. For example, Vanderwee et al. (2006) conducted an

experiment to investigate whether repositioning patients at specific time intervals reduced the incidence of pressure ulcers. This research is interesting, as the researchers accepted their null hypothesis, and found that more frequent repositioning did not lead to fewer pressure ulcers. They were able to conclude that the more frequent repositioning could not be considered as an effective preventive measure. In this study, the independent variable is the time periods for repositioning the patient, whereas the dependent variable is the incidence of pressure ulcers.

Methods of collecting data

Within quantitative research, a number of data collection methods are used, and their use is dependent upon the type of study that is being conducted. They broadly fall under five main headings. This includes physiological measurement, structured observation, self-reports like interviews and questionnaires, and documentary analysis.

Physiological measurement

Physiological or biological measurement is an objective way of obtaining data. A number of different approaches can by used within studies, for example taking blood pressure before and after exercise to determine the effects of exercise on blood pressure. The independent variable is the level of exercise, whereas the dependent variable is the blood pressure. Similarly, physiological measurement can be recorded to provide data for a study that seeks to determine the effect of psychological concepts like loss or bereavement upon individuals.

Structured observations

Some studies require structured observational measurement when the researchers are trying to determine how people behave or react under certain conditions. In quantitative research, the researchers must develop an observational tool to ensure that they are clear about what it is they are observing. LoBiondo-Wood and Haber (2001) argue that for observations to be scientific, they must fulfil four conditions:

1 The researchers must have a standardised, systematic plan for recording the data. This means that the researchers have to develop a plan that clearly indicates how the observations are going to be made, recorded and coded.
2 The observations must be consistent with the specific objectives of the study. Therefore, if the study is concerned with the number of times behaviour occurs, then that is what is measured, and inferences of behaviour or reasons why the behaviour occurred are not recorded.
3 All observations should be checked and controlled.
4 The observations must relate to scientific concepts and theories.

Structured interviews

Structuring interview schedules can enable the researcher to apply different degrees of control into the data collection. Because the schedules are designed prior to data collection, the researchers can specify the conduct of the interviewer. For example, in some studies, the researchers may allow the interviewers to clarify questions, whereas in other studies the interviewers have to order and control the manner in which they ask the questions.

While face-to-face interviews have been the norm in quantitative research, there has been a move towards telephone interviewing as a cost-effective and reliable form of structured interview. However, as with questionnaires, they are self-reporting methods of data collection and are dependent on truthful responses to the questions.

Questionnaires

Self-administered questionnaires can be offered in a number of different formats, ranging from a list of closed questions to a scale or questionnaires that require more detailed self-explanations. A researcher will use **closed questions** when they have determined a fixed number of responses. A number of scales, for example the **Likert scale**, use this strategy, requiring the respondent to choose between a selection of predetermined responses. **Open-ended questions** will be applied to a questionnaire by researchers who have not determined all the responses available.

Questionnaires and structured interviews are normally the main method of data collection of surveys. They tend to apply to methods of data collection that fall under the quantitative descriptive approaches. They can, however, be adopted in other research approaches where multiple methods of data collection are required.

Documentary analysis

This method of data collection enables the researcher to use existing records, and often apply a different perspective to the data they contain; for example, case notes of an individual will detail that individual's medical history. If the medical records of a population or geographical area are studied, descriptive data can be obtained to identify the incidence of specific conditions within that population, or geographical area.

Organisation and analysis of data

Once all the data have been collected, the researcher must make sense of, and organise in such a way that they can be analysed. The way data are organised is determined when the researcher specifies their research design. The type of analysis that the researcher engages with is, in turn, determined by the type and level of research conducted. Within quantitative designs, the emphasis is on measuring phenomena, therefore the data will be presented in the form of numbers.

Burns and Grove (2005) argue that nurses avoid statistics, as they do not have an understanding of statistical analysis or its meaning. There is a general tendency for readers of research to gloss over the data analysis section in a research report, when in fact it is possibly one of the most important sections.

Activity 18.1

Read a research report that employs some statistical analysis. Attempt to follow the way this analysis relates to the overall body of the research and how it informs the conclusions reached by the researcher.

To aid understanding of the analytical process, it is important to appreciate the following important concepts.

Hierarchy of measurement

When measurements are taken, they require a scale. These scales have been organised into a hierarchy of four levels to determine the type of statistical analysis that is applied to the data – **nominal scale**, **ordinal scale**, **interval scale** and **ratio scale**. Table 18.1 demonstrates the four levels of measurement with examples of how the scale is applied and the type of statistical analysis required.

Table 18.1 Levels of measurement

Level of measure-ment	How it is used	Examples of the type of data	Measure of central tendency	Measures of variance
Nominal	Organising data into categories/labels	Gender, hair colour, marital status, height, ethnicity (parametric data)	Mode	Range, percentage, frequency
Ordinal	You can assign to a category that information that can be ranked, but these intervals are unequal	Levels of wellness, intensity of pain (nonparametric data)	Mode and median	Range, percentage, frequency, semi-quartile
Interval	Ranking with equal intervals but no absolute zero	Measuring changes in temperature using Fahrenheit and Centigrade	Mode, median and mean	Range, percentage, frequency, semi-quartile, standard deviation
Ratio	Highest form of measurement, meeting the rules of nominal, ordinal and interval. Ratio has an absolute zero	Weight, length, reaction time, blood pressure, height, pulse	Mode, median and mean	The use of any statistical procedure is possible

4

Frequency

This is analysis at its most basic, in which the number of times each event occurs is counted. This analysis is often presented as a bar chart, graph or pie chart.

Measures of central tendency

In organising data, the researcher will begin to make sense of the data by summarising them, which can then lend itself to further statistical analysis. Often they will use measures of **central tendency**, which are the mode, the median and the mean:

1 The **mode** is represented as the score that occurs more frequently. For example, in the sequence of numbers below:

7 7 4 7 2 3 3 4 6 9 7

the mode = 7 as it occurs four times.

2 The **median** within the same values is calculated by putting the sequence in ascending order:

2 3 3 4 4 6 7 7 7 7 9

therefore, the median = 6.

The median is calculated by identifying the middle score in order of size. If an even number of values are presented, the median is calculated by taking the two middle values, adding them together and dividing by 2.

3 The **mean** is the average of the scores, and can be calculated by adding together all the values in the sequence and dividing it by the number of the values:

2 3 3 4 4 6 7 7 7 7 9 = 59 divided by 11

so the mean = 5.3.

The mode and the median are unaffected by a single extreme value, but the mean can be distorted if one of the values is greatly increased or decreased, known as an **outlier**.

Measures of variability

Not only are the measures of central tendency important in summarising data ready for further statistical analysis, but also the measures of **variability**, or dispersion. The two main methods of variability are the range and the standard deviation. The **range** is calculated by identifying the difference between the lowest and highest score. Referring back to the sequence of values used to explain the mean, mode and median, 2 3 3 4 4 6 7 7 7 7 9, the range is identified as 7.

The **standard deviation** is a measure of the distribution of scores around the mean. If the standard deviation of a group of scores is high, that means that more scores deviate from the mean. If the standard deviation is low, the group of scores bunch closely around the mean. Normally 68% of all scores in a distribution fall within one standard deviation. In this instance, this is referred to as a **normal distribution**.

Activity 18.2

From a basic research text, discover what a normal distribution bell curve looks like. Determine the ages of a cross-section of people on your course and from this data draw a simple bell curve showing the age distribution across your chosen population.

1 Was the curve skewed to the left or the right?
2 Did the majority of your subjects fall somewhere in the middle?
3 What inferences can you deduce from your results?

Inferential statistics

In considering the process of drawing statistical inference, be mindful that unless you are going to carry out a study, you will not necessarily need to understand how to carry out the different statistical tests. You do, however, need to understand the researcher's reasons for using the statistical tests. In nursing practice, you must use the best available evidence. You need to know that the study you are examining is both valid and reliable with the appropriate level of rigour.

The rationale for using statistical inference is twofold, according to LoBiondo-Wood and Haber (2005). First, the researcher may want to test a hypothesis about a population, or the researcher may want to estimate the probability that statistics found in the sample accurately reflect the population characteristic. When a researcher is designing a study to test a particular theory, they will develop a hypothesis, which is a predictive statement about the relationship between the independent and dependent variables.

In reality, the researcher attempts to disprove the hypothesis and prove a null hypothesis. The **null hypothesis** is an opposing statement, which states that there is no relationship between the variables. Mateo and Kirchoff (1999) claim that in 'research and therefore statistical analysis, nothing can be proved', arguing that the researcher is only studying a sample of a given population. However, statements about populations can be refuted. In effect, the researcher is unable to prove the hypothesis, but can show support for it by rejecting the opposing statement (null hypothesis) stating there is no relationship.

Before a researcher can generalise their findings from the sample they have used to the general population, their statistical testing must have taken account of a number of assumptions that underpin their use. Mateo and Kirchoff (1999) identify these assumptions to be:

1 The way in which the sample was drawn from the population
2 The level of measurement used
3 If the data suggest a normal distribution.

The last point is significant in terms of the type of **inferential statistics** to be used. There are two types of inferential statistics, parametric and nonparametric. These are demonstrated in Table 18.1 in relation to the level of measurement. In essence, **parametric tests** are used when the researcher is using the characteristics of a population that reflect a normal distribution. **Nonparametric tests** are tests that do not use the characteristics of a population and are therefore distribution free. These tests are normally applied when the measurements used are of nominal or ordinal scale.

The purpose of applying inferential statistics to the data is to find out whether or not the results have occurred by chance. In effect, the researcher is making an inference from their data, in that if the test highlights that the results were not due to chance, then if the research was repeated, the same results would be obtained and so the research results are significant. If, however, the test highlighted that the results were due to chance factors, then the researcher has been unable to factor in all small extraneous variables that have been too unpredictable to control, and so the research results are not significant.

Conclusion

This chapter has explored quantitative approaches to the collection and analysis of data that contributes to a body of knowledge within the discipline that it is conducted. A variety of different methods to collect data can be employed, including physiological measurement, structured observations, interviews and questionnaires, and documentary analysis. The approach adopted in quantitative research seeks to collect and analyse data primarily in numerical form. As such, the researcher can organise and summarise the data, and dependent upon the levels of measurement applied, can also make inferences about the data.

References

Burns, N and Grove, SK (2005) *The Practice of Nursing Research: Conduct, Critique and Utilisation* (5th edn), St Louis, MO: Elsevier Saunders

Duncan, CP and Dealey, C (2007) Patients' feelings about hand washing, MRSA status and patient information, *British Journal of Nursing*, **16**(1): 34–8

Graziano, AM and Raulin, ML (2004) *Research Methods: A Process of Inquiry* (5th edn), Boston: Allyn & Bacon

Lee, YY, Tsay, WL, Lou, MF and Dai, YT (2006) The effectiveness of implementing a bladder ultrasound programme in neurosurgical units, *Journal of Advanced Nursing*, **52**(2): 192–200

LoBiondo-Wood, G and Haber, J (eds) (2002) *Nursing Research Methods: Critical Appraisal and Utilisation* (5th edn), St Louis, MO: Mosby

Mateo, M and Kirchoff, KT (1999) *Using and Conducting Nursing Research in the Clinical Setting* (2nd edn), Philadelphia, PA: WB Saunders

Pharoo, K (2006) *Nursing Research Principles, Process and Issues* (2nd edn), Basingstoke: Palgrave Macmillan

Vanderwee, K, Grypdonck, MH, DeBaquer, D and Defloor, T (2006) The effectiveness of turning with unequal time intervals on the incidence of pressure ulcer lesions, *Journal of Advanced Nursing*, **57**(1): 59–68

Ware, LJ, Epps, CD, Herr, K and Packard, A (2006) Evaluation of the revised faces pain scale, verbal descriptor scale, numeric rating scale and Iowa pain thermometer in older minority adults, *Pain Management Nursing*, **7**(3): 117–25

4

19 qualitative research

Elaine Ball

In this chapter we will explore:

> What is meant by qualitative research
> The significance of qualitative methodology in research
> How qualitative data can be processed
> How one makes sense of data

What is meant by qualitative research?

Qualitative research is a methodological enquiry into social phenomena and its context. Detailed data are gathered from a series of collection methods usually comprising interview techniques, face-to-face interviews or **focus groups**. The conduct of the qualitative enquiry limits disruption of the natural environment of the phenomena of interest. The main feature of qualitative research is that its conveyance of an understanding of phenomena (findings) is reported in a literary style with participant commentaries. Unlike quantitative analysis, which measures outcomes and has strict controls, qualitative analysis is flexible and inductive, with its own logical processes that have to be accessible to the critical reader. This process is listed below (Hungler and Polit 1993):

> to *describe* a phenomenon
> to *explore* the scope and context of a phenomenon
> to *explain* why things happen the way they do
> to *generate* an outcome
> to holistically *report* an outcome.

Some qualitative studies adopt one or more of the above reasons, but all have at least one as their justification to carry out a study. Some examples below are given of research that principally fulfils these reasons.

The description of a phenomenon

This is a pretty straightforward goal of qualitative analysis in the traditional sense: it is to gain understanding of and answers to questions that have been posed from issues in the world around us. Traditional fields of qualitative methodology, such as ethnography, **phenomenology** (Husserl and Heidegger) and **grounded theory** (Glaser and Strauss 1967; Corbin and Strauss 1990), all have at their core a descriptive content that forms the building blocks of data collection, analysis and interpretation. Collectively, these terms can be described as three qualitative strategies concerned with real-world interpretation.

The exploration of a phenomenon

Sometimes, there exist issues that defy description in the literal, scientific sense and can only be described when placed into a context. Qualitative research is committed to a real-world approach that includes multiple viewpoints and contextual veracity. In 1984, a nurse researcher called Patricia Benner published her book, *From Novice to Expert*. In this qualitative work, Benner explores the notions of competence, experience and expertise. As isolated attributes, competence, experience and expertise mean very little. It is only when they are placed into a certain context and qualitatively analysed from a nursing perspective that they begin to have collective meaning.

Benner's work tries to capture the importance of experience, which is core to the qualitative pursuit, and defines certain steps of a nurse's development along a continuum, from 'novice' to 'expert' in the context of nursing practice. For the first time, experience is seen as a valuable component of nurses' experience and credentials for authoritative practice. This means that qualitative research begins to play a valuable role in the nursing profession. Benner explores how experience affects nursing work and the phenomenon of intuition emerges as a vital part of the journey towards expertise. This work has influenced nurse training in almost every sphere since. *From Novice to Expert* remains one of the bestselling books in nursing to date. Over 20 years later, it is still on many reading lists.

The explanation of a phenomenon

Qualitative research is a vital tool for questioning current thought on a particular area in time and describes how phenomena occur. A good example of this process is the work of a doctor called John Snow (1813–58), who turned his critical eye to the phenomenon of cholera. In the mid-nineteenth century, the spread of disease was attributed to 'miasma', or foul air. In particular, cholera was seen as being spread by this method. The science of microbiology had not developed at this time, and 'miasmatic theory' conveniently explained the spread of the disease.

Snow was a sceptic of the miasma theory, and published an essay *On the Mode of Communication of Cholera* in 1849. In 1854, he conducted a famous investigation into the Broad Street cholera outbreak, where he discovered that the source of cholera was, in fact, a water pump at this location. The story goes that he removed the handle from the pump, and the outbreak ceased. Snow was not one for conjecture, and he used detailed maps to plot the outbreak and statistical techniques to process his data. However, he also used qualitative

4

analysis to contextualise the problem and justify the results and, most importantly, disseminate the findings to the largely uneducated public. In so doing, he proved that water companies supplying water contaminated with sewage had an increased incidence of the disease. However, it was qualitative analysis, coupled with quantitative analysis that made the findings relevant and useful in terms of addressing the general public and the water company. This study was a ground-breaking event in the field of public health, saved thousands of lives and is a founding study for the discipline of qualitative **epidemiology**, the social study of illness and disease among populations.

The prediction of a phenomenon

Perhaps the most apt example of ground-breaking research in the area of disease causation can be attributed to Florence Nightingale (1820–1910). During her tenure as a nurse in the military hospitals in the Crimea, Nightingale was appalled at the unsanitary conditions of the care facilities for wounded soldiers. She discovered that more troops were dying of disease than actual wounds inflicted in battle, and set about proving this.

A noted statistician, Nightingale had already examined the data from Napoleon's disastrous Russian campaign, and had refuted the commonly accepted conclusion that the French troops had frozen to death. More likely, she argued, was that they had succumbed to disease because of unsanitary conditions. She thus used her mathematic understanding to support and develop theories to understand the social world in which she nursed.

In the Crimea, she famously compiled data on mortality, with seasonal variations. These findings were presented in a form of her own design, now called a 'polar area diagram'. This allowed people in influential positions with little or no statistical training to interpret her findings visually. It was the linking of quantitative and qualitative analysis that gave her such rich results. Like fellow epidemiologist John Snow before her, the use of qualitative social theory along with statistics justified her conclusions that sanitary conditions were a prerequisite to effective patient care. Consequently, there was a predictable link between the reduction of mortality and the quality of the care environment.

In her *Notes on Nursing*, Florence Nightingale was among the first recorded practitioners in Western healthcare who considered environmental elements and the means to manipulate them qualitatively when contemplating patient care. In her text, Nightingale (1859, p. 142) proposed that the environment plays a vital role in the nurse–patient relationship by stating: 'And what nursing has to do ... is put the patient in the best condition for nature to act upon him.'

From this observation, Nightingale argues that the patient's condition can be optimised by careful consideration to ventilation, noise, light and cleanliness, among other things. More importantly, she could prove this through social and statistical analysis. This work, along with the studies of hand washing by Ignaz Semmelweis (1818–1865) in the late 1840s and the promotion of aseptic technique by Joseph Lister (1827–1912) in the late 1860s, is the cornerstone of modern nursing practice today. Together, they prove the prediction that cleanliness reduces infection and mortality and also confirm that if cleanliness is neglected, then increased infection is a predictable outcome.

Key parts of any qualitative research study

Qualitative research studies are packaged differently, depending on who the audience is, what the subject matter is, what methods were used, and the social context. Each qualitative data method can be given a different look and feel because of this. For the moment, though, let's not concentrate on the things that make individual projects different, but what makes them the same. It may surprise the research novice to know that, in spite of different approaches, all research projects share some common features, shown in Table 19.1.

Table 19.1 Key elements common to all research studies

An investigator's agenda	Research term used to describe this
A problem or issue, research question or hypothesis	Same terms
The background of the issues to be investigated	Literature review
Identification of elements to examine	Variables
A population of subjects	Sample
Apply a method of investigation where the elements interact with the subjects	Methodology
Gather the information using the method	Collection
Look at the results	Analysis
Talk about the findings	Discussion

Activity 19.1

Identify two suitable research papers from any nursing journal. You could ask a tutor or mentor to help you. Look at them and see if you can identify all the elements in Table 19.1 in each paper.

4

The following sections look at each of these elements in greater detail.

Problems, questions and hypotheses in research

With all qualitative research, there is a starting point. Generally, this may be in the form of a statement to be tested (a hypothesis), a problem or real-world issue that needs investigation, or an appraisal-driven research question that requires sufficient investigation and evidence to answer satisfactorily. A research study may identify one or all of these starting points before setting out on the investigative journey.

Finding the problem

What, then, should we be looking for when we read a piece of qualitative research? We need to look for a strategy that is well thought out and shows that the researcher has used the most appropriate resources to answer the problem. In addition, we need to know what methodology has been employed.

Methodology

In a nursing context, a **methodology** is very much like a plan of care for a client. The researcher, having worked out *what* and *who* to ask, then needs to utilise a qualitative method of *how* to ask these questions. Traditionally, the qualitative researcher will choose a method of inductive or reflexive analysis. Sometimes, researchers can combine measuring and social engagement, as we noted above, but usually one is more dominant than the other. Some key differences in each of these methods are listed in Table 19.2.

Table 19.2 Differences between quantitative and qualitative methods

Quantitative	Qualitative
Tests ideas and/or develops theories through measurement	Develops ideas and concepts through questioning
By using measurement, can establish causation and interplay of phenomena	Develops meaning and significance by cognitive engagement with subjects
The researcher uses instruments to collect data, relying on impartiality and objectivity to elicit data	The researcher is the instrument of data collection, relying on communication and facilitation to elicit data

This list is by no means exhaustive, and each area is covered in more detail in this chapter and Chapter 18. Suffice it to say that, for the moment, the research method is a crucial part of any study, which should be theoretically sound and fit for the intended purpose.

In order to involve you in the qualitative research process, an exercise has been devised for you to involve yourself in. It is a qualitative research experience using a narrative research method.

Activity 19.2

You can do this exercise in groups of two or three. It also enables you to be personally involved in a two-way process – to be involved in the content of the research and also play the role of the researcher.

Confidentiality and moral obligation towards your sample is a given in any research. Please respect the confidentiality of the discussions and do not repeat anything you hear outside your group.

Bear in mind the following points:

• Aim to make your research narrative reflective rather than descriptive.

- The purpose of the exercise is to understand the event as it is interpreted.
- The values attached to the narrative should be understood and taken into account when recounting the research.
- Remember that you are the primary collection instrument; ask what are your values, biases and judgements on the research narrative.
- The results are focused on gaining real, rich and deep data.

To begin:

1 Look at the statements below
   - Recount an experience where you felt close to a patient or family member.
   - Recount an experience where you felt most supported by your nursing colleagues.
   - Recount an experience where you felt most let down by nursing or your team.
   - Recount an experience where you felt you had made your finest contribution, so far, to patients or the nursing team.

2 One of you acts as timekeeper – take one turn each, timing each speaker for two minutes as they recount their experience (be strict).

3 The person in the next seat but one writes up the story as it is being spoken.

4 As a researcher, your aim is to bring about dialogue and reciprocal exchange, so do not judge or challenge your subject.

5 Each take a turn in the three roles.

Narrative interpretation:

1 Try and understand the ways in which the sample's values and meanings influence how they construct, reflect upon and reiterate their story.

2 Feel free to draw upon the other shared stories and how a common narrative might be taking shape (is there an emerging group narrative?).

3 Is there a particular discourse emerging from the narratives, perhaps a caring discourse?

4 Narrative research is a constructive and reconstructive process, one which enables you to take a step back and see the cultural and contextual setting in which you exist.

5 Are there any main themes emerging?

6 Do not look for a consensus view, let differences emerge.

A particularly useful aspect of this research method is that it is a participatory process that has the potential to enrich the lives of those involved, while simultaneously enhancing the development of nursing practice.

4

Analysis of the data

Analysis is the detailed examination of gathered information. The whole aim of doing research is to yield information that can help the investigator answer the questions they began with. All this information needs to be processed, organised and examined rigorously. Any departure from this intention may introduce errors, which could ultimately lead the researcher to the wrong answer. Indeed, when one examines research that has been published, it is a major part of the critical process to question how the researcher has dealt with the data.

Typically, researchers use a variety of methods that can employ both numbers (statistics) and words to describe the findings. Exactly how these data are processed is dealt with in Chapter 20. Almost always, researchers offer a brief literature review near the beginning of a study. This helps them to tell the reader the key information to date about the topic in question, and places their issue under investigation into some sort of context.

Asking the right question

Remind yourself of the components of a research question by revisiting Chapter 17. You will see that supplementary to the hypothesis is the notion of the research question. This differs from the hypothesis, in that a question is something that needs to be answered and a hypothesis is a conjecture that can be either proven or refuted. Research questions also share common features but there are differences depending on the methodology in use. For example, typical questions that a qualitative study might seek to answer are:

> What is it like to have a certain condition?
> What does it mean for the patient?
> What has the experience been like?
> What do you think helped you through this experience?
> Has anything in particular made the experience better or worse?

Activity 19.3

Identify a suitable nursing research paper that examines any of the above questions and use the checklist below to test the meaning of the paper. You can ask your tutor or mentor to help you.

Table 19.3 The research consumer's checklist of critical questions

Key elements in a qualitative research paper	Questions to ask
Hypothesis, question or problem	Is the problem clearly stated?
Literature review	Is this relevant and up to date?
Goal characteristics	Are the data emergent, flexible and descriptive?
Sample	Is the sample small, nonrandom, theoretical? How many people were asked? How many people completed the study?
Methodology	Is the researcher also a primary instrument? Are there interviews and observations? Is it practical? Is it ethical?
Collection	What types of data did the method give? How were these data collected? What was done with the unprocessed data? How long did collection take? Who was involved?

Key elements in a qualitative research paper	Questions to ask
Analysis/reporting	Is the study inductive (by researcher)? Are any data missing? Does this reporting make sense to the reader?
Discussion	Do the data answer or address the issues identified at the start? Is the paper comprehensive and holistic? What does this have to do with me?

Discussion: do the data answer the original question posed?

After analysing the data, the researcher must come full circle and revisit the original questions asked. If the previous steps have been completed correctly, the researcher will not only be in a position to answer these questions, but also to say to what degree they are proven or refuted.

Whether or not the initial question or hypothesis is proven or not is, surprisingly, not the main priority. Principally, it is how these answers have been derived that is the most critical aspect of research – how rigorously the process has been followed. On this rests the possibility of applying credible findings to a wider population with confidence and certainty, or of the study being repeated in the future by another researcher.

Researchers will also refer back to the important literature surrounding their area of study. They would traditionally use this to form a background to the research at the start of the paper. This helps to place the issues in question in some frame of context, but also gives the writer the opportunity to say what is unique about their contribution to the field. Furthermore, the **discussion** allows the researcher to 'come clean' about any weaknesses of their study, and what, in retrospect, could have been done to fix these inconsistencies.

You can see in the example below how the four elements of hypothesis, sample, process and outcome are all present:

> *Hypothesis:* This could be put as: 'Surgical nurses on ward A1 react badly to a shift-pattern change initiative.'
> *Sample:* The staff on A1 surgical ward.
> *Process:* A 'focus group', asking them to describe their experiences during the change process.
> *Outcome:* A set of results is generated that can prove or disprove the hypothesis, and hopefully bring about a solution to the identified gap or problem.

You might also find other research elements in a paper. Although quality and description lie at the heart of all qualitative research, not all studies are performed in the same way. Each method has certain characteristics that lend it to answering a particular question or issue. How these are employed depends largely on whether the mode of investigation is:

4

> ethical
> practical
> workable
> timely
> cost-effective
> emergent (phenomena in a natural setting).

Example of a qualitative research method

This section looks at an example of a qualitative research method and why it is particularly suited to its application. That said, all qualitative studies set out to either observe or describe something, or describe the effect of one or more factors on another. The most obvious example of a qualitative study is one that immerses itself in a natural, ethnographic setting utilising participant observer research. Detailed data are gathered through open-ended questions that provide direct quotations, for example the case report. The interviewer is an integral part of the investigation and is often involved in the reflexive process.

Case series

A case control study is useful in examining questions about the experience or value-driven outcomes of a particular health issue/health problem/disease (Greenhalgh 2001). It is also useful in assessing changes in health service management or organisation; particularly when the researcher is involved in the **fieldwork** (Craig and Smyth 2002). A case report describes the medical history of a single patient and a number of case reports can be run together to form a case series. Its disadvantage is that it provides weak scientific evidence, but positively it provides a unique insight into the perceptions and experiences of patients; findings which can be utilised in patient-led initiatives featuring a unique personal narrative. The case series also has a number of other creditable points to recommend it:

> information can be conveyed that is subsumed in a trial or observational study
> information can be quickly written up
> the narratives can be understood by non-academics and lay readers.

Although the case series plays an important role in gaining patient perceptions, it is classified as low evidence and placed at the lower end of the hierarchy of evidence.

The hierarchy of evidence is a pyramid-shaped model employed to analyse critically and rank methodologies in order of scientific rigour and critical exactitude (Figure 19.1). Quantitative data in the form of systematic reviews and **randomised control trials** are placed at the top of the pyramid, while more qualitative studies are ranked below. As you can see, the case report comes at the bottom end. In terms of making evidence fact and influencing change, the

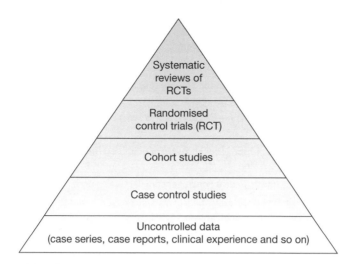

Figure 19.1 *Hierarchy of evidence*

case series has a specialist role based on verisimilitude rather than the scientific veracity that quantitative analysis generates. What this means is that quantitative analysis has more scientific authority than its qualitative counterpart; however, in terms of what we want to know as nurses, qualitative analysis supports many of the questions we pose as nurses, so that rather than shoehorning our ideas into the quantitative precision of statistical analysis, we are able to ask the right questions and be confident that the hopes, expectations, fears and experiences of patients and nurses are answered methodically employing the logical processes of qualitative methods.

Conclusion

Qualitative analysis is more than an agent in the mechanics of knowledge transfer; it is a method that, if used correctly, conveys answers to some of the most fundamental questions in health delivery today posed by nurses and others. It enables those who employ it as a means of quality enhancement to embed changes locally within their own real-world environment but also generate an evidence base that can support new knowledge, learning and, most importantly, improvement of patient care.

4

Further reading

Greenhalgh, T and Donald, A (2000) *Evidence Based Health Care Workbook*, London: BMJ

Muir Gray JA (1997) *Evidence-based Healthcare*, London: Churchill Livingstone

Polit, DF, Beck, CT and Hungler, BP (2001) *Essentials of Nursing Research: Methods, Appraisal and Utilisation*, Philadelphia: Lippincott

Sackett, DL, Straus, SE, Scott Richardson, W et al. (2000) *Evidence-based Medicine: How to Practice and Teach EBM*, London: Churchill Livingstone

References

Benner, P (1984) *From Novice to Expert: Excellence and Power in Clinical Nursing Practice*, Menlo Park, CA: Addison-Wesley

Corbin, J and Strauss, A (1990) Grounded theory research: procedures, canons, and evaluative criteria, *Qualitative Sociology*, 13: 3–21

Craig, JV and Smyth, RL (2002) *The Evidence-based Practice Manual for Nurses*, Edinburgh: Elsevier Science

Glaser, BG and Strauss, AL (1967) *The Discovery of Grounded Theory: Strategies for Qualitative Research*, New York: Aldine

Greenhalgh, T (2001) *How to Read a Paper*, London: BMJ

Hungler, BP and Polit, DF (1993) *Essentials of Nursing Research: Methods, Appraisal and Utilisation*, New York: Lippincott Williams & Wilkins

Nightingale, F (1859) *Notes on Nursing: What It Is, and What It Is Not*, London: Harrison & Sons

Snow, J (1849) *On the Mode of Communication of Cholera*, London: John Churchill

4

getting research into practice

Annette Jinks and James Richardson

In this chapter we will explore:

> How to keep up to date with nursing research
> Accessing the relevant literature
> Reading the literature
> Critiquing published research

Introduction

When caring for patients it is vital that nurses use best practice approaches. Evidence-based practice principles are geared towards providing best practice guidelines. An essential part of the evidence-based practice agenda is that nursing care has its foundations in sound, robust research findings. However, it is important to remember that a single research study rarely provides all the answers, which is why the findings of replicated studies and systematic **reviews** of the studies done in a particular research area are the bread and butter of evidence-based practice approaches. Opening sections of this chapter cover subject areas such as the importance of keeping up to date and how to access relevant research literature and synthesised information concerning the findings of systematic reviews. Later sections deal with reading research literature and guidelines for critically appraising research publications.

Keeping up to date

Imagine you have successfully finished your programme. You have now graduated and are working in the world of healthcare. There are no lecturers to chivvy you along and there are no assignments to make sure you keep up to date. You have settled in and are happy and comfortable in the practice area where you work. So how do you keep up to date with the ever changing world of clinical practice? How do you make sure you continue to give the best care possible?

National bodies in the UK such as the Nursing and Midwifery Council (NMC) give guidelines on how to keep up to date in order that you to continue to provide the highest standards of care. For example, **post-registration education and practice** (PREP) is a set of NMC standards and guidance designed to help you provide a high standard of practice and care (NMC

2008). PREP helps you to keep up to date with new developments in practice and encourages you to think about and reflect on your practice. These are legal requirements, which you must meet in order for your registration to be renewed. The NMC does regular audits of people's professional portfolios called 'revalidation' in order to ensure practitioners comply with these regulations.

Activity 20.1

Go to Chapter 15 and read the section on Clinical supervision. Reflect on the meanings stated here regarding the importance of practitioners maintaining their skills and knowledge through continuing professional development.

A wide-ranging number of activities count as continuing professional development. For example, it can be as simple as you listening to a colleague who is giving an updating session in your clinical area. It can also be a more formal activity such as attending an employer-organised study day, going to a conference or enrolling on a programme of study at your local higher education institute. However, these activities should be directed at improving your practice, usually by employing reflective learning approaches. A cornerstone to improving practice is through knowledge and understanding of the pertinent research in a particular area and applying the principles of evidence-based practice.

Starting out

One way of keeping up to date can be as simple as going to the local healthcare library or logging onto one of the many databases that give details of healthcare research and familiarising yourself with the latest research findings concerning an aspect of your practice. Your reflections on reading research-based journal articles and incorporating the findings into your practice help to get research into practice. It costs nothing and can be an effective way of improving the evidence base of practice.

However, the first two questions you may need to ask are: Do you need to look at a range of articles on the subject area you are interested in? Do you need to search the literature yourself from scratch or has this been done already? There are now many resources available to you that provide easily digestible information on the subject you are interested in, that is, the findings of systematic literature reviews that underpin a particular area of clinical practice. For example, the Cochrane Collaboration (http://www.cochrane.org/index.htm) gives free access to numerous systematic reviews on various aspects of clinical practice, known as Cochrane Reviews. As well as giving full reports of the systematic reviews undertaken, the Cochrane Collaboration also gives short, easily read abstracts that are designed for layperson consumption. Similarly, the Joanne Briggs Institution (http://www.joannabriggs.edu.au/

about/home.php) is an Australian-based organisation that undertakes evidence-based reviews on a variety of healthcare topics and gives short summaries of the findings of the review undertaken. Finally, Bandolier (http://www.medicine.ox.ac.uk/bandolier) is also a useful source for accessing information on various aspects of evidence-based healthcare. Bandolier presents its findings as simple bullet points of those things that worked and those that did not. The information used by the Cochrane Collaboration, Joanne Briggs Institute and Bandolier comes from systematic reviews, **meta-analyses**, randomised trials and high-quality observational studies. These sources give relatively short, easily accessible accounts of relevant research and the strength of evidence about particular aspects of clinical practice. For example, it may be that you are interested in tissue viability and compression bandaging for venous leg ulcers and would therefore find the Cullum et al. (2001) report summary on the Cochrane website a useful starting point to investigate.

Accessing the relevant literature

Assuming that a systematic review of the subject area you are interested in is not available and you need to find the relevant research articles yourself, you can of course just go to the library and browse through the available journals on the library shelves. It is certainly one way of keeping yourself abreast with the latest approaches and may be something you may decide to do in any case later on in your search of the literature. For example, hand searching of key journals or back-chaining from the reference lists of research papers you have located is useful but usually undertaken in later stages of a search. However, initially you may decide that it is very much a scattergun approach. You may find a more targeted approach is better as it makes more efficient use of your time.

If you have a relatively clear idea of the area you want to investigate, it may be quicker for you and more systematic if you initially search one of the many electronic databases that give publication details of the available research literature. This is the type of approach used by those who produce evidence-based guidelines such as the Cochrane Collaboration, Joanne Briggs Institute and Bandolier. There are lots of electronic databases to search. Some common ones used by healthcare researchers are CINAHL (Cumulative Index for Nursing and Allied Health), Proquest nursing journals, MEDLINE (PubMed), BNI (British Nursing Index), PsycINFO, the Social Science Citation Index and the Web of Science. These databases will give you the publication details of the papers you may be interested in. In some instances, they will also give you access to the paper's abstract or even the full text version of the paper. Initially, you will, however, also need to decide which search words to use to help you search the electronic database. For example, if you wanted to look for a paper that focuses on learning disability nursing, you will need to use all the possible variations of the term 'learning disability nursing'. Variations may well include, for example, learning disability, learning disabilities, learning difficulties, intellectual disabilities, mental handicap, or even, mental retardation.

4

Once you have selected the search words to use, it is advisable to choose more than one of the electronic databases mentioned earlier to search. This way you can be more certain that you are retrieving all the publication details in the area you are interested in. It is recognised, even today, when many more people are computer literate, that to undertake such activities for the first time may be daunting. Therefore if you are new to using these types of search approaches, the best person to help you decide where the most relevant research papers can be found, that is, which electronic databases to search, and how to develop your searching skills is your healthcare librarian. They are a useful resource not to be undervalued, who will be able to guide you in the right direction and have a wealth of subject-based knowledge. Don't, however, expect them to do the literature searching for you.

Another source of information you may decide you need to access is the grey literature. **Grey literature** is commonly defined as any documentary material that is not commercially published and typically comprises such things as government and organisational reports, unpublished research reports, working papers and conference proceedings (Coad et al. 2006). The greatest challenge to the use of grey literature is the proverbial 'finding a needle in a haystack' situation, as it first involves identifying and gaining access to the pertinent information. Those with access to the internet will find that grey literature is freely available on numerous websites as many organizations and individuals now provide access to their works online. There are also a number of commercial websites that provide access to selectively indexed information. For example, Wikipedia is a web-based encyclopedia, which may help give you some starting out information, and doing an internet search using a search engine such as Google will almost certainly give you access to lots of this type of information. However, the absence of editorial control and journal peer review systems, which are a feature of the majority of research-based health-care journals, raises questions about the reliability of information from these types of source. As such, these sources are not usually accepted as a reference source by higher education institutions for these reasons. Greater reliability may result by searching an agency or institution website that is more likely to produce robust research-based literature. For example, in the UK, a search of the Department of Health website http://www.dh.gov.uk/en/Researchand-development/Researchanddevelopmentpublications/index.htm gives access to Department of Health-funded research and development reports. The National Institute of Clinical Excellence (NICE) also provides free access to research-based clinical guidelines (http://www.nice.org.uk/Guidance/Type). Finally, the Royal College of Nursing website gives access to the abstracts of recent nursing research conferences (http://www.rcn.org.uk/newsevents/events). However, to return to the point made at the beginning of this section, a thorough search for the grey literature on a subject is not easy and may require you looking at a large number of different sources.

Reading the literature

Many novices and indeed even experienced researchers find reading some research papers is often heavy going as they are primarily designed for an academic audience. This obviously puts the uninitiated off reading this type of literature. However, one thing that may take the initial sting out of accessing this type of literature is knowing what to expect in the first place – what the common structure of a research paper may be and how to find your way around it. Table 20.1 presents a brief guide to how research articles are commonly presented.

Table 20.1 The common structure of a report of a research study

Abstract	An abstract should not be confused with the introduction, as it should give an overview of all the content of the paper. It may be useful to initially scan the abstract to establish the relevance of the paper to the topic area of your search
Introduction	This is the curtain-raiser and should give you a clear idea of what the article is about and the background of the topic area. A clear statement of the research problem or question is usually given and why the research topic area is important to improving clinical practice
Literature review	The literature review section usually covers what research has already been done into the topic area, the relationship of the study's focus to previous research and any omissions in the literature. A good paper will give an account of how the literature review has been undertaken – the literature review methodology – which will give you reassurances that a strong evidence base underpins the findings of the review. Gaps in the literature obviously give added justification for doing the research
Methods	This section of a research article focuses on the way the information or data have been gathered. Research design refers to how the study has been framed and research methods refer to how the data have been collected. So, for example, a researcher might use a survey design and a questionnaire method
	The principles of data analysis are also usually outlined at this point. In number-crunching-type research (quantitative methods), it may be the statistical data analysis undertaken that is described, whereas in narrative-type research (qualitative methods), a description of how the qualitative data analysis has been undertaken is described. Examples of qualitative data analysis approaches are, for example, thematic content analysis or grounded theory approaches
Results	The results are merely that, what the researchers have found out from their investigations
	In quantitative studies, the authors will present their findings in a neutral fashion and reserve comment until the discussion section. Statistical analysis may be illustrated by use of graphs and tables
	Qualitative researchers often use actual quotations from those who have been involved in the research to illustrate their findings. Commonly in qualitative research, authors merge results and discussion sections together where they will refer back to the literature and make comment on the study's findings in a merged results/discussion section

4

Discussion	In both qualitative and quantitative research, the discussion element of an article is probably the most significant, and this is an important reason why articles must be read from beginning to end and not just beginning and end. The discussion section should link back to the research question/s and the literature review findings. It will give the authors' understanding on the research conducted and is where analytical thought comes into its own. Suggestions for future research will also be given
References	These may be useful in giving an idea of the standard of research conducted. For example, if the reference list is thin or the articles cited are dated, this raises questions about the scholarship of the paper. Importantly, references may give pointers to how to find out more about the subject. For example, closer examination of the references may give you hints to which other articles may be important sources of information

If you wish to look at how these feature in a typical research paper, why not try accessing and reading Jinks and Chalder (2007), which describes a study looking at mental health consultant nurses.

Critiquing research

So you have got your research papers and feel happy with what to expect from your initial reading of them. The next step is to critically read and evaluate the worth of the evidence presented in the papers. Critiquing (or making a judgement) might seem to be an academic word and often incites anxiety; it is, however, an activity we all do frequently in our everyday lives. For example, many television programmes ask you to critique or judge the worth of an individual's performance in diverse programmes such as talent competitions, ballroom dancing or even cooking skills. Although we are looking at critiquing research papers, we are looking at similar processes – the content, level of performance and how it compares with others are being evaluated and judgements made on its worth. To give a more precise definition in the context of the subject matter of this chapter, critiquing research literature is 'the careful consideration of both the strengths and limitations of a published piece of research' (Rees 2003).

There is often a tendency for us to accept uncritically the conclusions of a piece of published research. It is hard to accept that authors with an impressive range of qualifications who have published in esteemed research journals may have got it wrong. There are examples in the history of science when a whole body of evidence is questionable. For example, although there is controversy around the exact details of Sir Cyril Burt's failings, it has been claimed that the method of factor analysis he was reputed to have developed in psychological testing was in fact the work of his mentor and predecessor as chair of the psychology department at University College London, Charles Spearman (Blinkhorn 1995). Burt is also known for his studies on the effect of heredity on intelligence. Shortly after he died, his studies of inheritance and intelligence came into disrepute after evidence emerged indicating he had falsified research data (Loring Brace 2005). However, instances such as this are relatively rare, and it is more usual to find that authors may not have got it all right rather than being entirely wrong. When you are reading a paper, what you need to discover is where authors perhaps have not got it all right and come to a balanced conclusion on the strengths and limitations of the paper you are reviewing.

In order to successfully critique a body of research, you will need:

> Some basic research knowledge and understanding of the research approaches being used
> A systematic critique framework.

The following sections look at these two points.

Basic appraisal of research approaches

Chapters 18 and 19 give an introduction to differing research approaches. The following gives a hierarchy of how the strength of research evidence for biomedical sciences interventions may be viewed. While primarily designed to help healthcare practitioners make decisions concerning which intervention is best for the patient, it may also help to give you some initial guidance to how the approaches taken in the various studies you are looking at may be classified.

Development of this hierarchy of evidence has been informed by a number of sources (including, for example, Closs and Cheater 1999; Polit and Beck 2008; Atkins et al. 2004). A simple version of the strength of evidence derived from various research designs is given in Table 20.2.

Table 20.2   Hierarchy of research evidence in the biomedical sciences

Grade	Design	Definitions
1	Systematic review and meta-analysis	Systematic review is appraisal of a body of literature. The use of explicit methods to locate the relevant papers and precise criteria to assess the quality of the papers are hallmarks of a systematic review Meta-analysis is a statistical analysis that combines or integrates the results of several clinical trials or randomised controlled trials
2	A single randomised control trial	Individuals are randomly allocated to either a control group or a group that receives a specific intervention – commonly a new form of treatment. Otherwise the two groups are identical. Differences in outcomes and the probabilities of any differences in outcomes occurring by chance are established using statistical analysis
3	Cohort studies	Groups of people are selected on the basis of their exposure to a particular treatment and followed up to establish what the outcomes are
4	Case control studies	'Cases' with the condition or illness are matched with 'controls' without the condition or illness. A retrospective analysis is used to look for differences between the two groups

Grade	Design	Definitions
5	Surveys	A questionnaire or interview study of a sample of the population of interest
6	Case studies	A report based on a single patient or subject; sometimes collected together into a short series of investigations
7	Expert opinion	A consensus of experience from well-known, respected scholars. Journal editorials often fit into this category

You will have noticed that in the above hierarchy there is virtually no mention of qualitative research designs or methods. This stems partly from opinions as to the relative worth of qualitative research and that it is less widely valued as a source of evidence. However, in nursing, qualitative research may often be the most suitable approach, owing to the nature of the research questions being addressed. This is because nurses are often concerned not only with the effectiveness of an intervention – where the biomedical hierarchy of evidence comes into its own – but also the patients' and their families' experiences of the illness for which they are being treated. Understanding these illness experiences is where deploying qualitative research designs and methods can be most useful.

Nevertheless, there are obviously good and poor qualitative research studies. While less common, some authors do give an overview of what to look for generally in assessing the quality of qualitative research studies. For example, Willis (2007) describes four levels of a qualitative hierarchy that may be applied to assessment of quality of the evidence for practice. A summary of the hierarchy adapted from Willis's findings is given in Table 20.3.

Table 20.3 *Hierarchy of research evidence in qualitative research*

Grade	Definitions	Features
1	Generalisable studies	Conceptual frameworks are developed from detailed analysis of data. An appropriately diversified sample is used in the study
2	Conceptual thematic approach	Detailed description of both analysis and findings. The findings are used to develop a conceptual framework but are limited due to lack of diversity in the sample group
3	Descriptive study only	Detailed description of data is given with helpful quotations illustrating the findings but little detail of analysis is given
4	Single case study	Limited description and analysis of a single case study. Often these types of studies are small, locally based investigations

You may find it useful to refer to Chapter 19 where the relevant methods are described.

Using a systematic critique framework

Well, we are nearly there. You have located some research papers that focus on your area of interest, scan read your papers, decided generally how the papers are structured and how they fit into a hierarchy of research evidence – or have started to assess the quality of the studies being described. The final step in your quest to keep up to date and improve your practice through reading research literature is to use a more detailed and systematic framework to structure your reading and critique the individual papers you are reviewing.

There are many research critique guides available. Some, such as those of Polit and Beck (2006), give a number of differing guides that are appropriate for reviewing different types of studies. For example, not only do Polit and Beck describe the principles of critiquing quantitative research methods but they also give a guide for appraising just one type of research design such as a meta-analysis. Such guides are useful especially when you get more experienced but can be a bit off-putting when you are first starting out. It is hoped that Tables 20.4–7 give an easily applied structure, which conforms to the usual areas given in most other similar guidelines.

First you need to assess the credibility and relevance of the paper. The questions given in Table 20.4 may be useful here.

Table 20.4 Critiquing the credibility and relevance of a paper

Elements	Checklist
Author/s	Who is/are the author/s? Do the authors' qualifications and position indicate detailed knowledge of the subject area? Are the authors based at a university or clinical research centre with a well-established track record of research into the topic or is the research part of a whole programme of research activities?
Journal	Which journal has the paper been published in? Has the journal got a reputation of publishing high-quality, internationally significant research? Has the journal got high-impact value? Impact value is based on journal citation record and gives an indication of the quality of the journal but is not an indication of the quality of individual paper
Funding	Is the research a commissioned piece of research? If so, who is the funding body? If it has been funded by one of the research councils such as the Medical Research Council, it would indicate that the **research proposal** and conduct of the research has been rigorously reviewed. Even small, locally funded projects will have been the subject of review, as it is rare to receive money for a project where value for money and robust, credible findings are not important. You may also want to consider the converse. Funding provided by a pressure group may have introduced an inherent bias into the study's findings
Title	What is the title of the publication? Does the title adequately describe the study? Is the title concise and free from distracting phrases? Beware of catchy titles that are used for effect that may not necessarily be an indication of quality
Abstract	Does the abstract clearly summarise the study's purpose, methods and findings? Does the abstract provide you with sufficient information to determine whether the article fits with the area of practice you are interested in?

4

Presentation

Another earlier feature of the article you need to assess is how it is presented and 'sold' to the audience. Table 20.5 gives questions that may be useful to ask yourself about how the paper is presented.

Table 20.5 *Critiquing the presentation of a paper*

Elements	Checklist
General impressions	Is the report well written? Is it concise, grammatically correct and is the use of jargon avoided wherever possible? It is important not to be put off by the language of research. While in good reports the use of jargon is avoided, it is still important to use the correct words that precisely describe an aspect of the study. Words like phenomenology or quasi-experimental may be off-putting but do give an accurate description of the study design. When all is said and done, much of the language of clinical practice is inaccessible to the layperson. So it is important to use a resource such as Wikipedia to check out the meaning of words you don't understand
Introduction	How is the article introduced? Is it a good curtain-raiser? Is the research problem and its relevance to clinical practice clearly identified? Is the problem significant enough to warrant the study that has been conducted?

Rationale

By now you are getting into the meat of the article. Such things as the evidence in the subject area are presented, which may well lead on to the rationale for the study. The questions you may wish to pose are given in Table 20.6.

Table 20.6 *Critiquing the rationale of a paper*

Elements	Checklist
Literature review	Are the methods given of how the literature was retrieved? This will give reassurances that rigorous methods have been used to retrieve all the available literature on the topic area and that the author is not selectively using the literature and thereby giving a biased account. Other questions to ask are: Is the review logically organised? Is the majority of recent origin and mainly from empirical sources? Finally, a critique of the literature should be given, which gives an overview of the limitations of the literature reviewed and identifies any gaps in the body of research reviewed. This leads to justification for the study and research questions or aims that are being posed

Robustness

The final and probably most important area of your critique of the paper is establishing how robust the methods used in the study are. Questions that you may want to ask yourself are given in Table 20.7.

Table 20.7 Critiquing the robustness of a paper

Elements	Checklist
Aims/objectives/ research questions/ hypotheses	Are these clearly stated and logically presented and do they marry well with the research problem? You will need to return to the aims/objectives/ research questions/hypotheses of the study when you have read the article and use your judgement as to whether or not the authors have achieved what they set out to do
Operational definitions	In quantitative research, it is important that tight definitions of the concepts being used in the study are given so the reader understands the implications of all the terms being used
Sample	Is the sample (usually identified as research participants in qualitative research) clearly described in terms of size (n = numbers), relevant characteristics, selection and assignment procedures? Has a probability or nonprobability sample been used in the study? Have randomisation methods been used in assignment procedures? In qualitative research, have purposive sampling methods been used or is it simply a convenience sample? Is the sample size adequate? Usually, in quantitative research studies, the larger the sample size, the more robust the study's findings, whereas in qualitative studies, often small numbers of participants take part in the study. Frequently, the more homogeneous the characteristics of the participants, the greater the generalisation properties of a qualitative study's findings. It is the experiences of the participants that provide an in-depth insight into the phenomena being studied that qualitative researchers are most interested in
Research design	Is the research design clearly identified? Do research methods and analysis conform to the research design philosophy? Are the ways data have been gathered adequately described? In quantitative studies, is sufficient information given on the reliability and validity of the data collection instruments? Was a pilot study undertaken? Qualitative researchers normally do not use a standardised tool. In fact, a feature of qualitative studies is the fluid nature of the ways data were obtained, which may make some readers uncomfortable with the lack of standardisation. Within qualitative research, the researcher and participant often have 'close relationships', especially if data collection spans several months. This is typical in ethnographic studies, thus researchers must be careful not to introduce bias and 'go native'. In some phenomenological approaches, researchers must separate out their feeling by a process called 'bracketing'. How such safeguards have been incorporated into the study are the types of question you may wish to pose
Ethics	Have the researchers gained ethical approval for their study? Nearly all studies involving patients and NHS staff or research conducted on NHS premises will require local NHS ethical approval. Similarly, most studies conducted by academic staff will require university ethical approval. Other questions you may wish to ask yourself are: Have the rights of the participants been protected? Is adherence to the principles of anonymity and confidentiality evident? Remember, it is not just about gaining ethical approval, it is about the researchers considering the ethical dimensions of their study at every step of the research process. Note that ethics approval may be a lengthy process

4

Elements	Checklist
Data analysis	Are the ways data analysis has been undertaken adequately described? In quantitative research, this is often seen as the most daunting part of the critique, especially for those not comfortable with the complex language and principles of statistical analysis. A rule of thumb is that descriptive studies use descriptive statistics, whereas correlation and experimental studies use inferential statistics. An important thing to look out for is reports on differences in the various population groups. These are usually reported as significant differences that have not occurred by chance and are established by reporting of measures of **probability** (p = probability). Concerning qualitative studies, are the reports of qualitative data analysis clear and rigorous? Remember, qualitative data analysis is time-consuming, as researchers need to be immersed in the data over a long period of time. Also, if more than one researcher has been involved in undertaking the analysis and the qualitative analysis procedures could be duplicated, would it give greater reassurances of the truth value and confirmability of the study's findings?
Findings	Are the findings presented in an easily understood fashion? In quantitative reports, graphs and tables will be used to report on the findings, so ask yourself if the graphs and tables are clearly labelled and easy to follow. Do look at the figures and try and work out what they mean – don't always assume that they are right. In quantitative research, response rates are important. A good response rate (usually over 50%) is needed if response bias is to be avoided (Polit and Beck 2008). In a qualitative study, you may wish to establish if the data themes are adequately illuminated by quotations from the original data, which also gives the impression that rich, in-depth data has been collected
Discussion	Does the discussion draw on the findings to come to some conclusions? Does the discussion return to the literature to compare the findings to other similar studies? Do the authors address any limitations of their study? Importantly, do the authors give new insights into the subject area studied?
Conclusions	Do the study's findings have implications for your practice? An important activity here is for you to decide to what extent the research may be useful to your practice. Are the findings trustworthy? Do you agree with the conclusions, although this would need to be objectively and not subjectively considered? Do the authors say anything that is new? Are the limitations of their study described? Do they highlight any research in the subject area that needs to be conducted in the future?
References	Is an accurate list of all the reference sources given? Are the sources cited up to date? Is a broad range of original sources given, including all the most important papers on the topic area? It may be useful to go back to the original sources to check that there is no misinterpretation of accidental misreporting

So you have taken the first step in reading and appraising a piece of research literature. It is important to remember in your critique that often the word limits imposed by journals do not allow the research to report all aspects of the research or their findings – you may even need to consider going back to the full report. Also, it does not stop there, as it is rare to find one article that will give you all the answers to your questions. You need to read other articles on the subject area to gain a balanced view.

Conclusion

In conclusion, we hope we have taken some of the mystique away from reading and critiquing research. We hope you find the content of this chapter useful when you consider how you can keep up to date and by doing so improve your practice. One last thing to remember is that there is no such thing as a perfect piece of research. All researchers get it wrong sometimes. It can be fun discovering just how wrong (or how right) researchers have got it. Crossword or sodoku enthusiasts will know what we mean when we say how satisfying it is to solve a difficult puzzle because that is really what critiquing research is often about.

References

Atkins, D, Best, D and Briss, PA (2004) Grading quality of evidence and strength of recommendations, *British Medical Journal*, **328**(7454): 1490

Blinkhorn, SF (1995) Burt and the early history of factor analysis, in NJ Mackintosh, *Cyril Burt: Fraud or Framed?*, Oxford: Oxford University Press

Closs, SJ and Cheater, FM (1999) Evidence for nursing practice: a clarification of issues, *Journal of Advanced Nursing*, 30: 10–17

Coad, J, Hardicre, J and Devitt, P (2006) Searching for and using grey literature, *Nursing Times*, **102**(50): 35–6

Cullum, N, Nelson, EA, Fletcher, AW and Sheldon, TA (2001) Compression for venous leg ulcers, *Cochrane Database of Systematic Reviews,* Issue 2. Art. No.: CD000265. DOI: 10.1002/14651858.CD000265

Jinks, AM and Chalder, GE (2007) Consensus and diversity: an action research study designed to analyse the roles of mental health consultant nurses, *Journal of Clinical Nursing*, **16**(7): 1323–32

Loring Brace, C (2005) Sir Cyril Burt: scientific fraud, in C. Loring Brace, *Race is a Four-lettered Word: The Genesis of the Concept*, Oxford: Oxford University Press

NMC (Nursing and Midwifery Council) (2008) *The Prep Handbook,* London: NMC

Polit, DF and Beck, CT (2006) *Essentials of Nursing Research*: *Methods, Appraisal and Utilizations* (6th edn), Philadelphia, PA: Lippincott, Williams & Wilkins

Polit, DF and Beck, CT (2008) *Nursing Research: Generating and Assessing Evidence for Nursing Practice* (8th edn), Philadelphia, PA: Lippincott, Williams & Wilkins

Rees, C (2003) Critiquing research, in C Rees, *An Introduction to Research for Midwives* (2nd edn), Oxford: Books for Midwives

Willis, KF (2007) A hierarchy of evidence for assessing qualitative health research, *Journal of Clinical Epidemiology*, **60**(1): 43–9

4

part 4 glossary

Case study Research that attempts to achieve in-depth understanding of a single situation.

Cause and effect Measurable consequences resulting from a certain course of action.

Central tendency A single score that represents all the scores.

Closed question A question that requires a specific response, often in the form of rankings, scaled items and categorical responses.

Control Managing extraneous influences that could affect the dependent variable.

Convenience sample A sampling technique where a research population is selected because of ease of access and proximity to the researcher.

Correlation The extent to which two or more things are related.

Data Information obtained during the course of a study.

Dependent variable A variable that is the observed result of the influence exerted by one or more of the independent variables; said to be the presumed outcome of the study.

Discussion Chapter or section of a report that explains what the results mean.

Epidemiology The study of disease, injury and health in a population.

Experimental research Type of research that involves the manipulation of treatments in an attempt to establish cause and effect relationships.

Fieldwork Research in which data are gathered in natural settings.

Focus groups Qualitative approach using small groups of individuals concerning a specific topic.

Grey literature Literature that is either 'semi-published' or not published and/or is not available through the usual bibliographic sources such as databases or indexes. It is often information that has been conveyed by another route such as an oral presentation or an internal report.

Grounded theory Qualitative approach that starts with a non-theoretical perspective and develops theory that is grounded in the information gathered.

Hypothesis The anticipated outcome of the study – anticipates change, difference, association.

Independent variable The part of the study that the researcher manipulates.

Inferential statistics Statistics concerned with testing hypotheses and using sample data to make generalisations concerning populations.

Interval scale Scale/level of data that provides not only the order of the scores but also the magnitude of the distance between them.

Likert scale Closed question that requires the subject to respond by choosing one of several scaled items with the assumption that there are equal intervals between them.

Limitation A possible shortcoming or influence that either cannot be controlled or is the result of delimitations imposed by the researcher.

Mean The average score of the group.

Median The middle score of the group.

Meta-analysis A technique of literature review that contains a definitive methodology, in which the results from the various studies are converted to a standard metric that allows the use of statistical techniques as a means of analysis.

Methodology A technique of enquiry that, when applied to a sample of subjects in a certain context, yields useful data.

Mode Most frequently occurring score of the group.

Nominal scale Scale/level of measurement in which scores are classified by name.

Nonparametric tests Statistical tests that do not meet the criteria for parametric tests.

Normal distribution Frequency distribution of data in which the mean, median and mode are at the same point.

Null hypothesis The anticipated outcome of the study – anticipates no change, no difference or association.

Open-ended question A question that allows the respondent latitude to express opinions, feelings and to expand on ideas.

Ordinal scale Scale/level of measurement in which scores are classified by ranks.

Outlier Unrepresentative score, one that lies outside the range of normal scores.

Parametric tests Statistical tests based on assumptions of interval/ratio level of data, normal distribution, equal variance and independence of observation.

Phenomenology Qualitative approach, the purpose of which is to describe some aspect of life as it is lived by the participants.

Population The larger (complete) group from which the sample is taken.

Post-registration education and practice (PREP) Nurses continue to update and develop their knowledge and skills throughout their careers. This is done formally every three years through PREP. There are two elements to PREP:

1 The *practice standard*, the aim of which is to ensure that nurses are current in their practice which in turn will safeguard the health and wellbeing of the public.

2 The *continuing professional development standard*.

'Nurses are required to practice in some capacity by virtue of their nursing qualification during the previous 3 years for a minimum of 450 hours' (NMC 2008, p. 11).

4

Probability The odds that a certain event will occur.

Qualitative research Type of research that involves intensive, long-time observation in a natural setting; precise and detailed recording of what happens in the setting.

Quantitative research Type of research that measures the affiliation that exists between two or more variables.

Quasi-experimental research Research that is based on the experimental design, but subjects are not randomly assigned to groups or control groups are not used.

Randomised control trial Study in which clinical treatment is compared with a control. Subjects are randomly assigned to groups.

Random sample A simple random sample gives each member of the population an equal chance of being chosen.

Range A variation between the uppermost and lowest numbers.

Ratio scale Scale/level of data with all the characteristics of interval scale, plus a true zero that represents a complete absence of the characteristic.

Reliability The degree of consistency with which an instrument measures a variable.

Research proposal Formal preparation that includes the introduction, review of literature and proposed method for conducting the study.

Review A research paper that is a critical evaluation of research on a particular topic.

Sample A group of subjects, treatments or situations selected from a larger population.

Standard deviation An estimate of the variability of scores around the mean.

Validity Degree to which a test or instrument measures what it purports to measure.

Variability The degree of difference between each individual score and the central tendency score.

4

Reference

NMC (Nursing and Midwifery Council) (2008) *The Prep Handbook,* London: NMC

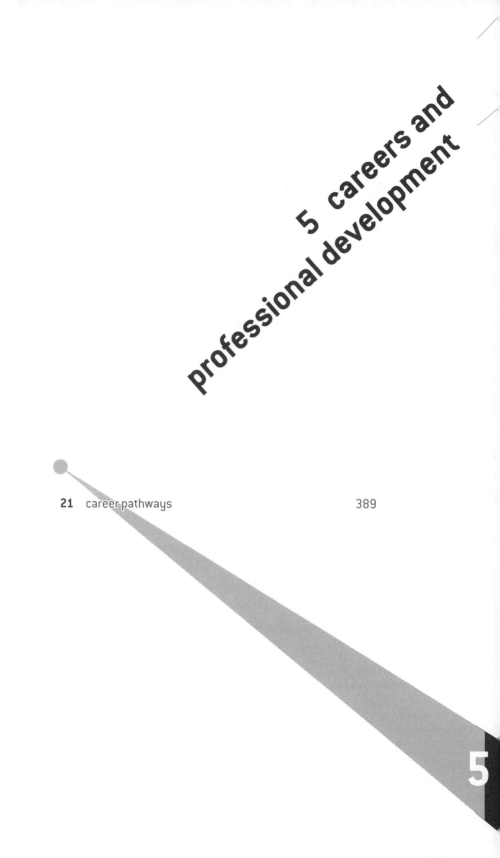

5 careers and professional development

5

Introduction

Part 5 of *The Nursing Companion* looks at the many career options open to you upon qualification. As you progress through your course of study, different pathways will emerge. You may already have preformed ideas of what you wish to specialise in. For example, you may wish to develop a career in nursing children and young people or spend your professional life working with people who have a learning disability. Whatever you choose to do, it is well worth considering all the career options open to you. Perhaps as your career progresses, you may develop a taste for management or moving to a higher academic level in order to become a lecturer. There are also possibilities for advancement within organisations outside the NHS and these are discussed here.

This wide-ranging part of *The Nursing Companion* equips you with the essential knowledge necessary for developing a professional profile through which you can present yourself to prospective employers in the best possible light. The job market is competitive and employers will be looking for the 'complete package' when seeking to fill posts. Throughout this book, you will discover many links to career development, for example maintaining a portfolio of professional and academic development achieved through continuing education or being aware of current research. Your CV will need to reflect more than just a list of qualifications and job experience. Should you need help in any aspect of your career, it is available here.

21 career pathways

James Richardson

In this chapter we will explore:

> Long-term conditions
> The nurse's role
> Lifelong learning
> *Agenda for Change*
> Career opportunities outside the NHS
> How to get on in your career

Introduction

Nursing careers are responsive to the changing nature of healthcare delivery in the UK and continued change will be needed for the future. Nursing is a dynamic profession that is adaptive to meeting the needs of the public in a changing society, where:

> there is an increasingly ageing population
> health inequalities persist
> there is growing sociocultural diversity
> there is an increase in the public's expectations of healthcare delivery
> there are advancing treatments and technologies.

Modernising Nursing Careers (DH 2006, p. 16) anticipates that nursing staff will be able to move between clinical, management and academic careers, between different organisations and between the three sectors – the health service, the independent sector, and local community and voluntary groups, charities, foundations, social enterprises and cooperatives, collectively known as the 'third sector'. It should encourage movement and progression, but also provide opportunities for those who choose to stay where they are comfortable and work locally. Nurses are caring for an ever growing ageing population, the members of which will often need higher levels of care and support, especially those with long-term conditions (DH 2006). As increasing services are offered in or closer to home, there will be opportunities for nurses to follow patients from acute settings into the community. Indeed, some nurses will choose to start their working career in the community. We will therefore start by examining long-term conditions, before moving on to examine the nurse's role.

5

Long-term conditions

Long-term conditions (LTCs) are conditions that cannot at present be cured, but can be controlled by medication and other therapies. These include diabetes, renal disease, respiratory disease, stroke, neurological conditions, depression and dementia. Over 15 million people in the UK are living with an LTC. The government's priority is to improve care for people with LTCs by moving away from reactive care based in acute systems towards a systematic, patient-centred approach. People with LTCs are the most intensive users of the most expensive services and the numbers are increasing due to an ageing population, health inequalities and the lifestyle choices that people make. People with LTCs are not just high users of primary and specific acute services but also social care and community services and urgent and emergency care (DH 2005). Therefore the nature of future nursing careers will require changes to where care will be delivered, namely in the community or in people's homes. To meet the needs of this ageing population, it is important that health and social care services are able to work in partnership. Many older people have complex health and social care needs and account for most of the current spend on health and care services.

The key outcomes for older people with complex needs are (DH 2001a):

> improved health and wellbeing
> improved experience
> care delivered closer to home.

The nurse's role

There are four elements to a nurse's role (DH 2006):

1 Practice (clinical skills development)
2 Education, training and development (educational)
3 Quality and service development
4 Leadership, management and supervision (managerial).

Career development pathways in all four elements are possible. For example, in practice, there is scope to become an advanced practitioner or specialist. In education, training and development, there are opportunities as:

> staff development officers
> manual handling coordinators
> resuscitation officers
> policy advisers
> researchers
> lecturers.

As leaders, managers or supervisors, there is scope to become a ward manager, director or chief executive, or work for regulatory bodies or professional organisations. The opportunities are endless but it will depend on individual circumstances, opportunities and motivation.

The four elements of the nurse's role are integrally linked to the *National Health Service Knowledge and Skills Framework* (KSF) (DH 2004a) and as such relate to your future career development, whether a lateral career journey or an escalating career is chosen.

Nurse careers will continue to change in tandem with changing health reform and the nature of nursing will change from that of the traditional role. In future, nurses are likely to work in a range of settings, crossing hospital and community boundaries, with new types of practitioner, for example assistant practitioners, for diverse employers, as leaders of multidisciplinary teams in and out of hospital, and across health and social care. Nurses will develop skills to work with patients and carers of those with long-term conditions, using health promotion and preventive interventions. They will need to come to terms with new technology such as telemedicine and become care or case managers. Despite these changes, there will always be a need for nurses to deliver hands-on, basic care and advances and developments in healthcare management should never overshadow this.

The nurse of the future will require a career structure that enables the development of a mix of skills both generalist and specialist. This will occur in a variety of care settings, taking on changing roles and responsibilities and pursuing education and training as necessary. Each of the four elements are considered below.

Practice/clinical skills development

In recent years, nurses have played a vital role in improving the quality of patient care by taking on new and enhanced roles and responsibilities, such as:

> advanced practitioners
> clinical specialists
> nurse prescribers
> modern matrons
> community matrons
> nurse consultants.

The chief nursing officer of England's 'ten key roles' (DH 2002) provide authority to take on the following new responsibilities:

1 To order diagnostic investigations such as pathology tests and X-rays
2 To make and receive referrals direct, for example to a therapist or pain consultant
3 To admit and discharge patients for specified conditions and within agreed protocols
4 To manage patient caseloads, for example for diabetes or rheumatology
5 To run clinics, for example for ophthalmology or dermatology

5

6 To prescribe medicines and treatments
7 To carry out a wide range of resuscitation procedures including defibrillation
8 To perform minor surgery and outpatient procedures
9 To triage patients using the latest information technology to the most appropriate health professional
10 To take a lead in the way local health services are organised and in the way they are run.

In Scotland (DH 2006, p. 12), clinical quality indicators were introduced to enable clinical leaders to demonstrate the impact of the nursing team on the delivery of safe and effective practice, as well as reviewing the role of the senior charge nurse to enable frontline leaders to maximise their contribution to safe and effective care.

Advanced practice/specialist practice

There is currently a lack of clarity concerning the career pathway to advanced and specialist roles, but *Agenda for Change* (DH 2004b) and the KSF have been developed to enable healthcare professionals to demonstrate career development. The NMC does not currently register advanced practice and the multitude of job titles can be confusing to the general public. There are nurses who hold job titles that imply an advanced level of knowledge and competence, but who do not in reality possess such knowledge and competence. In addition, their practice may not be subject to the scrutiny of another professional as they often act as independent practitioners.

The specialist practice qualifications leading to health visiting, school nursing and occupational health nursing have been phased out and replaced with the specialist community public health nursing (SCPHN) qualification. The SCPHN qualification became the third part of the NMC register from 2004 after nursing and midwifery. Specialist community practice qualifications in practice nursing, mental health, learning disability, community children's nursing and district nursing are not affected (NMC 2006).

The NMC (2007) has recognised that there are now significant changes in the way that services are delivered to patients, with nurses and midwives undertaking treatment and care that was once the domain of other healthcare professionals. The title of 'advanced nurse practitioner' is likely to become a registerable qualification in the future and appear as a sub-part of the nurses' part of the register.

Nurse prescribers

The numbers and categories of nurses who can prescribe have grown significantly since prescribing by certain groups of nurses began in 1994. In addition, new legislation has been introduced that enables nurses and midwives to supply and administer medicines via patient group directions (NMC 2005).

Prescribers are first-level nurses or midwives who have completed an

5

extended, supplementary or independent nurse prescribing programme at an accredited university, or specialist practitioners (formerly district nurses, health visitors or practice nurses with a district nurse or health visitor qualification). Strict guidelines are in place as to the extent of what can and cannot be prescribed.

The National Prescribing Centre's (2001) *Maintaining Competency in Prescribing: An Outline Framework to Help Nurse Prescribers* is a tool to aid reflection on prescribing practice and identify continuing professional development (CPD) needs.

Education, training and development

From September 2001, in respect of the lecturer/practice educator role, there has been only one teaching qualification recorded by the NMC. Teacher programmes prepare appropriately qualified and experienced practitioners for the role of lecturer in the higher education sector. The lecturer role involves curriculum design, programme/module management, and curriculum evaluation and development to ensure the provision of appropriate learning experiences for students to meet specified learning outcomes. The lecturer works as a member of the teaching team with a range of responsibilities, including programme leadership/directorship, pathway leadership/directorship, module leadership, personal tutor responsibilities and developing professional knowledge. In carrying out these responsibilities, lecturers draw on expertise in their professional disciplines and education management. As a member of the teaching team, the lecturer identifies appropriate resources to support learning and works in partnership with other professionals, lecturers, practice educators, nurses and other healthcare consultants and mentors to ensure that the learning experiences and assessment strategy enable students to meet the identified learning outcomes of modules and programme as a whole in institutional and practice settings (ENB/DH 2001a).

In order to achieve NMC teacher standard, a teaching qualification, which has been approved by the NMC as leading to lecturer/practice educator status, must be undertaken. Study should be at postgraduate level. Programmes for the preparation of lecturers will enable the NMC's outcomes for stage 4 to be achieved (NMC 2008a).

Approved institutions in partnership with the NHS ensure the strategic management of the lecturer's practice role, including acknowledging teaching in practice hours, as part of the lecturer's contracted teaching hours. Institutions should give due recognition to the practice element of the lecturer's role and provide dedicated time for lecturers in the practice environment to ensure that they are confident and competent to undertake their roles (ENB/DH 2001b, p. 13). CPD should be provided to support the practice role, including reviewing and updating skills and knowledge related to the role (ENB/DH 2001b).

5

In order to enter a programme leading to a recordable teaching qualification, the registered practitioner must:

> be registered in the same part or sub-part of the register as the students they support
> have completed at least three years post-registration experience, gained additional professional knowledge and skills, and have experience in an area where students are gaining practice experience relevant to their registration
> have extended their professional knowledge, relevant to their field of practice, to at least first degree level
> be able to lead programme development and coordinate others in assessing and delivering programmes of learning in academic and practice settings
> be able to support interprofessional learning and working
> be able to generate and use cross-professional assessment criteria to supervise mentors, practice teachers and teachers from all professions
> be able to teach and assess in practice and academic settings
> be able to provide leadership in education in practice and academic settings.

Lecturer/practitioners

Lecturer/practitioners are seen as experts within their own field of speciality and often hold a jointly funded position between a university and an employer. The clinical aspect of their work usually refers to a speciality such as infection control, care of the elderly or tissue viability. The educational aspect of their role is to organise, deliver and teach on a range of pre- and post-registration courses.

Research

Research is a fundamental part of many nursing roles nowadays and underpins all aspects of nursing. Nursing is no longer based on tradition, customs and practice, but on evidence-based practice, that is, there is a measurable and justifiable reason why procedures are carried out the way they are. All policies and practices are based on best practice guidance, so perhaps, without appreciating it, most duties undertaken nowadays are based on research findings. Nurses involved in research may have negotiated their roles based on local recognition of the value of their contribution to research, or pursue research in their own time, leading to published articles in journals, chapters in books or presented papers at conferences. (The relevance of research to practice and different approaches to research can be found in Chapters 17–20.)

Many organisations and trusts have research and development units or departments or clinical trials units employing research nurses or nurse researchers.

Research nurses

The role of research nurses will depend on how they are employed; some posts are for fixed periods while involved in specific studies. Research nurses may work with or under the supervision of academics or medical practitioners. All studies relating to patients must meet strict research ethics frameworks, good clinical practice and the *Research Governance Framework for Health and Social Care* (DH 2001b). While roles will vary, the posts may include collecting, interpreting and processing data, screening of patients, running clinics and obtaining informed consent. A degree or research experience is not always necessary.

The nurse consultant role was one of the first NHS posts where research was built into the national job description.

Nurse consultants

Nurse consultant posts were first established in 1999 and are central to the modernisation of the NHS, helping to provide patients with services that are fast and convenient. Nurse consultants are experienced registered nurses, who specialise in a particular field of healthcare such as critical care, infection control, learning disabilities or forensic mental health. Every role is different, depending on the needs of the service, and is designed to create a professional career path in nursing by empowering senior nurses to take on broader responsibilities. Nurses working at this level are among the highest paid of their professions (www.nhscareers.nhs.uk). Nurse consultants are responsible for developing professional practice, research, evaluation and contributing to education, and service development, but spend approximately half of their time working directly with patients. Their medical responsibilities might include prescribing, case management and key roles in specialist units, ensuring that those using the NHS benefit from the very best nursing skills.

Quality and service development

These types of post are inextricably linked to management and supervision, so are included below.

Leadership, management and supervision (managerial)

Modern matrons

The matron role was reintroduced into the NHS following the implementation of *Modernising Matrons: Improving the Patient's Experience* (DH 2003).

Matrons were recruited from senior sisters and charge nurses with a track record of strong, visible clinical leadership. They are easily identifiable to patients and deal with the patient all the way through their clinical journey, leading by example in the drive for the highest possible standards of care, making the difference at ward level. Modern matrons are a key part of the plan to transform the NHS into a patient-centred service, that is, making the system fit the patient – not the other way round. Improving the patient experience is central to the reputation of the NHS and not just about meeting targets. A

5

matron's fundamental role therefore is to provide better care faster, which means making hospitals cleaner, more comfortable, friendlier places, and providing patients with better information and more choice (DH 2003, pp. 4–5).

Community matrons

The NHS Improvement Plan (DH 2004c) described a new clinical role for nurses to be known as 'community matrons'. These experienced, skilled nurses use case management techniques with patients who meet criteria denoting high intensity use of healthcare. With special intensive help, these patients are able to remain at home longer and have more choice about their healthcare (DH 2004c). The case management work of community matrons is central to the government's policy for the management of people with long-term conditions.

Lifelong learning

This section describes the relevance of CPD to career progression. Nurses and midwives practise in an environment of constant change. This involves new and expanding roles for health professionals, increasing technological advances in treatment and care, continuing reorganisation and the redirection of resources. It is vital that they develop their professional knowledge and competence to cope with these demands and the complexities of modern professional practice. This requires demonstrating responsibility for learning through the development of a portfolio of learning and practice and being able to recognise when further learning and development may be needed. The principle of lifelong learning in nursing comprises an essential conceptual shift from the notion of the registered nurse or midwife merely being a competent health service employee to one who engages in professional learning in order to keep their knowledge and skills up to date. Lifelong learning is more than simply keeping up to date, as it requires an inquiring approach to nursing and midwifery practice as well as to issues that impact on that practice. The principles and values of lifelong learning are increasingly important to all registered practitioners as the pace of change in the delivery of healthcare and the public's expectations of registered practitioners continue to increase.

Pre-registration education prepares for practice at the point of registration, while CPD is linked to the registration renewal process through the post-registration education and practice (PREP) standards (NMC 2008b). PREP represents an important part of lifelong learning linked to professional practice and builds upon the requirements for continued entry to the register and is explained below.

Post-registration education in practice

All nurses and midwives are required by law to renew their registration every three years and must meet the PREP requirements in order to renew their registration (NMC 2008b). There are two separate PREP standards that affect registration:

1 The PREP *practice standard* requires nurses and midwives to have worked in some capacity by virtue of their qualification during the previous three years for a minimum of 450 hours. They can only meet the practice standard for nursing by practising nursing, and similarly for midwifery. If they have been out of practice, they must have undertaken an approved return to practice course.

2 The PREP *continuing professional development standard* requires them to have undertaken and recorded CPD over the three years prior to registration renewal.

The PREP CPD standard requires that you:

> undertake at least 35 hours of learning activity relevant to your practice during the three years prior to your renewal of registration
> maintain a personal professional profile of your learning activity
> comply with any request from the NMC to audit how you have met these requirements (NMC 2008b).

PREP allows nurses and midwives to decide for themselves how they meet the standards. In some cases, nurses will find that the learning activities are free or that they must self-fund activities or attend in their own time due to financial and staffing problems. In order to renew the registration, you will also need to provide a signed notification of practice (NOP) form and pay the renewal of registration fee. The NOP requires a declaration of meeting the PREP requirements and that they are of good health and good character. Registration is not renewed until all documentation and fees have been received.

Midwives will need to give notice of their intention to practise, in accordance with Rule 3 of the *Midwives Rules and Standards* (NMC 2004a). Submitting a completed 'annual intention to practise' form every year to their named supervisor of midwives is required. The number of hours needed to meet the practice standard to renew registration(s) is given in Table 21.1.

Table 21.1 Hours needed to meet the practice standard to renew registration

Registration	Hours required
Nursing, or midwifery, or nursing and specialist community public health nursing (SCPHN)	450
Nursing and midwifery, or midwifery and specialist community public health nursing, or nursing, midwifery and specialist community public health nursing	900

Nurses and midwives who don't comply with these requirements and who let their registration lapse will not be able to work as a registered practitioner. In future, it is possible that there will be a system of revalidation by employers to take responsibility for ensuring that staff are keeping their practice updated, which would replace PREP.

The easiest way to demonstrate how these requirements are being met is to maintain a professional portfolio similar to that developed as a student (see examples in the section How to get on in your career). From August 2004, anyone entering the NMC register or renewing their registration is required to provide a declaration of their good health and good character. This requirement should help to strengthen public protection and confidence (NMC 2004b).

Agenda for Change

Agenda for Change (DH 2004b) involved a radical revision of the NHS pay system. It applies to over one million NHS staff across the UK, including nurses, midwives and allied health professionals but excludes doctors, dentists and most senior managers. *Agenda for Change* introduced a new pay system to ensure fair pay and a clearer system for career progression and staff are paid on the basis of the jobs they do and the skills and knowledge required for those jobs. There are nine levels, ranging from 1 (initial entry posts) to 9 (senior management) (see Table 21.2). This pay reform is underpinned by a job evaluation scheme specifically designed for the NHS. The process of matching jobs to national profiles, or evaluating jobs locally, determines in which pay band a post should sit. The NHS job evaluation scheme (DH 2004d) made provision for most NHS jobs to be matched to nationally evaluated profiles on the basis of information from job descriptions, person specifications and additional information. National job profiles also provide a framework against which to check the consistency of local evaluations. One of its aims is to remove rigid professional demarcation allowing staff to move between roles in a pay band. The KSF (DH 2004a) is used to assess development so that staff can progress within pay bands. This competency-based framework has driven role and service design. The KSF is a key part of the NHS *Agenda for Change* pay system and applies to all staff employed under its terms and conditions. In future, all NHS nursing and midwifery posts will be subject to the *Agenda for Change* pay reform and posts will be matched to the job profile undertaken by the individual, not merely the job itself. Within *Agenda for Change* and the KSF, CPD is an important requisite for nurses and midwives to maintain their registration. Traditional occupational boundaries have been broken down, enabling greater transferability of skills, which will provide better career opportunities for all staff.

5

Table 21.2 Agenda for Change *pay scales (2009/10), job examples and qualifications*

Pay band	Job examples	Qualifications
Band 1 £13,233–£13,944	Nursing auxiliary	
Band 2 £13233–£16,333	Nursing assistant Clinical support worker (endoscopy, community)	NVQ level 2 in direct patient care, therapy or health. Good level of general education. Basic literacy and numeracy skills
	School health support worker	NNEB
Band 3 £15,190–£18,157	Clinical support worker nursing higher level (hospital, mental health, learning disabilities) Pharmacy support worker nursing higher level	NVQ level 2/3. Good level of secondary education equivalent to AS level or higher
Band 4 £17,732–£21,318	Associate practitioner (acute care/community/mental health/learning disabilities)	NVQ level 3/4
	Maternity care assistant	Foundation degree
Band 5 £20,710–£26,839	Staff nurse Aesthetic/cosmetic nurse Theatre nurse	Current NMC registration. Diploma in operating department practice
Band 6 £24,831–£33,436	Junior sister or charge nurse	Leadership or management qualifications
	Nurse team leader	Post-registration qualification
	Senior staff nurse	ENB 998/mentorship
	Resuscitation trainer	ILS/ALS provider/instructor
	Clinical teacher	Good first degree/teaching qualification
	Health visitor	Specialist community public health nurse (school nurse)
	Moving and handling trainer	Qualification in back care. Training/teaching qualification
Band 7 £29,789–£39,273	Senior sister or charge nurse	Leadership qualification
	Clinical practice educator	Postgraduate Certificate in Education
	Donor transplant coordinator	Relevant post basic qualification in critical care
	Community practice teacher – district nursing	Specialist practitioner – district nursing. Nurse prescribing
	Lecturer/practitioner	Stage 4 teacher

5

Pay band	Job examples	Qualifications
Band 8A £37,996–£45,596	Modern matron	Evidence of extensive post-registration professional development. Diploma in management
	Cognitive behaviour therapist	Doctoral-level qualification in clinical or counselling psychology
Band 8B £44,258–£54,714	CAMHS/learning disability consultant	Masters degree related to nursing. Post-registration qualification in CAMHS
Band 8C £53,256–£65,657	Nurse consultant Associate chief nurse	Nonmedical prescriber. Honorary academic post at an appropriate higher education institution
Band 8D £63,833–£79,031	Assistant director of nursing Deputy director of nursing and quality	Masters-level qualification or equivalent
Band 9 £75,383–£95,333	Director of operations	Masters degree in appropriate management discipline

Source: *NHS Terms and Conditions of Service Handbook* © Crown copyright material is reproduced with the permission of the Controller of HMSO and Queen's Printer for Scotland. Reproduced under the terms of the Click-Use Licence
Note: Please see www.nhsemployers.org for further information and the most up-to-date information

Career opportunities outside the NHS

Third sector employment

Services that incorporate voluntary, private and independent healthcare services along with charities are known as the 'third sector'. This sector has huge potential capacity to address a wide variety of social problems and public service delivery challenges. The third sector is an essential employer and partner in service provision. It offers scope to involve people in solving their own problems and may have expertise in particular issues of concern such as substance misuse, mental health, community care and learning disabilities (Longley et al. 2007). Independent sector organisations are managed privately by individuals or consortia to make profit and may include individual or group nursing homes and treatment centres. Commercial sector organisations again work to make profit and may include general practice groups, private schools or occupational health organisations. Charities provide services on a non-profit-making basis including religious organisations.

It is likely that this sector will continue to expand, assuming that they will maintain enhanced roles in providing public services encouraging market competition, strengthening communities by building wide social networks in disadvantaged communities, and acting as recognised advocates for vulnerable groups. They can bid for service contracts from service commissioners such as primary care trusts (PCTs).

Self-employment, franchised services or small business

You might consider setting up your own business to include teaching and training and nursing services or nursing agencies. The numbers of nurses involved in aesthetic nursing continues to grow, with some nurses setting up their own clinics offering nonsurgical cosmetic services, beauty therapies and treatments.

The armed forces (regular or territorial)

The Ministry of Defence (MOD) offers a variety of opportunities for suitably qualified and experienced nurses who are physically very fit. Nurses with mental health, intensive care or emergency nursing qualifications are particularly welcome and there are also a limited number of vacancies for midwives and children's nurses. These positions are better paid than the NHS and offer opportunities for working and travelling overseas, as well as excellent pension schemes, but posts are subject to age restrictions. There is a good prospect of career progression within the armed forces. You could find yourself working as part of a humanitarian aid team in areas affected by conflict or natural disaster. The role may require more responsibility than most regular staff nurses and you may find yourself working as an autonomous practitioner treating and discharging patients and not always working for or under the guidance of a medical doctor.

Career opportunities for each of the armed forces are described on the MOD websites, which are detailed at the end of the chapter.

Within the armed forces, you can be offered professional development courses provided by the MOD, which could be up to and include PhD level, as well as external courses in areas of specialist practice provided by universities and healthcare establishments throughout the UK, but funding may be subject to selection. Some examples of the career opportunities include:

> *Registered mental health nurses* manage a range of mental health issues for personnel providing psychiatric care in departments of community mental health and in the field. They are also deployed on operations in times of conflict and peacekeeping situations, so must have the knowledge and skills to work in a variety of challenging situations.

> *Staff nurses* (adult nurses) help look after the health and fitness of everyone in the armed forces or other support staff. Nurses also provide care for entitled civilians and personnel from other services. They have three main areas of responsibility: primary healthcare, secondary healthcare, based at one of the MOD hospitals or in the Defence Medical Rehabilitation Centre at Headley Court, and an operational role, which involves assisting in the evacuation of casualties from overseas to hospitals in the UK for treatment.

> *Nursing officers* posts require at least two years' full-time experience following registration as a registered nurse in either adult or mental health. All

5

officer jobs call on the ability to lead and motivate the personnel under your command, and officers need the maturity and sense of responsibility necessary for a role in which the wellbeing of services personnel and civilians can depend on the outcome of their decisions. Officers must also be able to act on their own initiative and take orders if and when the situation calls for it.

Bank work and agency work

Many student nurses also work as bank or agency healthcare assistants to supplement their income. Indeed, many registered nurses who have jobs also work bank and agency hours to supplement their salary. However, student nurses must be aware that any additional work should not impinge on the academic and practice placement expectations of their course. Indeed, some higher education institutions will not actively support extracurricular work of students.

The Prison Service

The Prison Service employs nurses to work within secure settings to look after prisoners who may have complex needs, often with multiple diagnoses and a significant number may have mental health problems, addictions or drug or alcohol dependencies. Some prisons have clinics, ward areas, sick bays and even offer minor surgery and nurse-led clinics. As such, there is considerable variation in the career prospects available but skills needed may include counselling, assessment, referral, advice and treatment. Due to high numbers of prisoners with mental health problems, mental health nurses are often required, and for those with drug addictions, substance misuse workers are often required. Working as an occupational health adviser, you would provide an occupational health service to prison employees and contribute to the development, implementation and evaluation of the Prison Service occupational health policies and procedures. Further careers advice on the prison service can be found at the website provided at the end of the chapter.

Complementary and alternative medicines

Complementary and alternative medicines (CAMs), for example acupuncture, aromatherapy, chiropractice, homeopathy, hypnotherapy, massage, reflexology and osteopathy, are now becoming available on the NHS and the numbers of people opting for a CAM as their main treatment or therapy, or indeed an adjunct to support this, is likely to continue to increase. Complementary therapy is therefore an alternative career choice to make. CAMs are defined as (DH 2000):

> a broad domain of healing resources that encompasses all health systems, modalities and practices, and their accompanying theories and beliefs, other than those intrinsic to the politically dominant health system. CAM

includes all such practices and ideas self-defined by their users as preventing or treating illness or promoting health and well-being.

Treatments can be made available via the NHS or privately through private practitioners, health centres or clinics, or NHS homeopathic hospitals. PCTs are responsible for making the decisions on what services or treatments to commission to meet their community's health needs. Nurses may wish to train in any of these therapies as part of their nursing role or to become a private practitioner. For further information, you are recommended to consult the *Complementary Medicine Information Pack for Primary Care Groups* (DH 2000).

Ships nurses

If you like a sense of adventure, like to travel and do not suffer from seasickness, then there are opportunities on the expanding networks of cruise liners. Nurses are required to work within a small medical team providing both emergency and general care for a confined population with a wide variety of clinical conditions in modern, well-equipped, on-board medical centres. A range of illnesses are dealt with, from occupational health issues to the emergency care of trauma, anaphylaxis, cardiac emergencies, orthopaedic injuries and surgical cases. Nurses are required to be physically fit, and with experience of acute medical or emergency care such as accident and emergency, intensive care, practice or occupational health nursing. Further details can be found at cruise companies' websites.

Medical evacuation companies

Medical evacuation companies provide nurses to escort injured and ill patients to repatriate them to their country of origin. While this may seem exciting and involve flying abroad, it may not be as glamorous as being a flight attendant and insists upon serious responsibility for the patient's welfare.

Working abroad and overseas

The nursing press constantly has adverts for staff to go and work abroad. Opportunities to work overseas are varied, ranging from unpaid voluntary work with charities in remote, rural conditions, to paid employment in developed countries in highly technical environments. Nursing abroad can enhance your development and increase your confidence personally and professionally. There are, however, many issues to consider before taking a job overseas. There will be many positive reasons for wanting to nurse overseas, including the challenges of working and living in a culturally different country. There may be higher salaries and a better standard of living or warmer climate in some of the developed countries. However, nursing abroad may not be as glamorous as it first appears, and the reality of overseas work may be very different from what was expected. A more realistic view of the positive and negative aspects of working in a particular country could be to consider informal sources of

5

information such as from friends or colleagues who have worked in that country or networking at conferences or study days. It is important to understand how the health sector in a country is organised as there may be very different working practices for nurses, even in developed countries. Learning the language of the country will be important as it will be difficult to practise safely and competently without a good command of the host language. It will also make the work more interesting and enjoyable.

Preparing to work overseas needs careful organisation. Bear in mind that some agencies will charge a joining or annual subscription fee and that some countries require entrance exams to be taken before posts are offered and that visa and registration requirements and so on must be met. You must consider practical details such as employment conditions, visas, work permits, income tax, NHS pensions, national insurance, medical insurance and personal health abroad. In developed countries, there is usually assistance with insurance, air fares and accommodation.

The Royal College of Nursing (RCN, www.rcn.org.uk or email international.office@rcn.org.uk) and the Royal College of Midwives (RCM, www.rcm.org.uk) have immigration advisers who can provide their members with a comprehensive information pack containing details on general topics on nursing overseas, including nursing in specific countries, employment contracts, work permits, registration requirements and so on.

Working in the European Economic Area (EEA)

Free movement within the European Union states and the mutual recognition of qualifications have led to greater opportunities in Europe. The practicalities of employment in each country vary but nurses and midwives are entitled to full registration in any EEA country providing they are a citizen of a member state and have completed primary training in a member state and hold a recognised qualification.

Voluntary organisations

Voluntary work can be very personally and professionally rewarding and allow the opportunity to travel to unusual destinations. Some choose to do this as a short UK career break or during their holidays, others might avail themselves at times of natural disaster. Depending on the organisation you choose to volunteer for, there may be costs and expenses incurred. Consider the information available from each organisation as well as from the overseas information officers of the RCN and the RCM before committing yourself. Remember that this may involve expenditure from your own pocket including food and flights. The websites of a few voluntary organisations can be found at the end of the chapter.

5

Newly qualified profile pools or national talent pool

A national talent pool for newly qualified professionals was implemented in England in April 2007 for newly qualified nurses and midwives who did not have a job. It was set up and is managed by NHS employers with contributions from partner organisations, including the 10 strategic health authorities (SHAs) across England. Individuals are required to register via the NHS Jobs website (www.jobs.nhs.uk) for three-monthly periods, during which time they will be provided with information on the availability of posts. Individuals post their profile on the NHS Jobs website to search and apply for positions within the NHS and to enable them to benefit from additional job-seeking support. Newly qualified profile pools have been developed for the 10 SHAs in England, but the profile can only be posted in the SHA pool where the student's course was commissioned (NHS Jobs n.d.). Once registered, the profile can be viewed by all the employing organisations within that SHA region, who may even contact the individual directly with job opportunities. A full list of SHAs, including contact details, can be found at www.nhs.uk/England/AuthoritiesTrusts/Sha/list.aspx.

How to get on in your career

Portfolio of professional development

All pre-registration students should be compiling a portfolio of professional development, to demonstrate to practitioners and academic staff how well they are progressing during the course. This portfolio is beneficial for interviewers to gain an overview of the student's development and progress and may be required at interview. As a new registrant, you should always make it available to interviewers. Refer to it during your interview to evidence the care and commitment you have taken to maintain it. It is, after all, a true reflection of your progress and performance during your pre-registration education. Getting used to maintaining an up-to-date portfolio as a student will enable you to continue developing your post-registration portfolio as part of your CPD. While there are no specific guidelines as to its contents, the following are suggested as a minimum:

> curriculum vitae (CV) (see example format below)
> list of placement experiences
> feedback from academic assessments
> practice learning
> attendance and absence information (both academic and theory time)
> professional development undertaken during the course, for example statements/certificates of attendance at conferences or workshops
> formal reflection or critical incident analysis
> special achievements
> feedback from patients/service users

5

> clinical skills development/competences.

While the work market is so competitive, sickness and absence rates may determine which of two similar candidates is offered a position.

Students' ongoing achievement record

From September 2007, all students undertaking pre-registration nursing and midwifery education are required to have an ongoing achievement record (NMC 2008a). This may be a stand-alone document or perhaps incorporated into the student's portfolio. It should also be available to interviewers as a means of demonstrating a profile of skills, knowledge and ongoing professional development.

Applying for jobs and interview preparation

There are numerous ways in which you can find out about job vacancies, but note that the employment market changes continuously based on factors such as service reconfiguration, retirement and staff movement. Many trusts and organisations advertise their jobs on their own websites and via other media. A list of websites, which may be beneficial, can be found at the end of the chapter.

Curriculum vitae

There are many different formats for CVs available. Many nursing posts will not request a CV, but it should be available within your portfolio. Keep your CV clear, up to date and succinct, preferably only on one side of A4 paper, or use two sides if you have a lot of relevant work experience or qualifications – supplementary information and evidence can be made available if and when requested. Only relevant and important information is necessary, so you do not need to include your marital status, how many children you have, your date of birth or age. A CV is useful for sending off to potential employers ad hoc, who just might have forthcoming vacancies or some may keep your details on file. Photographs should not normally be attached.

Ensure your CV is well written, up to date, and presented to sell your personal and professional skills and qualities. Use the contacts from the university and local trusts to assist you, and ensure you have the correct contact details and titles of anyone you wish to be a referee. It is always polite to ask them first if they are happy to be a referee. If you are applying for your first position, your referees should consist of one from your university and one from practice, for example your mentor from your final placement or your manager if you have part-time job. Check your CV and covering letter (as well as application form) carefully before you send them, use the spellchecker on the computer (set the language to British English rather than American English) and ask a native English speaker to proofread what you have written and ask this person for any comments.

While there are many examples of CV formats to be found, here is a basic one that should encompass most organisations' requirements.

> ### Box 21.1 CV format example
>
> **Name**
> Full name including your title
>
> **Contact details**
> Address: (make sure that you will be able to receive mail at this address, and include the full postcode)
> Telephone numbers: home, office and mobile, starting with area code
> Email address: work and private
> (Check your voicemail and email messages regularly)
>
> **Personal details**
> Work status where relevant, for example student visa or EC citizen (no work permit required)
>
> **Interests**
> Include three or four main hobbies or interests, especially those which may show the interviewer that you have good social or teamworking skills, or that may be useful in the job, for example computer or language skills
>
> **Employment**
> List the most recent jobs first
>
> **Education**
> Remember that the person reading your CV may not be familiar with the education system in your country
>
> **Other skills**
> List other skills or qualifications that you believe may be relevant

Application forms

If possible, do not handwrite your application forms, as they can be messy or difficult to read, especially if they have had to be photocopied for the selection process. Many are now available electronically, so word-processed forms look neater and demonstrate your ability to use IT skills. It is also easier to save copies that can easily be adapted and updated for future applications.

Do not append a CV to an application form if not requested to do so, it looks like you have not followed the guidance given to you, or not taken the time or effort to do what was asked of you.

The application form should be written such that you address each of the points in the person specification in your supplementary information. Do not rely on the fact that you have gained a particular skill or qualification, make it clear on the application. The rule is always to be explicit, and not implicit.

Note the deadline time or date for submission of the application and if you are struggling to meet the postal deadline, ring the appropriate administrator and ask if you can send an electronic version (via email or fax) to meet the deadline, with the original to follow immediately by post. It is unlikely that

5

anyone would check postal applications before the Monday morning for Friday afternoon deadlines.

You must always keep a copy of your application form, job description and person specification in case you are called to interview. If some of the required specification criterion is to be assessed at interview, don't be put off applying even if you do not have all the essential criteria.

If submitting a postal application, send it first class or recorded rather than second class, as this can show you care about getting the job. Telephone to make sure any electronically submitted applications have been received and send an application in the post as well. Many organisations do not allow for applications to be handed in personally.

Work experience

During your placements, always try to make a good impression on the staff you work with. Enthusiasm, timekeeping, professionalism and taking an interest in the speciality, the staff and the patients will be noticed. Ensure you are reliable and trustworthy, be punctual for your shifts and turn up for the correct shifts at all times. After all, who would look after the patients if everyone turned up late for the start of a shift? Sickness is allowed occasionally, but make sure it is just for that reason and any missed time is authorised and explained. Offer to make up any missed time at the employer's convenience. Remember this will show up on your overall attendance record. Each placement during your training can be considered as a potential employment opportunity, so utilise it to your benefit even though it is not exactly what you want. Once in employment, it can be easier to secure further employment. In the current situation of a lack of jobs, you could find yourself in a catch-22 situation where you cannot secure employment without experience, yet cannot gain that experience without employment. If you get on well with staff and patients, show an interest and convey a professional image, then you could potentially be informed unofficially about pending opportunities.

If you are allowed to choose your final placement, which will prepare you for your first staffing post, think about areas where you would potentially like to work, don't merely choose it because you simply like the idea of working there. The final placement should enable you to meet the requirements/ outcomes for your final placement, as well as develop your all-round nursing experiences. Such feedback will be evidence in your portfolio.

Research the post and the employer

Ensure you research a post before an interview. Look at their websites or any pertinent documents such as quality assurance reviews or performance indicators relating to the post or the employer, so that you are familiar with the attributes of a potential employer. Employers will be impressed you have done your research. If you are able to, request an informal visit prior to the interview to familiarise yourself with the placement area and even get to know the staff. Remember that first impressions count and there will be many others applying for that post, so make your mark and stand out from the crowd.

Turn up in plenty time for an interview, ensuring you are appropriately dressed. Appear enthusiastic. Have a list of written questions you want to be answered at the interview. Mark them off as they are answered during the interview. At the end, when you are asked if you have any questions, you should hopefully have some left to ask. Always ask a couple of questions of them, for example: What are the prospects of being supported for further development and training?

Presentations or demonstrations

Some posts require a brief presentation or practical demonstration to be given. Ensure you have read the presentation or demonstration brief carefully. Research the subject, prepare by practising, in front of friends or family may be useful. This can help with timing, and always use a grammar and spellchecker. Using a PowerPoint presentation can show off your IT and teaching skills, but make sure you always have a back-up in case of technical difficulties (this may be on a disk, a handout, acetates or on your USB pen). If you have been asked to demonstrate a particular skill, then demonstrate it and don't merely talk about it.

Finally, always be on the lookout for job fairs and conferences where employers are represented.

Conclusion

This chapter has equipped you with the essential knowledge necessary for developing a professional profile. It has also looked at the many career options open to you upon qualification. We hope this has given you some fresh ideas and wish you the best of luck in your chosen career path, safe in the knowledge that you have elected to work in a caring profession that is well regarded by society at large. Good luck!

Useful resources

Armed forces

www.armyjobs.mod.uk

www.rafcareers.com

www.royalnavy.mod.uk/careers

Prison Service

www.hmprisonservice.gov.uk/careersandjobs

Voluntary organisations

Voluntary Service Overseas www.vso.org.uk/

Medical Emergency Relief International (MERLIN) www.merlin.org.uk/

5

Medecins Sans Frontières www.uk.msf.org

Starfish Ventures www.starfishventures.co.uk

Job seeking

www.nhsjobs.uk

www.nhsprofessional.nhs.uk

www.jobcentrplus.gov.uk

www.fish4jobs.co.uk

www. monster.co.uk

www.jobsearch.co.uk

www.jobsinhealth.co.uk

www.nursingtimes.co.uk

www.careerbuilder.co.uk

www.jobs4medical.co.uk

www.nursingnet.com/job

www.rcn.org

www.rcm.org

www.nhsemployers.org

www.wales.nhs.uk/careers/

www.careers-scotland.org.uk/careersscotland/

References

DH (Department of Health) (2000) *Complementary Medicine Information Pack for Primary Care Groups*, London: DH

DH (2001a) *National Service Framework for Older People*, London: DH

DH (2001b) *Research Governance Framework for Health and Social Care*, London: DH

DH (2002) *Developing Key Roles for Nurses and Midwives: A Guide for Managers*, London: DH

DH (2003) *Modernising Matrons: Improving the Patient's Experience*, London: DH

DH (2004a) *The Knowledge and Skills Framework (NHS KSF) and the Development Review Process*, London: DH

DH (2004b) *Agenda for Change: Final Agreement*, London: DH

DH (2004c) *The NHS Improvement Plan: Putting People at the Heart of Public Services*, London: DH

DH (2004d) *NHS Job Evaluation Handbook* (2nd edn), London: DH

DH (2005) *National Service Framework for Long Term (Neurological) Conditions*, London: DH

DH (2006) *Modernising Nursing Careers: Setting the Direction*, London: DH

ENB/DH (English National Board/Department of Health) (2001a) *Preparation of Mentors and Teachers: A New Framework of Guidance*, London: ENB/DH

ENB/DH (2001b) *Placements in Focus: Guidance for Education in Practice for Health Care Professions*, London: ENB/DH

Longley, M, Shaw, C and Dolan, G (2007) *Nursing: Towards 2015: Alternative Scenarios for Healthcare and Nurse Education in the UK in 2015*, Pontypridd: Welsh Institute for Health and Social Care

National Prescribing Centre (2001) *Maintaining Competency in Prescribing: An Outline Framework to Help Nurse Prescribers*, Liverpool: National Prescribing Centre, available online at http://www.npc.co.uk/prescribers/resources/maint_comp_prescribing_nurs.pdf, accessed 16/6/2010

NHS Jobs (n.d.) *Newly Qualified Profile Pools: A Guide for Job Seekers*, available online at http://www.nhsemployers.org/SiteCollectionDocuments/jobs_newly_qualifed_profile_pools.pdf, accessed 18/6/2010

NMC (Nursing and Midwifery Council) (2004a) *Midwives Rules and Standards*, London: NMC

NMC (2004b) *Requirements for Good Health and Good Character*, Circular 19/2004, London: NMC

NMC (2005) *Nurse Prescribing and the Supply and Administration of Medication: Position Statement*, NMC: London

NMC (2006) *Phasing out of Specialist Practitioner Qualifications Leading to Health Visiting, School Nursing and Occupational Health Nursing*, Circular 29/2006, London: NMC

NMC (2007) *Advanced Nursing Practice*, update 19 June, London: NMC

NMC (2008a) *Standards to Support Learning and Assessment in Practice*, NMC: London

NMC (2008b) *The Prep Handbook,* London: NMC

index

Page numbers in *italics* denote glossary reference